D1565986

MOTIVATIONAL INTERVIEWING
IN GROUPS

Applications of Motivational Interviewing

Stephen Rollnick, William R. Miller, and Theresa B. Moyers, *Series Editors*

www.guilford.com/AMI

Since the publication of Miller and Rollnick's classic *Motivational Interviewing*, now in its third edition, MI has been widely adopted as a tool for facilitating change. This highly practical series includes general MI resources as well as books on specific clinical contexts, problems, and populations. Each volume presents powerful MI strategies that are grounded in research and illustrated with concrete, "how-to-do-it" examples.

Motivational Interviewing in the Treatment of Psychological Problems
Hal Arkowitz, Henry A. Westra, William R. Miller, and Stephen Rollnick, Editors

Motivational Interviewing in Health Care: Helping Patients Change Behavior
Stephen Rollnick, William R. Miller, and Christopher C. Butler

Building Motivational Interviewing Skills: A Practitioner Workbook
David B. Rosengren

Motivational Interviewing with Adolescents and Young Adults
Sylvie Naar-King and Mariann Suarez

Motivational Interviewing in Social Work Practice
Melinda Hohman

Motivational Interviewing in the Treatment of Anxiety
Henny A. Westra

Motivational Interviewing: Helping People Change, Third Edition
William R. Miller and Stephen Rollnick

Motivational Interviewing in Groups
Christopher C. Wagner and Karen S. Ingersoll, with Contributors

Motivational Interviewing in Groups

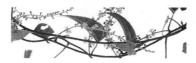

Christopher C. Wagner
Karen S. Ingersoll
with Contributors

Series Editors' Note by
Stephen Rollnick and William R. Miller

THE GUILFORD PRESS
New York   London

© 2013 The Guilford Press
A Division of Guilford Publications, Inc.
370 Seventh Avenue, Suite 1200, New York, NY 10001
www.guilford.com

Printed in the United States of America

This book is printed on acid-free paper.

Last digit is print number: 9 8 7 6 5 4

The authors have checked with sources believed to be reliable in their efforts to
provide information that is complete and generally in accord with the standards
of practice that are accepted at the time of publication. However, in view of the
possibility of human error or changes in behavioral, mental health, or medical sciences, neither the authors, nor the editors and publisher, nor any other party who
has been involved in the preparation or publication of this work warrants that the
information contained herein is in every respect accurate or complete, and they are
not responsible for any errors or omissions or the results obtained from the use of
such information. Readers are encouraged to confirm the information contained
in this book with other sources.

Library of Congress Cataloging-in-Publication Data

Wagner, Christopher C.
  Motivational interviewing in groups / Christopher C. Wagner,
Karen S. Ingersoll.
    pages cm. — (Applications of motivational interviewing)
  Includes bibliographical references and index.
  ISBN 978-1-4625-0792-4 (hardback)
  1. Group psychotherapy. 2. Motivational interviewing.
I. Ingersoll, Karen S. II. Title.
  RC488.W33 2013
  616.89′152—dc23
                                                    2012040523

To my son, Jason Wagner,
who continues to inspire and teach me,
and to my ever-expanding extended family

Thank you to my mentor, Don Kiesler,
and to other early supervisors in individual
and group practice, for their inspiration and guidance:
Jim McCullough, Jack Corazzini, Jim Schmidt, Sandy Colbs,
Kathy Scott, Deb Haller, Bill Riley, and David M. Young

Finally, thank you to my colleagues and students,
past and present,
at Virginia Commonwealth University

—CCW

With love and gratitude to my first group,
the sources of such motivation—my family of origin:
my father, the late James Ross Schneider;
my mother, Emilie Tuma Schneider;
and my brother, Christopher James Schneider

Thank you to my sons,
Jamie Ingersoll and Tristan Ingersoll,
for continually refreshing my view of groups,
and of the possibilities of this world

—KSI

About the Authors

Christopher C. Wagner, PhD, is Associate Professor of Rehabilitation Counseling, Psychology and Psychiatry at Virginia Commonwealth University. A clinical psychologist, he has led psychotherapeutic, psychoeducational, and support groups targeting addictive behaviors, sexual behaviors and identity, HIV disease coping, schizophrenia, and organ transplant, as well as general adult mental health and development. Dr. Wagner is a past president of the Society for Interpersonal Theory and Research and is a member and former steering committee member of the Motivational Interviewing Network of Trainers (MINT). His research interests include interpersonal processes in motivational interviewing and other therapies, and comparing motivational interviewing with other therapeutic approaches.

Karen S. Ingersoll, PhD, is Associate Professor of Psychiatry and Neurobehavioral Sciences at the University of Virginia School of Medicine. A clinical psychologist, she has conducted psychotherapeutic, psychoeducational, and support groups targeting intimate partner violence, smoking cessation, relapse prevention for addictive behaviors, HIV treatment adherence, and women's health. Dr. Ingersoll is a corecipient of the Charles C. Shepard Science Award from the Centers for Disease Control and Prevention, for a study that reduced the risk of alcohol-exposed pregnancies using a motivational interviewing intervention. She is a MINT member whose research tests motivational interviewing as a foundational approach to improve health for people with health and addiction concerns.

Contributors

John S. Baer, PhD, is Research Professor of Psychology at the University of Washington in Seattle. He is also Associate Director for Training and Education at the Center of Excellence for Substance Abuse Treatment and Education at the Veterans Affairs Puget Sound Health Care System. Dr. Baer's research and clinical interests include the assessment, prevention, treatment, and relapse of substance use and abuse, with specific focus on the development and evaluation of brief interventions and motivational interviewing. He is a member of the Motivational Interviewing Network of Trainers.

Susan Butterworth, PhD, MS, is Associate Professor at Oregon Health and Science University and a member of the Motivational Interviewing Network of Trainers. Through her consulting practice, Q-consult, she assists health care organizations in integrating behavior change science into their programs, interventions, and training activities.

Ann Carden, PhD, is a private-practice consultant and trainer in Bowerston, Ohio. In her 30-year career as a mental health and addiction professional, Dr. Carden has served as psychotherapist, educator, researcher, author, and consultant. Her expertise in the dynamics of intimate partner abuse and in the use of motivational interviewing approaches with men who have been adjudicated for spousal battery inform her chapter. She is a member of the Motivational Interviewing Network of Trainers.

Sandra S. Downey, MS, LPC, has extensive experience as an outpatient therapist at the Harrisonburg–Rockingham Community Services Board in Virginia. She conducts trainings in motivational interviewing and has been a member of the Motivational Interviewing Network of Trainers since 2004.

Kelli L. Drenner, PhD, is a research scientist with the Institute for Community Health Promotion at Brown University. Dr. Drenner has experience with the development and delivery of interventions that integrate motivational interviewing principles and strategies with behavior change theories such as the transtheoretical model and social cognitive theory. She is also a motivational interviewer trainer.

Erin C. Dunn, PhD, is a registered psychologist in British Columbia, Canada, and the coordinator of an intensive inpatient eating disorders treatment program at St. Paul's Hospital in Vancouver. She is a member of the Motivational Interviewing Network of Trainers.

Mark Farrall, PhD, is Director of Ignition, an independent agency providing specialized training and consultancy in the areas of domestic violence and abuse and of motivational interviewing. He is a chartered and forensic psychologist and psychotherapist and has developed and delivered several innovative program models based on motivational interviewing. He is a member of the Motivational Interviewing Network of Trainers.

Sarah W. Feldstein Ewing, PhD, is a licensed clinical psychologist, Assistant Professor of Translational Neuroscience at the Mind Research Network, and Assistant Professor in the University Honors Program at the University of New Mexico. Dr. Feldstein Ewing has been dedicated to conducting translational research, specifically investigating the connection between basic biological mechanisms (e.g., genetic risk factors, functional brain activation) and health risk behavior (e.g., treatment outcome, behavioral symptoms). Her goal is to improve health outcomes and reduce current health disparities for high-risk adolescents of all backgrounds. She is a member of the Motivational Interviewing Network of Trainers.

Jacki Hecht, RN, MSN, Senior Research Associate at Butler Hospital, has a research affiliation in the Department of Psychiatry and Human Behavior at the Alpert Medical School of Brown University. She is a member of the Motivational Interviewing Network of Trainers.

Winnie Hunt, MEd, is a Trager practitioner and somatic movement educator who specializes in embodied transformational change. As a published poet, licensed counselor, and life skills coach trainer, she facilitates groups and individuals to expand their sense of health and well-being.

Frances Jasiura, BPHE (Hons), BSW, cofounder of Change Talk Associates, offers training and coaching across Canada in evidence-based and trauma-informed communication practices that increase engagement and build motivation for health-related change. She is a member of the Motivational Interviewing Network of Trainers and Spiritual Directors International, and an instructor at Okanagan College in British Columbia, Canada.

Wendy R. Johnson, PhD, is a clinical psychologist with the Portland VA Medical Center. She has worked extensively with substance-using clients, beginning her addictions career with mandated clients in an Oregon state prison. Dr. Johnson has consulted in motivational interviewing internationally with a variety of criminal justice fields and has been a member of the Motivational Interviewing Network of Trainers since 2003.

Jonathan Krejci, PhD, is Director of Clinical Programs, Training and Research at Princeton House Behavioral Health in Princeton, New Jersey. He is a member of the Motivational Interviewing Network of Trainers.

Claire Lane, PhD, is a trainee clinical psychologist at the University of Birmingham, United Kingdom, who has extensive research experience teaching, practicing, and integrating motivational interviewing within health care contexts. She has been a member of the Motivational Interviewing Network of Trainers since 2005, and regularly trains physical and mental health practitioners in motivational interviewing.

Steve Martino, PhD, is Associate Professor in the Department of Psychiatry at the Yale School of Medicine and Chief of the Psychology Service at the VA Connecticut Healthcare System. He practices, trains, and researches motivational interviewing, with specific foci on adaptations of motivational interviewing for people with co-occurring substance abuse and psychiatric conditions and strategies for training, disseminating, and implementing the approach in community program and health care settings. He is a member of the Motivational Interviewing Network of Trainers.

David S. Prescott, MSW, LICSW, is Director of Professional Development and Quality Improvement for the Becket Family of Services. He has produced nine books on the topic of sexual aggression and is a past president of the Association for the Treatment of Sexual Abusers. A member of the Motivational Interviewing Network of Trainers, he has trained around the world on issues related to sexual abuse.

Marilyn Ross, PhD, LCSW, LSOTP, is a motivational interviewing trainer and clinician in private practice. Dr. Ross specializes in working with people who have been sexually abused. She is a member of the Motivational Interviewing Network of Trainers.

Elizabeth J. Santa Ana, PhD, is Assistant Professor in the Clinical Neuroscience Division, Department of Psychiatry and Behavioral Sciences, at the Medical University of South Carolina. She is the recipient of a VA Clinical Science Research and Development (CDA-2) Career Development Award for her role as Principal Investigator on a study that investigates the impact of group motivational interviewing and in-home-messaging devices on dually diagnosed veterans. She is a member of the Motivational Interviewing Network of Trainers.

Linda Speck, DClinPsy, is a consultant clinical health psychologist and head of health psychology services at Abertawe Bro Morgannwg University Health Board, Wales, United Kingdom. She is a member of the Motivational Interviewing Network of Trainers. Dr. Speck trains health professionals in methods of health behavior change and nationally with the British Association for Cardiovascular Prevention and Rehabilitation.

Nanette S. Stephens, PhD, a licensed clinical psychologist, is a research scientist and Director of Training at the Health Behavior Research and Training Institute, School of Social Work, University of Texas at Austin. Dr. Stephens has extensive experience integrating the transtheoretical model and motivational interviewing principles and strategies in her work as a trainer, supervisor, teacher, researcher, clinician, and consultant. She is a member of the Motivational Interviewing Network of Trainers.

Cristine Urquhart, MSW, RSW, cofounder of Change Talk Associates, offers training and coaching across Canada in evidence-based communication practices that increase engagement and build motivation for health-related change. She is a member of the Motivational Interviewing Network of Trainers, an instructor at the University of British Columbia, and a contributing author to the book *Motivational Interviewing in Social Work Practice.*

Mary Marden Velasquez, PhD, is Professor, Associate Dean for Research, Director of the Center for Social Work Research, and Director of the Health Behavior Research and Training Institute at the University of Texas at Austin. She has been involved in the conceptualization, design, and implementation of research studies using the transtheoretical model of behavior change, specializing in the development and implementation of interventions using the model's stages and processes of change and motivational interviewing. She is a member of the Motivational Interviewing Network of Trainers.

Scott T. Walters, PhD, is Professor of Behavioral and Community Health at the University of North Texas Health Science Center. His research focuses on the use of motivational interviewing and other brief interventions to help people make changes in substance abuse and other problem behaviors. He is a member of the Motivational Interviewing Network of Trainers.

Series Editors' Note

The question arose in our earliest training workshops in the 1980s: "Can you do motivational interviewing in groups?" As this volume reflects, the answer now is clearly "Yes." There is sufficient research evidence at this point to show that motivational interviewing can be delivered well in group formats. Beyond potential cost-effectiveness benefits, groups allow participants to benefit from each other's wisdom and mutual support.

The spirit and method of motivational interviewing endure across individual and group formats. Yet, as is clear from Wagner and Ingersoll's book, skillful practice is not just a matter of using individual motivational interviewing with a group of people. We have recommended that providers first develop good clinical skills in motivational interviewing with individuals before attempting to use it in groups, precisely because there is so much more to manage in a group context. Additional skills are needed to balance individual progress with that of the group, to encourage members to help each other to approach change, and to avoid dysfunctional exchanges that can arise.

There is a definite art as well as science to offering motivational interviewing in groups, and that art is beautifully described here. The authors convey with wisdom and heart their extensive experience in developing, providing, and evaluating motivational interviewing groups. In many settings, treatment or health education is conducted in group rather than individual sessions. The authors offer sound perspectives and advice that are likely to be helpful across a range of professions and settings.

Of course, there is still much to learn. The technology for studying motivational interviewing processes in groups is at a relatively early stage. More is known about group motivational interviewing for some target problems and settings than for others. We do not anticipate the appearance of one "gold-standard" method for group practice of motivational interviewing. What will become clearer as research continues are the components of effective practice that predict subsequent positive change. No doubt there will be some surprises, as has been the case throughout the history of this very organic clinical method. With this timely new volume in an emerging field, Wagner and Ingersoll provide a state-of-the-art account of how to do motivational interviewing when working with groups. We are delighted to have this important book in the Applications of Motivational Interviewing series.

STEPHEN ROLLNICK
WILLIAM R. MILLER

Acknowledgments

We wish to thank Bill Miller and Steve Rollnick for their inspiration, guidance, support, and generosity. Thanks also to our many colleagues around the world in the Motivational Interviewing Network of Trainers (MINT), who have contributed immeasurably to the ongoing development of motivational interviewing through the years.

We also thank Jim Nageotte, Jeannie Tang, Jodie Beecher, Paul Gordon, Judith Grauman, Jane Keislar, Katherine Lieber, and the rest of The Guilford Press staff for polishing and shaping the book into its final form, and Marian Upton, Rachel Green, and numerous counseling students for feedback on earlier drafts of the book. We thank Dwight McCall for his leadership in bringing motivational interviewing to public sector services in Virginia in the 1990s, and Sandy Gharib for collaborating with us on an earlier motivational interviewing group guide that was part of that initiative. We also thank Jim May, Karen Redford, and the Richmond Behavioral Health Authority for providing the practice site at which many of our early ideas about motivational interviewing groups were piloted. Finally, we thank Paula Horvatich and the Mid-Atlantic Addiction Technology Transfer Center for supporting our development as motivational interviewing trainers and group developers, and for supporting motivational interviewing and the MINT network with a website for several years.

Without all of them, this work would be less than it is.

Contents

PART I

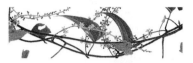

Foundations of Motivational Interviewing Groups

This book is arranged into three parts. The first part lays the foundation for adapting motivational interviewing (MI) to group interactions. Chapter 1 reviews the need for orienting our perspectives to group-level interactions and dynamics, then considers how MI differs and complements other current group approaches. Chapter 2 reviews key aspects of theory and research related to therapeutic groups, including elements such as group climate, cohesion, and other group processes, therapeutic factors, group development, and the functions of group leaders. Chapter 3 provides a working overview of MI, including the role of ambivalence and change talk, the spirit behind the MI approach, common communication methods, and typical therapeutic processes and strategies. Chapter 4 focuses on integrating evidence-based group practices with MI methods to create coherent MI groups. Chapter 5 reviews the current evidence base around MI in groups.

The second part focuses on MI groups in practice. Chapters 6 and 7 focus on designing and implementing MI groups, training and supervising practitioners, and enhancing the effectiveness of services offered. Chapters 8 through 12 focus on conducting MI groups across the four phases of development.

The third part of the book (Chapters 13–21) includes contributed chapters that provide diverse examples of MI groups with various difficulties and settings. Practitioners will find a wealth of therapeutic experience and ideas that can inspire their own work in developing and running MI groups to benefit the people they serve.

CHAPTER 1

Introduction

In Western cultures, we tend to see ourselves as separate from others—as individuals first and only secondarily as members of groups. We learn to think and act on our own. We carry our family's surname but typically consider the successes and failures we experience in life as our own, not as products of our families, networks, and communities. When we describe ourselves, we mostly use individualistic terms rather than the interpersonal descriptors more commonly used by those in non-Western cultures, such as societal roles or membership in cultural or ethnic groups (Triandis, McCusker, & Hui, 1990). Even our models of ourselves are individualistic, including concepts such as separation and individuation to signify appropriate psychological maturation.

In this context, most of the helping services we offer are individually oriented as well, focused on the challenges and opportunities of individuals, and interpreted through a lens that focuses on individuals' characteristics, dysfunctions, or pathologies. Even strengths-based approaches focus more on individual strengths than on interpersonal opportunities or supports.

Although we may see ourselves as separate, we are inextricably linked to others in groups. Our species evolved through the support and protection of the group. Our identities are shaped by the feedback we receive from family, peer, and social groups, as are our thoughts, decisions, attitudes, and values (Forsyth, 2011). Working together, we accomplish more, because the diverse knowledge and skills of the entire group can benefit each individual. Thus, most of us work with others; join others in families, friendships, peer groups, and communities; and rely on society to provide us with access to shelter, food, and other necessities. We rely on groups for many aspects of our existence, because groups can do for us what we cannot always do for ourselves. When we align ourselves with supportive groups, we are less stressed, less lonely, and we have greater self-esteem, are healthier, and may even live longer (Forsyth, 2011).

3

In recognition of the power of groups, therapeutic services have been developed for couples and families, as well as groups created solely to enable people to achieve together what they may struggle to achieve on their own. More than just serving as efficient delivery mechanisms, group services offer benefits that individually based services cannot provide. In therapeutic groups, members provide each other support, understanding, enlightenment, protection, and the opportunity to grow through contributing to the growth of others.

Group services are more complex than individual services. In a dyadic interaction, there is one relationship between two individuals. By adding a third person, there become seven possible relationship configurations (three one-on-one relationships, three one-on-two relationships, and one whole group relationship). With a group of only four people, there are 25 combinations of possible subgroup relationships, in addition to the group as a whole. As groups continue to grow in size, the potential relationships and subgroups for leaders to track and attend to increase exponentially, requiring leaders to develop high sensitivity in order to build upon subtle interaction patterns or minimize their influence on the group as a whole, whichever is appropriate.

Group services are unable to give individuals as much direct attention and floor time as individual services, and there are group processes that can inhibit or even hurt. Given the potential for both harm and benefit from subgroup relationships in therapeutic groups, careful adaptation of services initially developed for individuals is necessary to capitalize on possibilities and minimize potential problems.

Motivational interviewing (MI) has been developed as a client-centered, goal-oriented, individual therapeutic approach. MI focuses on client perspectives rather than framing issues from a professional viewpoint. Practitioners avoid directing clients toward specific solutions in ways that may elicit resistance. Instead they evoke clients' own interests in change and steer the conversation toward commitment to specific actions that lead toward clients' change goals, using the four general processes of engaging, focusing, evoking, and planning to achieve these aims (Miller & Rollnick, 2013).

> MI *focuses more on client perspectives than on framing issues from a professional viewpoint.*

MI is a descendent of Rogerian client-centered therapy and has a humanistic orientation. From this perspective, people are naturally inclined to pursue growth and wellness. The role of the practitioner is to help them to more clearly sort out what they believe and who they experience themselves to be, not by providing education, but by helping them feel more comfortable with who they are and hear their own voices more clearly.

Practitioners view clients positively, accepting and embracing them as the unique people they are. By reflecting an accurate view of who clients see themselves to be, along with optimistic reflections of their strivings toward growth and their ability to become who they want to be, client-centered helpers assist clients in moving forward toward more fulfilling lives, while not attempting to set a particular path for them. As clients become more who they truly are (vs. being constrained by the limiting things they have been told about themselves), they begin to perceive and act in different, more congruent ways.

MI also has roots in behavioral therapy and the behaviorist tradition. From this angle, people's behaviors (and thoughts) are identifiable, measureable, and can be influenced toward more positive or useful patterns. By helping people identify (and track) unproductive patterns of thinking and acting, practitioners help them to establish and maintain more productive habits or patterns. Thus, behavior therapy helps people become more clearminded and purposeful in living.

MI integrates elements of humanistic, client-centered therapy with those of behavior therapy—deeply valuing people for who they are while helping them identify specific ways they'd like to change and develop plans to implement those changes. MI practitioners talk with clients about the aspects of their lives that are dissatisfying and the ways that they'd like things to be better. They honor clients' ambivalence about making changes and strategically focus on those elements that provide momentum for positive change. They then help to develop plans that clients feel confident about implementing.

This book adapts the evidenced-based practice of individual MI to group format by integrating MI and core group therapy concepts into coherent MI groups. The model benefits from the ideas of colleagues working alongside us in this venture as practitioners, developers, and researchers, and those who have previously written MI group treatment manuals or descriptions (W. G. Anderson, Beatty, Moscow, & Tomlin, 2002; Beatty & Tomlin, 2002; Ingersoll, Wagner, & Gharib, 1999; Krecji, 2006; Murphy, 2008; Noonan, 2001; Velasquez, Maurer, Crouch, & DiClemente, 2001). We also integrate our understanding of MI with our group leadership experiences and the evidence-based recommendations of other developers and researchers in group therapy and the positive psychology movement.[1]

---

[1]While MI is not a part of the positive psychology movement, we have drawn significant inspiration from positive psychology and have integrated ideas from it into the MI group model presented in this book. Like Peterson (2006), we see positive psychology and humanistic psychology as close relatives, with more similarities than differences. MI incorporates elements of humanistic, behavioral, social, and cognitive psychology, and its proponents are fully committed to the scientific study of MI, as well as to updating the approach as conclusive findings accrue.

Groups at an Impasse

Before exploring what MI groups are, it may be useful to consider some challenges in providing group services that may be helped by incorporating MI concepts and strategies. Consider the following four scenarios.

Diabetes Support Group

A nurse and dietician facilitate a semimonthly diabetes support group. Although they facilitate group conversations in tandem, each has a specific focus. The nurse makes sure that participants understand the normal physiological processes of the kidney and pancreas, how disease interrupts these processes, and the appropriate use of insulin to compensate for the body's inability to manage insulin levels in a healthy fashion. The dietician focuses on managing insulin levels and overall health through careful and deliberate eating habits, and on making specific lifestyle choices regarding exercise, sleep, and alcohol use. As this is intended to be a support group, they also facilitate discussions about difficulties that patients experience. Because they are not trained as counselors, however, they ask group members to keep the discussion focused on specific difficulties in managing their illness, and they regularly steer the conversations back to this focus when members veer into more personal or emotional topics. Members were initially highly tuned in to the discussions, but over time their involvement seems to have diminished, and fewer attend each meeting. The leaders are unsure what they might do to reenergize the group.

Cognitive–Behavioral Therapy Group

A psychologist and an intern lead a group with a cognitive-behavioral focus for members who are struggling with anxiety. The group is well-structured, teaching members to identify cognitive errors, to become more aware of their automatic thoughts and internal dialogue, to do functional analyses, and to make behavioral plans. Group members regularly express that the cognitive-behavioral model helps them make better sense of their lives and possibilities. Still, week after week, only a few complete homework assignments, despite their continued confidence that next week will be better.

Addiction Psychoeducational Group

A substance abuse counselor runs an intensive outpatient group focused on interesting members in recovery and helping them rebound from relapse, using a psychoeducational approach with instruction, handouts, and practice exercises. The counselor's engaging, informal, and supportive style is sometimes blunt and direct when participants disown responsibility for their difficulties or paint a prettier picture of their lives than reality may support. Some members confront others on their attempts to manipulate the group into supporting their unhealthy perspectives, and others offer practical advice based on their own experiences and things they have learned from community support groups. One thing these group members have in common with the counselor is a belief that people need to admit their problems and accept some truths about being an alcoholic or an addict. Other members doubt that they are truly addicted, and point toward the ongoing struggles of those who identify themselves as addicts as proof that "it's not much help anyway to knock yourself down or call yourself names." One member believes that Alcoholics Anonymous (AA) is a brainwashing religious group that is "almost cult-like." Group members continue to struggle with each other and conversation reaches a standstill, prompting one member to reflect, "Sometimes it seems like a combat zone in here."

Process-Oriented Psychotherapy Group

A social worker conducts a process-oriented psychotherapy group in which members are encouraged to focus on issues that are important to them and to use the time to define their own perspectives, identity, and values. Several members have identified specific issues on which they want to work, and a few already have focused on certain changes they want to make. Others who are not sure what to focus on just know they are not happy and feel like something is missing from their lives. The group runs smoothly and is never at a loss for conversation. The group leader skillfully reflects member perspectives and facilitates greater depth of dialogue. Members speak openly during the sessions, sharing useful feedback and support. A few months into the weekly sessions, however, a few members begin to question whether this is "all there is" to group therapy. A feeling of discontent seems to settle over the group. Conversations seem to go in circles, and a few members express frustration that others just complain about their lives rather than do something to make them better. The group leader affirms both the honesty of those who are frustrated and the autonomy of those who are targets of complaints in order to lead all members to define their own perspectives and goals for therapy. Still, the group seems to have reached an impasse, and the leader decides to consult with a colleague for input.

How MI Might Help These Groups

MI has something to offer to each of these groups experiencing a therapeutic impasse. In the diabetes support, cognitive-behavioral therapy (CBT), and recovery group examples, the group facilitation is more counselor-centered and directive than is typical of MI groups. The psychotherapy group uses the client-centered style, but the facilitation is closer to nondirective following than to guiding. The MI combination of client-centered attitudes and goal-oriented processes can help establish momentum toward positive change, while avoiding some of the pitfalls of becoming overly directive or nondirective when leading a group.

In the diabetes group, knowledge of MI might influence the leaders to reduce the amount of information they provide in order to improve retention of the key facts members need to know to manage their illnesses. Instead of providing copious information, they might elicit what members already know, then "fill in the blanks" where there are gaps in knowledge, while helping members personalize health information to their own lives. This eliciting approach helps members better focus on their own important changes and can make sessions more interesting as discussions rather than lectures. MI may also help the leaders be more comfortable working with a broader array of life issues, that may indirectly relate to the goal of managing diabetes. By attending to related issues, while remaining focused on health goals, these practitioners can weave change strategies into the broader fabric of patients' lives.

In the CBT group, cognitions and behavior seem disconnected. The group members see how the CBT model can help them understand their problems and provide strategies for reducing those problems, yet they don't seem to use the model to change things. Incorporating MI strategies might help members "back up" a bit. Before they prompt members to implement changes based on the CBT model, the leaders might spend time eliciting members' goals, hopes, and values, helping them envision a more satisfying future and connect to goals they want to achieve, then return to examining dysfunctional cognitions, only now with greater clarity on how these thoughts and reactions get in the way of achieving their goals. In this way, MI strategies may help members see connections between their specific thoughts and behaviors, and their more general hopes and wishes. When members perceive that CBT strategies not only address problems in perceiving and thinking but also help them lead happier lives, their investment in doing homework will likely increase, as they come to perceive homework as a helpful step down a more fulfilling path.

Another issue is that members see the leaders as experts who teach the group about thinking errors and ways of analyzing behavior. This tends to reduce the extent to which group members talk to each other or feel committed to each other's growth and development. By adding thematic linking of similar issues, thoughts, and behaviors through reflecting these on a "meta" level, the leaders can increase group cohesion and the likelihood that members will see themselves as drivers of change rather than as mere passengers.

In the substance abuse group, the leader has taken a stance on issues that cause ambivalence for group members. Because some members have ambivalence about the traditional recovery model, when the leader argues for one side of ambivalence they naturally defend the other side. In taking sides, the leader has externalized the ambivalence that members experience and inadvertently split the group into two camps rather than focusing the group on individually tailored changes that members may achieve in different ways. MI practice would suggest that the group leader should elicit and explore members' ambivalence rather than argue against it. Additionally, MI practice would guide the leader to model acceptance of the idea that "many roads may take you there" so that group members feel safe in expressing their views and do not fear being attacked for being wrong. Thus, the MI spirit of partnership, acceptance, compassion, and evocation can become a core part of group interactions. This can lead to fewer conflicts, more support, and more excitement about participating.

The psychotherapy group has skilled client-centered facilitation by the social worker. What MI can offer this group is more direction. By adding directional strategies to already skilled empathic responding, the group leader could help members focus on doing in addition to being and guide them to move toward more fulfilling lives, while deepening their understanding of themselves and their peers.

While MI can help these groups avoid or move past their therapeutic impasses, no approach can eliminate every challenge or obstacle. Some impasses and conflicts perhaps shouldn't be eliminated even if it were possible, because they can lead to transforming a set of individuals into a more meaningful, cohesive working group. During these transformative moments, many group members find their voices and increase ownership of their own lives.

Challenges of Running MI Groups

Providing high-quality, productive group leadership is more difficult than providing individual services. There are more ways for things to go wrong, and it can be harder to set things right again once negative cycles begin. Rather than having only one client to help along a productive path, you must help many people make progress. This requires facilitating focused and productive interactions between members with different histories, beliefs, values, and communication styles, while simultaneously processing your own internal impulses to focus on some members more than others.

Group leadership is more difficult than conducting individual therapy. There are more ways for things to go wrong, and they're harder to fix when they do.

Given the challenges of running groups well, why should you consider groups at all? Although empirical support for MI groups lags behind that established for individual MI, the available evidence is both positive and promising. The evidence base is modest at present partly because MI groups are a more recent development than individual MI (and are still developing), and partly because groups are more difficult to research than individual services. Some controlled studies show promise for MI groups, but it is too soon to determine how they compare to MI with individual clients.

While studies of MI groups are only about a decade old, group services have been a reality far longer. In many settings, groups are firmly embedded into the array of services offered, and this is unlikely to change, even without strong evidence to support their use. And MI groups may have several benefits that are more difficult to achieve in individual services.

Potential Advantages of MI Groups

One benefit of MI groups is that they reduce the social isolation of members and increase recognition of the universality of suffering (Yalom & Leszcz, 2005). Often people who are struggling feel as if they are alone, different, and less competent or worthy than others. This perspective robs them of both self-esteem and *self-efficacy,* the belief that they can successfully make changes. Groups can remedy these problems more directly than individual services, because groups bring people together to share concerns and support one another, increasing their hope and confidence. By "going through it together," members inspire one another through their progress and successes, without the isolation they might continue to feel in individual treatment.

Another potential advantage of MI groups is their flexibility. There are several complementary ways to go about translating MI to the group format, with different methods to achieve success across different settings and populations. Groups can be developed in context, adapted to members' needs and goals, and to the setting in which they are run.

MI groups may focus on support, education, psychological change or behavior change. MI groups may incorporate different conversational strategies, depending on what is most useful in the moment. Thus, MI groups may help clients to consider things more broadly or deeply, to think ahead, to focus more narrowly on specific actions they can take, and to restore their healthy defenses when sessions close. There are many options for running groups as they develop through their natural phases of engaging, exploring perspectives, broadening perspectives, and moving into action. Although some groups may meet only once and others have revolving sets of participants, we aim our discussion toward the prototypical group that involves a mostly consistent set of members over a period of time.

Our Hopes for This Book

While a body of supportive evidence about MI groups is still accumulating, we are impressed by the wealth of ideas and therapeutic innovation shared by our collaborators. The richness of MI group descriptions for many diverse concerns presented in later chapters will likely inspire further innovations. Additionally, we hope that this book encourages researchers to develop a more comprehensive knowledge base on MI group models. This process will extend our understanding of the possibilities of MI groups, offer guidance toward further adaptations, and pose new challenges regarding the ongoing practice of MI groups.

We hope this book is useful for a broad audience, including both those who do therapeutic work informed by MI and are considering expanding their work to groups, and those who lead groups and are interested in learning what MI might have to offer. We want the book to be helpful to those whose work is primarily psychotherapeutic in nature, and to those who work in professions such as health care and corrections, in which traditional psychotherapy may be tangential to their core missions. Thus, we have written a book that can be read sequentially or in piecemeal fashion, depending on readers' background and interests.

References

Anderson, P., Beatty, J., Moscow, S., & Tomlin, K. (2002). *Exploring change group*. Portland, OR: West Interstate Clinic, Kaiser Permanente Northwest Region, Department of Addiction Medicine.

Beatty, J., & Tomlin, K. (2002). *Engaging youth in treatment: Group and family curriculum*. Portland, OR: West Interstate Clinic, Kaiser Permanente Northwest Region, Department of Addiction Medicine.

Forsyth, D. R. (2011). The nature and significance of groups. In R. K. Conyne (Ed.), *The Oxford handbook of group counseling* (pp. 19–35). New York: Oxford University Press.

Ingersoll, K. S., Wagner, C. C., & Gharib, S. (1999). *Motivational groups for community substance abuse programs*. Richmond, VA: Mid-Atlantic Addiction Technology Transfer Center.

Krecji, J. (2006). *Motivational interviewing group treatment in behavioral health settings*. Princeton, NJ: Princeton House Behavioral Health.

Miller, W. R., & Rollnick, S. (2013). *Motivational interviewing: Helping people change* (3rd ed.). New York: Guilford Press.

Murphy, R.T. (2008). Enhancing combat veterans' motivation to change posttraumatic stress disorder symptoms and other problem behaviors. In H. Arkowitz, H. A. Westra, W. R. Miller, & S. Rollnick (Eds.), *Motivational interviewing in the treatment of psychological problems* (pp. 57–84). New York: Guilford Press.

Noonan, W. C. (2000). Group motivational interviewing as an enhancement to outpatient alcohol treatment. *ProQuest Digital Dissertations Database*, Publication No. AAT9998849.

Peterson, C. (2006). *A primer in positive psychology*. Oxford, UK: Oxford University Press.

Triandis, H. C., McCusker, C., & Hui, C. H. (1990). Multimethod probes of individualism and collectivism. *Journal of Personality and Social Psychology, 59,* 1006–1013.

Velasquez, M. M., Maurer, G. G., Crouch, C., & DiClemente, C. (2001). *Group treatment for substance abuse: A stages-of-change therapy manual*. New York: Guilford Press.

Yalom, I., & Leszcz, M. (2005). *The theory and practice of group psychotherapy* (5th ed.). New York: Basic Books.

CHAPTER 2

Therapeutic Groups

Groups can powerfully influence their members' attitudes, values, and perceptions (Forsyth, 2011). Most people rely on social interaction to process information (Fishman, Ng, & Bellugi, 2010), and considerable information processing—conceptualizing, evaluating, brainstorming, problem solving, deciding, planning—is done in groups. Groups can result in more effective decision making, because group processing allows people to hear and consider new ideas and perspectives from others grappling with the same concern rather than having to generate all possibilities themselves (Kerr & Tindale, 2004). Group processing also can require less effort than individual processing. When a majority of group members converges on a perspective or idea, individual members tend to accept it with less exploration and processing than when each person has to consider all ideas individually. Over time, if members come to perceive groups as being reliably helpful, they become satisfied with using "good-enough" ideas generated by the group to move forward, rather than continuing to search for the best possible ideas (Tindale & Kameda, 2000), reducing rumination time and increasing time spent actively moving toward a goal.

Groups can also influence both the type and strength of members' emotional reactions, as emotions become "contagious" among members of a shared group. This can be negative, as with a mob, but it can also influence members in positive ways, such as in successful product development teams or sports teams, where members converge upon similar enhancing moods and motivational levels over time to achieve synergistic outcomes (Kelly, 2004). In therapeutic groups, emotional expression in a supportive context can increase members' awareness of emotions, sense of responsibility for their behavior, consideration of others' feelings, and control of aggression toward others (Giese-Davis et al., 2002; Whelton, 2004).

13

Finally, groups influence members' actions, as is evident by observing the impact of family and peer groups on individuals' behavior. This influence may become strong enough that individuals' actions in groups become unpredictable based on their usual patterns and habits outside the group—a process referred to as the *discontinuity effect* (Wildschut, Pinter, Vevea, Insko, & Schopler, 2003). This process is regularly overlooked, however, as we tend to attribute people's actions to their individual dispositional traits, and miss the power of situational attributes and reinforcers (Gawronski, 2004). The magnitude of a group's influence on individual members' behavior is affected by the strength of relationships within the group and boundaries around the group, the structure and cohesion of the group, and the group members' perceptions of the interdependence of their fates (Forsyth, 2011). We consider these group properties later in the chapter.

Types of Therapeutic Groups

Groups have varying goals and methods depending on setting, logistical issues, and theoretical orientation. Over time, many different types of groups have evolved—from top-down, hierarchically delivered classes to expert-interpreted long-term treatment intended to re-create early family structures and conflicts, to time-limited, highly interactive, group-centric approaches that focus more on discrete change than on personality reconstruction (Barlow, 2011; Barlow, Burlingame, & Fuhriman, 2000). Typically, groups are ongoing, although single-session groups are common in some settings. Ongoing groups can provide support to those dealing with a life transition or situation requiring ongoing maintenance, such as adjusting to a new illness, dealing with grief and loss issues, or managing recovery among those who are addicted to a substance or have a destructive habit. These *support groups* are sometimes peer-led, and when they have a professional leader, that person often focuses on presenting information or leading general discussion, typically focusing the group on adjustment and support rather than using the group for more intensive purposes.

Alternatively, groups can focus on a particular problem or condition, led by a trained psychotherapist or counselor who focuses more on individual issues than group processes. These problem-focused, *psychoeducational groups* may focus on behavior change or cognitive and emotional aspects of the problem, with the group providing support and the opportunity to explore new information or practice new skills. Whether members are learning relapse prevention, assertiveness, or anger management skills, the group serves as an efficient, convenient setting in which to develop more functional behaviors. Leaders may capitalize on some group processes to facilitate learning and change, but a focus on process remains secondary to content and skills development.

Finally, groups may focus on interpersonal processes and personal growth. Emerging primarily out of the psychodynamic and humanistic traditions, these *psychotherapeutic groups* explore more ingroup interactions and dynamics in comparison to the other approaches. Typically facilitated by practitioners trained specifically in group leadership, these groups often address identity, psychological development, emotional conflict, and dysfunctional interpersonal patterns. Rather than focusing on problems only as they exist outside the group, problems are viewed as embedded in social interactions, and the ingroup dynamics are used directly as an agent of change in helping individual members learn and grow in the here and now.

Evidence about Therapeutic Groups

Therapeutic group services are common in health, mental health, addiction, and criminal justice settings. Group therapy is effective overall (Burlingame, Fuhriman, & Mosier, 2003), and as effective as individual services for many problems (Barlow, 2011; Bernard et al., 2008; Burlingame, MacKenzie, & Strauss, 2004; McRoberts, Burlingame, & Hoag, 1998; Minniti et al., 2007; Oei, Raylu, & Casey, 2010; Weiss, Jaffee, de Menil, & Cogley, 2004). Some recent studies of group therapies found them to be more cost-effective than individual or standard care in the areas of health (Befort, Donnelly, Sullivan, Ellerbeck, & Perri, 2010; Howard, Dupont, Haselden, Lynch, & Wills, 2010; Lamb et al., 2010) and mental health (Marchand, Roberge, Primiano, & Germain, 2009; Muroff et al., 2009; Niccols, 2008; Oei & Dingle, 2008; Siskind, Baingana, & Kim, 2008). Some analyses suggest that groups have efficiency advantages such as lower dropout rate (Minniti et al., 2007), fewer empty time slots in practitioners' schedules, and lower overall costs resulting from serving more people at once (Sobell, Sobell, & Agrawal, 2009).

Several group-specific processes relate to positive outcomes. At the simplest level, group members who participate more, exploring both positive and painful feelings, benefit to a greater degree (Fielding, 1983; Piper, Ogrodniczuk, McCallum, Joyce, & Rosie, 2003). When members believe that they are the agents of change, they engage more in group processes and are more likely to achieve positive outcomes (Delsignore, Carraro, Mathier, Znoj, & Schnyder, 2008). The "interpersonal field," comprising the environment and its social actors, is broader and deeper in group therapy than in individual treatment. There are more opportunities to experience others who may spark desires to be close or stay away, and to lead the interaction or to follow. Therefore, the interpersonal environment and focus on others are more relevant in group therapy than in individual therapy (Holmes & Kivlighan, 2000). Some factors related to outcome are exclusive to groups, such as vicarious learning, universality, and altruism (Bernard et al., 2008).

Focus is also important. Groups that focus on the full range of issues facing participants versus single issues driven by program focus may be more effective (Weiss, Griffin, Kolodziej, Greenfield, Najavits, et al., 2007), as are groups that focus more on identifying solutions than on understanding problems (Smock et al., 2008).

Moving beyond the question of whether groups are effective, and into defining best practices, things become somewhat less clear. However, two recent sources provide useful summaries of the empirical literature and evidence-based practice recommendations. The American Group Psychotherapy Association (AGPA) convened an expert panel to make evidence-based practice recommendations (Bernard et al., 2008; Klein, 2008). Although the focus was on "dynamic, interactional and relationally-based group psychotherapy" (p. 456), many of their recommendations are relevant to MI groups as well. The *Oxford Handbook of Group Counseling* (Conyne, 2011) also compiled literature summaries by many group counseling experts. We draw from both of these sources to introduce issues related to therapeutic factors and mechanisms, group processes, and leader functions here, and we return to them in later chapters as they relate to specific MI group phases.

Group Climate

The influence of therapeutic groups on members is a result of several (overlapping) factors. Perhaps the most basic element is the *group climate*. Also described as the group's "feeling tone," the climate of the group establishes the atmosphere in the group (McClendon & Burlingame, 2011). The initial climate is often established in the pregroup orientation, or as the group members walk into the group room the first time. From the leader's welcome and orientation to the group through the establishment of group guidelines and the work of the group, a positive climate promotes increased engagement and decreased conflict over the life of the group (MacKenzie, Dies, Coche, Rutan, & Stone, 1987). In groups with a positive climate, members care about one another, try to understand themselves and each other, disclose personal information and feelings, feel that the group is important and worth participating in, and encourage one another to make progress toward goals (MacKenzie, 1983). As with individual therapeutic work, group leaders must always balance technical or task-oriented elements with tending to relationships and maintaining a safe environment.

Although both are important, a safe, engaging, and active group climate predicts positive outcomes, while focusing too much on the tasks of therapeutic work can harm the climate and limit the effectiveness of

> *Focusing too much on tasks can limit effectiveness by harming the group climate.*

the group (Kivlighan & Tarrant, 2001). We review specific group leader functions that promote positive outcomes later, but first we turn to several group aspects and processes that are more specific than the generalized group climate but less discrete than leader behaviors. Among the most important of these is group cohesion.

Alliance and Cohesion

Alliance and cohesion are considered crucial for productive therapeutic work, and necessary for positive outcomes (Johnson, 2007). Yet despite their presumed importance, neither seems to be easily captured by formal definitions or measurements.

In individual therapy, *alliance* is generally viewed as the the bond between client and therapist, agreement on the goals of working together, and agreement on the tasks involved in achieving those goals (Bordin, 1979). Alliance is a robust predictor of outcome, despite problems with defining and measuring it, and even questions about whose perspective to take when examining it—therapist, client, or observer (Martin, Garske, & Davis, 2000).

Cohesion is more complex than alliance. *Cohesion* can include member–member connections, member–subgroup or member–whole-group connections, or even member–leader connections (although it may be more useful to continue to consider member–leader connections as alliance). Group cohesion fosters a safe environment in which members experience belonging, allegiance to the group, and commitment to group outcomes (Yalom & Leszcz, 2005). The AGPA Working Group (Bernard et al., 2008) focused on intrapersonal, intragroup, and interpersonal cohesion. They defined *intrapersonal cohesion* as "members' sense of belonging, acceptance, commitment and allegiance to their group" (p. 467). *Intragroup cohesion* involves "mutual liking/trust, support, caring and commitment to

> *Group cohesion fosters a safe environment in which members experience belonging, allegiance to the group, and commitment to group outcomes.*

work as a group" (p. 467) among members, and *interpersonal cohesion* focuses on positive interactions between individuals or informal subgroups within the group.

Cohesion develops over time. *Immature cohesion* early in group development involves superficial agreement and sense of unity among group members, and can provide a basis for group discussion but ultimately inhibit sharing of vulnerable issues and divergent perspectives if it does not deepen over time. *Mature cohesion* involves true intimacy that allows divergent viewpoints and healthy conflict (Robbins, 2003). In a mature, cohesive atmosphere, group members lower their defenses, become open to new ideas and experiences, disclose and reveal themselves, seek and provide mutual support, and take emotional risks.

Cohesion positively relates to a number of other group processes, including increased attendance, participation, openness, harmony, ability to tolerate conflict, and commitment to and satisfaction with the group. Cohesion also relates to greater symptom reduction in diverse symptoms such as anxiety, depression, binge eating, complicated grief, addictions and severe mental illness across various types of group therapy, including brief and long-term psychodynamic and interpersonal process groups, time-limited CBT groups, and support groups. Not all studies find cohesion to be a positive predictor, but some null studies appear to be based on groups that have relatively low overall cohesion. A challenge for leaders is that group members who may gain the most from cohesion often have the most difficulty developing it, such as those with interpersonal problems, severe mental or physical illness, or relationship problems related to aggression (Marmarosh & Van Horn, 2011).

Several leader and member factors that increase or decrease group cohesiveness are summarized in Table 2.1 and discussed in later chapters.

TABLE 2.1. Leader and Member Factors that Affect Cohesion

Positive influence	Negative influence
Leaders	
• Encouraging sharing	• Failing to encourage interaction
• Modeling self-disclosure focused on responsibility	• Defensiveness
	• Anxious or avoidant attachment style
• Providing nonjudgmental feedback	• Judgmental or competitive attitudes
• Warmth and eye contact	• Being unable to share genuine warmth
• Acknowledging mistakes	• Failing to screen out toxic members
• Facing one's own and others' anger	• Allowing scapegoating and subgrouping without exploration
• Drawing attention to positive moments	• Failing to address absences and tardiness
	• Disallowing negative emotions

(*continued*)

TABLE 2.1. (*continued*)

Members	
• Turn taking	• Judgmental/evaluative responses
• Support/acceptance	• Interpersonal problems such as being nonassertive, vindictive, intrusive
• Self-disclosing	
• Psychological mindedness or higher educational experience	• Anxious or avoidant attachment styles
	• Inaccurate perceptions of others
• Willingness to experience emotions	• Lack of disclosure/risk taking
	• Being easily overwhelmed by emotions
	• Lateness or missing sessions

Beyond Alliance and Cohesion: Other Group Processes

Hornsey, Dwyer, and Oei (2007) suggest that the construct of cohesion has been conceptually intertwined with other variables such as risk taking and self-disclosure, which are sometimes included as elements of cohesion, and at other times are seen as antecedents or consequents of cohesion. They suggest that "because the definition of cohesiveness is so broad, it becomes very difficult to isolate predictors from mediators, and so the causal path between group processes and outcomes is not clearly delineated" (p. 573). Consistent with calls to integrate conceptualization of therapeutic processes with the broader scientific study of individuals, dyads, and groups (Forsyth & Strong, 2004; Kivlighan, 2008), they review three other common constructs in the social-psychological literature: group identification, homogeneity, and task interdependence. To understand the relevance of these, it is helpful to summarize social identity theory.

Social identity theory, a social-psychological model regarding the relationship between individuals and groups, suggests that our identities are formed and maintained partially through our participation in social groups (Turner, Brown, & Tajfel, 1979). According to this theory, we define ourselves partly in terms of an "us" relating to internalized membership in various groups that are important to us (member of a social or religious group, part of a family, etc.), giving us a sense of belonging and pride, and increased self-esteem (Forsyth, 2011). While our personal identity is defined largely in contrast to others, as unique and separate, our social identity is defined in relation to others, as similar and connected. In some cultures, a social identity is more prominent than a personal identity.

Group identification may be an important element of therapeutic groups. People feel loyalty to the groups with which they most closely identify, and in return, gain self-esteem through those groups' positive appraisals of them. Identification with the therapeutic group can increase members' commitment to group norms and values, providing a potential resource for engaging them in group processes and helping them move from talk into action. Commitment to change can be enhanced when it is based on more than individual striving and becomes intertwined with loyalty to the group and a source of pride and esteem among group members. Group identification can also decrease dropout, because leaving the group is perceived as a form of withdrawing support for others, which can be a powerful social reinforcer for retention. Members also develop a kind of *depersonalized trust* (Brewer, 1981), which they extend to others in their group. Assuming that acts of other group members come from helpful intentions through depersonalized trust can lower their defensiveness to others' comments. This may be especially important among clients with histories of dysfunctional relationships or treatment histories involving coercion or demand.

> *Identification with the group can increase members' commitment to group norms and values, helping them to move from talk into action.*

Another element of therapeutic groups is *group homogeneity*. Homogeneity is often thought of as similarity on preexisting variables such as demographics, clinical condition, or interpersonal style (Hornsey et al., 2007). However, through group interactions, members often develop a subjective sense of similarity even when there is a considerable range of ages, cultural backgrounds, clinical difficulties, and personality styles.

Thus, not only do we identify with the groups in which we participate and extend depersonalized trust to group members, but we are also more inclined to perceive similarities between ourselves and other members than if we met those same individuals outside the context of a group. This enhanced sense of connectedness and solidarity among group members increases the attractiveness and perceived value of other group members, and can lead to greater empathy and perspective taking. Group leaders can promote this process by linking members together through shared themes, strivings, and experiences.

A third element is *perceived task interdependence,* in which we believe that working with others can help us achieve our goals, and that we contribute to their efforts as well. Perceived task interdependence is related to greater cooperation and self-disclosure among group members, as well as helpfulness regarding others' concerns. Over time, these processes can become self-perpetuating. As group members move beyond self-interest to genuine investment in other members' outcomes, they begin to experience the increased self-esteem and sense of social competency that are the rewards of extending themselves in altruistic ways. This investment can be further enhanced when members perceive that their efforts truly contribute to others' growth or greater fulfillment.

Faris and Brown (2003) describe three other social psychology constructs relevant to group therapy and MI groups. *Elaboration likelihood* is the extent to which people explore their emerging ideas and perceptions in depth. When people have low elaboration likelihood, they process the group at reduced and more superficial levels. *Production blocking* occurs when people experience an obstacle between developing and communicating an idea. *Social loafing* is the tendency to put less effort toward tasks when in the presence of others who can also put effort toward achieving goals. Faris and Brown describe how these obstacles often occur at greater levels in groups versus individual interactions and how explicitly addressing them enhances group processes.

We draw from these group psychology constructs and evidence throughout this book.

Therapeutic Factors

Groups and individual services share several therapeutic factors and mechanisms of action (causal agents) in common. Group outcomes may be significantly influenced by nonspecific factors (i.e., those that are not specific to particular approaches but operate across therapeutic approaches) in addition to the effects of specific therapeutic tasks. Certain clients may be predisposed to benefit more from therapy due to their psychological mindedness, verbal processing abilities, comfort with self-disclosure, and other individual characteristics. Other client factors are more specific to the therapeutic situation, such as acceptance of the therapeutic rationale, commitment to participating in therapy and trying new behaviors, and positive expectations about likely outcomes. Relationship factors are also viewed as nonspecific factors, although different treatment approaches advocate different kinds of relationships among group members. But in general, across therapeutic approaches, development of a strong therapeutic alliance between practitioner and client improves outcomes. Practitioner competence is another nonspecific factor. Finally, extratherapeutic events can affect outcome by influencing client readiness to participate in therapeutic tasks, or by moderating treatment effects.

Certain therapeutic factors promote positive outcomes in group counseling and therapy. Since at least the 1940s, various theorists and researchers have proposed lists of therapeutic factors numbering one to 12 or more. At present, researchers are working to determine how these lists fit together, most likely in three or four overarching categories (Joyce, MacNair-Semands, Tasca, & Ogrodniczuk, 2011). Yalom's list of 11 therapeutic factors in open-ended interpersonal process groups is probably the best known (Yalom & Leszcz, 2005), itself an update of an earlier list of 10 factors (Corsini & Rosenberg, 1955). Bloch and Crouch (1985) revised this list, developing a (largely similar) list of factors based on an analysis of group members' perceptions of critical incidents in the life of time-limited groups. We use the Bloch and Crouch list for consideration of MI groups, because the deleted items from Yalom's list have relatively little to do with MI (e.g., corrective recapitulation of the family experience; existential factors) or are already considered separately (e.g., group cohesiveness), while the added factors appear related to MI (acceptance, self-disclosure, self-understanding). Because the definitions are fairly obvious, Table 2.2 focuses instead on the potential benefit of the factors to group members. Some of these therapeutic factors are directly related to MI; others are not. We focus on how MI groups draw from them in Chapter 4.

Group Development

Group members' investment in the group evolves over time, as do trust and intimacy, the depth of relationships, and the maturity of group processes.

TABLE 2.2. Group Therapeutic Factors

Therapeutic factor	Potential outcome
Acceptance	Members feel valued, understood, and cared for.
Altruism	Members gain self-esteem and greater appreciation of helping others.
Catharsis	Members learn to "let go" of negative emotions or perspectives that keep them stuck.
Guidance	Members gain knowledge from group participation.
Instillation of hope	Members develop greater optimism about change.
Learning from interpersonal interactions	Members learn more about their impact on others, learn to give better feedback, and learn to interact in more productive ways.
Self-disclosure	Members learn to be more open and genuine.
Self-understanding	Members gain greater knowledge of themselves and greater access to personal experiences.
Universality	Members recognize they are not alone or uniquely damaged.
Vicarious learning	Members adopt more productive ways of perceiving, thinking, and acting from observing others' examples.

Many models have been proposed to summarize these changes in group development, with most including the concept that groups pass through various linear phases or stages. No model can explain all groups due to differences in length, composition, stability of membership and theoretical grounding, but some basic elements are shared by most group models. MacKenzie (1994) identifies common assumptions across models that best fit longer-term outpatient groups but have some relevance to all group endeavors. First, groups develop in recognizable patterns, allowing better-than-chance predictions of near-term events. Second, these patterns are similar across comparable groups. Third, the development of later patterns or stages flows from successful passage through earlier patterns or stages. Fourth, group dynamics become more complex and subtle over time, and recycle through earlier patterns during periods of rapid change or stress.

Many stage models include variations of Tuckman's "forming–storming–norming–performing–adjourning" model proposed several decades ago (Tuckman & Jensen, 1977). Although the number of stages varies across models, most include four or five. Of the general group development models, MacKenzie's (1997) model of shorter-term groups, including stages of engagement, differentiation, interpersonal work, and termination, is closest to the four-phase model of MI groups we present in this book.

Leader Functions

Many group experts have described leadership functions. Yalom and Leszcz (2005) suggest that the leaders have three primary tasks—creating and maintaining the group, building the group culture, and activating/illuminating the here-and-now interactions between members. Trotzer (1977) considered the leaders' primary tasks to be process-oriented—promoting, facilitating, initiating, and guiding member interactions.

Several descriptions bear resemblance to recent conceptualizations of MI. For example, Bales (1958) suggested that leaders are responsible for task and maintenance functions, similar to the conceptualization offered by Miller and Rose (2009) of MI as having technical and relational elements. Dinkmeyer and Muro (1979) describe several leader tasks—promoting interaction, promoting cohesiveness, summarizing, resolving conflicts, "guiding" the elements of tone setting, structuring and limit setting, linking, providing support, reflecting, protecting, questioning, blocking, and regulating. Similarly, the therapist style in MI is also considered "guiding"—a midpoint between directing and following—with descriptors such as collaborating, eliciting, encouraging, enlightening, and supporting (Miller & Rollnick, 2013). Schutz (1961) proposed four leader functions: (1) establishing group goals and values; (2) negotiating a range of cognitive styles; (3) evoking skills and abilities; and (4) helping resolve problems. This model provides the closest parallel to both the four-phase model we offer in this book and the four processes of MI described by Miller and Rollnick (2013): engaging, focusing, evoking, and planning.

Although leaders' responsibilities vary depending on group goals and theoretical orientation, the AGPA practice guidelines (Bernard et al., 2008) suggest several central tasks for leaders to maximize the benefit of therapeutic factors and guide groups through their developmental course. AGPA guidelines include four functions for group leaders that have emerged in the literature over several decades: executive functions, caring, emotional stimulation, and meaning attribution (e.g., Lieberman, Miles, & Yalom, 1973). The AGPA Task Force added three other functions: fostering client self-awareness, shaping group norms, and displaying transparency. Leaders may approach these functions differently over the course of group development—perhaps giving more direct input early on and eliciting more at later stages—but throughout, leaders retain the responsibility to facilitate optimal outcomes.

Leaders serve as the group's executives. Leaders are responsible for organizing the group, setting general goals and parameters, managing development and maintenance of guidelines and limits, making sessions productive and timely, keeping records, and managing member turnover. These *boundary management* tasks are crucial. Bernard and colleagues (2008) describe several boundaries that leaders are responsible for, including boundaries around membership, time, subject matter, affective expression, and anxiety level. Failure of leaders to maintain these boundaries can lead to failure of the therapeutic enterprise. For example, groups can implode if leaders do not limit strong displays of anger, and can cause harm if clients feel coerced into specific beliefs or goals, or become too anxious to return to the next session. As the group executives, leaders are also responsible for productively focusing group conversations. While nonprofessional groups can promote temporary improvements through a positive therapeutic relationship, members of professionally led groups achieve longer-lasting change through careful and productive focusing by the leaders (Barlow, Burlingame, Harding, & Behrman, 1997). In MI groups, the therapeutic focus tends to be on positive change, similar to positive psychotherapy groups (Seligman, Rashid, & Parks, 2006).

It is important to communicate an investment in the well-being of group members and in the potential helpfulness of the group endeavor. *Communication of caring* helps to deepen the therapeutic alliance and models the value of investing in fellow human beings. It is also helpful to engage group members emotionally (*emotional stimulation*). Groups are likely to be less effective in helping members change if they focus exclusively on cognitive elements such as information provision, problem analysis, weighing pros and cons, decision making, and so on. Engaging groups emotionally may not require much from leaders in some groups, but at other times it may require considerable effort to elicit members' emotional expressions or model emotion-infused communication. There are probably both lower and upper boundaries of emotionality for effective group functioning. With low emotional involvement, groups are likely to be flat and unengaging. With high emotionality, groups may become too intense for certain members to open up to others, and it may be difficult for members to step out of emotional interactions to process and learn from them.

Stimulating group participation is of limited value, however, if members don't gain greater understanding of themselves, the possibilities in front of them, and the means to achieve their goals. Through personalizing general information provided by leaders and adapting ideas from the examples offered by other members, the process of *attributing personal meaning* to group experiences provides clients with a framework for proactive intentional change. While emotional involvement engages members in the process of change, insight helps set a direction and maintain longer-term pursuit of meaningful goals. Leaders can promote meaning attribution by broadening conversation from specific experiences toward more general themes, and by eliciting clients' thoughts on what they learn from group interactions. An important focus is *fostering client self-awareness* of patterns that tie life experiences together, as well as patterns in their interpersonal interactions.

Beyond helping the group establish general guidelines for functioning, leaders have a responsibility to *shape group norms,* implicitly building upon key group interactions or more explicitly guiding or eliciting group sensibilities about a number of issues. How often should each person talk, for how long, focusing on what content? How should members interact with each other? How much focus should be given to events in clients' lives outside the group versus events that happen within the group? How much focus is given to the past, the present, the future? Should members stick to discussing their own concerns, comment on concerns of others, offer advice or support, or challenge one another to be more honest or invested? Should members provide feedback on what they see in others' nonverbal behavior? What, if anything, should the leader do if a member misses a session or several sessions? How much do members have a say in shaping the direction and norms of the group itself? Is it acceptable for members to provide feedback about leaders' performance or is commenting on leaders off limits? Leaders can provide direct instruction regarding norms, use evocative questions to elicit certain patterns, and model the norms through their own behavior. Group norms develop whether group leaders tend to them or not. The careful leader intentionally develops normative patterns for the therapeutic benefit of members and tends to any developing patterns that may inhibit group effectiveness, rather than hoping that they will change on their own.

A final leader function is that of *transparency,* which includes self-disclosure, feedback, metacommunication, and openness in regard to internal processing. *Self-disclosure* can be valuable, yet risky, and novice leaders are often advised against it because of the difficulty in differentiating disclosure that serves a therapeutic purpose from disclosure that serves a momentary personal motive of the leader. It is challenging to use self-disclosure judiciously, to share relevant information that helps clients to feel comfortable opening up or to learn by example. Judicious self-disclosure can include sharing appropriate but not excessive detail, keeping the focus on clients, and avoiding self-aggrandizing stories (Bernard et al., 2008). *Feedback* involves sharing perspectives on client situations or choices, and *metacommunication* involves discussing relevant issues about clients' communication styles and their impact upon the leader or other group members—how they make others feel, think, or feel pulled to act in response. *Openness about internal processing* includes sharing internal reflections about group processes, internal deliberations about where to go next with the group, as well as how to help individual members. The leader may at times give voice to the "unspeakable" when members seem deliberately to ignore a negative process, such as a group member ignoring group guidelines, dominating conversation, or sitting passively. Like other interventions, leaders may start with relatively limited transparency, favoring discretion over disclosure, and become increasingly open as the group develops and deepens.

Successful leaders find a balance between providing structure and allowing spontaneity, between managing group interactions through direct involvement and standing outside of ongoing interactions to provide reflective feedback. Leaders serve as a kind of ballast for the group, steadying the group while it travels through deeper waters. Successful leaders have different styles, some more didactic or hierarchical, others more inspirational, and still others more facilitative, but all generally have the wisdom and flexibility to provide what is useful in the moment, even as that changes across phases of group development.

Successful leaders provide a balance between structure and spontaneity, between direct involvement and reflective feedback.

Leaders of MI groups may borrow selectively from the array of available group strategies, limiting the directions that might be pursued in service of keeping the group focused on the key tasks of MI. For example, exploration of the impact of historical events on current functioning is generally kept to a minimum in MI, which focuses more on the future than on the past. However, having knowledge of other approaches allows group leaders to creatively adapt their style to best support members' change efforts. We return to a focus on how to adapt and apply these general group practice guidelines in an MI format in Chapter 4, after we first review the MI approach more generally.

References

Bales, R. F. (1958). Task roles and social roles in problem-solving groups. In E. E. Maccoby, T. M. Newcomb, & E. L. Hartley (Eds.), *Reading in social psychology* (pp. 437–447). New York: Holt, Rinehart & Winston.

Barlow, S.H. (2011). Evidence bases for group practice. In R.K. Conyne (Ed.), *The Oxford handbook of group counseling* (pp. 207–230). New York: Oxford University Press.

Barlow, S. H., Burlingame, G. M., Harding, J. A., & Behrman, J. (1997). Therapeutic focusing in time-limited group psychotherapy. *Group Dynamics: Theory, Research, and Practice, 1,* 254–266.

Barlow, S. H., Burlingame, G. M., & Fuhriman, A. (2000). Therapeutic application of groups: From Practt's "Thought Control Classes" to modern group psychotherapy. *Group Dynamics: Theory, Research, and Practice, 4,* 115–134.

Befort, C. A., Donnelly, J. E., Sullivan, D. K., Ellerbeck, E. F., & Perri, M. G. (2010). Group versus individual phone-based obesity treatment for rural women. *Eating Behaviors, 11,* 11–17.

Bernard, H., Burlingame, G., Flores, P., Greene, L., Joyce, A., Kobos, J. C., et al. (2008). Clinical practice guidelines for group psychotherapy. *International Journal of Group Psychotherapy, 58,* 455–542.

Bloch, S., & Crouch, E. (1985). *Therapeutic factors in group psychotherapy.* Oxford: Oxford University Press.

Bordin, E. S. (1979). The generalizability of the psychoanalytic concept of the working alliance. *Psychotherapy: Theory, Research, and Practice, 16,* 252–260.

Brewer, C. L. (1981). Something for everyone. *PsycCRITIQUES, 26*(11), 872–874.

Burlingame, G., Fuhriman, A., & Mosier, J. (2003). The differential effectiveness of group psychotherapy: A meta-analytical perspective. *Group Dynamics: Theory, Research, and Practice, 7,* 3–12.

Burlingame, G. M., MacKenzie, D., & Strauss, B. (2004). Small group treatment: Evidence for effectiveness and mechanisms of change. In M. J. Lambert (Ed.), *Bergin and Garfield's handbook of psychotherapy and behavioral change* (5th ed., pp. 647–696). New York: Wiley.

Conyne, R. K. (Ed.). (2011). *The Oxford handbook of group counseling.* New York: Oxford University Press.

Corsini, R. J., & Rosenberg, B. (1955). Mechanisms of group psychotherapy: Processes and dynamics. *Journal of Abnormal and Social Psychology, 51,* 406–411.

Delsignore, A., Carraro, G., Mathier, F., Znoj, H., & Schnyder, U. (2008). Perceived responsibility for change as an outcome predictor in cognitive-behavioural group therapy. *British Journal of Clinical Psychology, 47*(Pt. 3), 281–293.

Dinkmeyer, D. C., & Muro, J. C. (1979). *Group counseling: Theory and practice* (2nd ed.). Itasca, IL: Peacock.

Faris, A. S., & Brown, J. M. (2003). Addressing group dynamics in a brief motivational intervention for college student drinkers. *Journal of Drug Education, 33*(3), 289–306.

Fielding, J. M. (1983). Verbal participation and group therapy outcome.*British Journal of Psychiatry, 142,* 524–528.

Fishman, I., Ng, R., & Bellugi, U. (2010). Do extraverts process social stimuli differently from introverts? *Cognitive Neuroscience, 2,* 67–73.

Forsyth, D. R. (2011). The nature and significance of groups. In R. K. Conyne (Ed.), *The Oxford handbook of group counseling* (pp. 19–35). New York: Oxford University Press.

Forsyth, D. R., & Strong, S. R. (2004). The scientific study of counseling and psychotherapy: A unificationist view. *The interface of social and clinical psychology: Key readings* (pp. 290–300). New York: Psychology Press.

Gawronski, B. (2004). Theory-based bias correction in dispositional inference: The fundamental attribution error is dead, long live the correspondence bias. *European Review of Social Psychology, 15,* 183–217.

Giese-Davis, J., Koopman, C., Fobair, P., Butler, L. D., Classen, C., Cordova, M., et al. (2002). Change in emotion-regulation strategy for women with metastatic breast cancer following supportive–expressive group therapy. *Journal of Consulting and Clinical Psychology, 70,* 916–925.

Holmes, S. E., & Kivlighan, D. M. (2000). Comparison of therapeutic factors in group and individual treatment process. *Journal of Counseling Psychology, 47,* 478–484.

Hornsey, M. J., Dwyer, L., & Oei, T. P. (2007). Beyond cohesiveness: Reconceptualizing the link between group processes and outcomes in group psychotherapy. *Small Group Research, 38,* 567–592.

Howard, C., Dupont, S., Haselden, B., Lynch, J., & Wills, P. (2010). The effectiveness of a group cognitive-behavioural breathlessness intervention on health status, mood and hospital admissions in elderly patients with chronic obstructive pulmonary disease. *Psychology, Health and Medicine, 15,* 371–385.

Johnson, J. (2007). Cohesion, alliance, and outcome in group psychotherapy: Comments on Joyce, Piper, & Ogrodniczuk (2007). *International Journal of Group Psychotherapy, 57,* 533–540.

Joyce, A. S., MacNair-Semands, R., Tasca, G. A., & Ogrodniczuk, J. S. (2011). Factor structure and validity of the Therapeutic Factors Inventory—Short Form. *Group Dynamics: Theory, Research, and Practice, 15,* 201–219.

Kelly, J. R. (2004). Mood and emotion in groups. In M. B. Brewer & M. Hewstone (Eds.), *Emotion and motivation* (pp. 95–112). Malden, MA: Blackwell.

Kerr, N. L., & Tindale, R. S. (2004). Group performance and decision making. *Annual Review of Psychology, 55,* 623–655.

Kivlighan, D. M., Jr. (2008). Comments on the practice guidelines for group psychotherapy: Evidence, gaps in the literature, and resistance. *International Journal of Group Psychotherapy, 58*(4), 543–554.

Kivlighan, D. M., Jr., & Tarrant, J. M. (2001). Does group climate mediate the group leadership–group member outcome relationship?: A test of Yalom's hypotheses about leadership priorities. *Group Dynamics, 5,* 220–234.

Klein, R. H. (2008). Toward the establishment of evidence-based practices in group psychotherapy. *International Journal of Group Psychotherapy, 58,* 441–454.

Lamb, S. E., Hansen, Z., Lall, R., Castelnuovo, E., Withers, E. J., Nichols, V., et al. (2010). Group cognitive behavioural treatment for low-back pain in primary care: A randomised controlled trial and cost-effectiveness analysis. *Lancet, 375*(9718), 916–923.

Lieberman, M., Miles, G., & Yalom, I. D. (1973). *Encounter groups: First facts.* New York: Basic Books.

MacKenzie, K. R. (1983). The clinical application of a group climate measure. In R. R. Dies & K. R. MacKenzie (Eds.), *Advances in group psychotherapy: Integrating research and practice* (pp. 159–170). New York: International Universities Press.

MacKenzie, K. R. (1994). The developing structure of the therapy group system. In H. S. Bernard & K. R. MacKenzie (Eds.), *Basics of group psychotherapy* (pp. 35–59). New York: Guilford Press.

MacKenzie, K. R., Dies, R. R., Coche, E., Rutan, J. S., & Stone, W. N. (1987). An analysis of AGPA institute groups. *International Journal of Group Psychotherapy, 37,* 55–74.

Marchand, A., Roberge, P., Primiano, S., & Germain, V. (2009). A randomized, controlled clinical trial of standard, group and brief cognitive-behavioral therapy for panic disorder with agoraphobia: A two-year follow-up. *Journal of Anxiety Disorders, 23,* 1139–1147.

Marmarosh, C. L., & Van Horn, S. M. (2011). Cohesion in counseling and psychotherapy groups. In R. K. Conyne (Ed.), *The Oxford handbook of group counseling* (pp. 137–163). New York: Oxford University Press.

Martin, D. J., Garske, J. P., & Davis, M. K. (2000). Relation of the therapeutic alliance with outcome and other variables: A meta-analytic review. *Journal of Consulting and Clinical Psychology, 68,* 438–450.

McLendon, D. T., & Burlingame, G. M. (2011). Group climate: Construct in search of clarity. In R. K. Conyne (Ed.), *The Oxford handbook of group counseling* (pp. 164–181). New York: Oxford University Press.

McRoberts, C., Burlingame, G., & Hoag, M. (1998). Comparative efficacy of individual and group psychotherapy: A meta-analytic perspective. *Group Dynamics: Theory, Research, and Practice, 2,* 101–117.

Miller, W. R., & Rollnick, S. (2013). *Motivational interviewing: Helping people change* (3rd ed.). New York: Guilford Press.

Miller, W. R., & Rose, G. S. (2009). Toward a theory of motivational interviewing. *American Psychologist, 64,* 527–537.

Minniti, A., Bissoli, L., Di Francesco, V., Fantin, F., Mandragona, R., Olivieri, M., et al. (2007). Individual versus group therapy for obesity: Comparison of dropout rate and treatment outcome. *Eating and Weight Disorders, 12,* 161–167.

Muroff, J., Steketee, G., Rasmussen, J., Gibson, A., Bratiotis, C., & Sorrentino, C. (2009). Group cognitive and behavioral treatment for compulsive hoarding: A preliminary trial. *Depression and Anxiety, 26,* 634–640.

Niccols, A. (2008). "Right from the start": Randomized trial comparing an attachment group intervention to supportive home visiting. *Journal of Child Psychology and Psychiatry and Allied Disciplines, 49,* 754–764.

Oei, T. P., & Dingle, G. (2008). The effectiveness of group cognitive behaviour therapy for unipolar depressive disorders. *Journal of Affective Disorders, 107,* 5–21.

Oei, T. P., Raylu, N., & Casey, L. M. (2010). Effectiveness of group and individual formats of a combined MI and cognitive behavioral treatment program for problem gambling: A randomized controlled trial. *Behavioural and Cognitive Psychotherapy, 38,* 233–238.

Piper, W. E., Ogrodniczuk, J. S., McCallum, M., Joyce, A. S., & Rosie, J. S. (2003). Expression of affect as a mediator of the relationship between quality of object relations and group therapy outcome for patients with complicated grief. *Journal of Consulting and Clinical Psychology, 71,* 664–671.

Robbins, R. N. (2003). Developing cohesion in court-mandated group treatment of male spousal abuses. *International Journal of Group Psychotherapy, 53,* 261–284.

Schutz, W. C. (1961). On group composition. *Journal of Abnormal and Social Psychology, 62,* 275–281.

Seligman, M. E. P., Rashid, T., & Parks, A. C. (2006). Positive psychotherapy. *American Psychologist, 61,* 774–788.

Siskind, D., Baingana, F., & Kim, J. (2008). Cost-effectiveness of group psychotherapy for depression in Uganda. *Journal of Mental Health Policy and Economics, 11,* 127–133.

Smock, S. A., Trepper, T. S., Wetchler, J. L., McCollum, E. E., Ray, R., & Pierce, K. (2008). Solution-focused group therapy for level 1 substance abusers. *Journal of Marital and Family Therapy, 34,* 107–120.

Sobell, L. C., Sobell, M. B., & Agrawal, S. (2009). Randomized controlled trial of a cognitive-behavioral motivational intervention in a group versus individual format for substance use disorders. *Psychology of Addictive Behaviors, 23,* 672–683.

Tindale, R. S., & Kameda, T. (2000). "Social sharedness" as a unifying theme for information processing in groups. *Group Processes and Intergroup Relations, 3,* 123–140.

Trotzer, J. P. (1977). *The counselor and the group: Integrating theory, training, and practice.* Monterey, CA: Brooks Cole.

Tuckman, B. W., & Jensen, M. A. C. (1977). Stages of group development revisited. *Group and Organizational Studies, 2*(4), 419–427.

Turner, J. C., Brown, R. J., & Tajfel, H. (1979). Social comparison and group interest in ingroup favouritism. *European Journal of Social Psychology, 9,* 187–204.

Weiss, R. D., Griffin, M. L., Kolodziej, M. E., Greenfield, S. F., Najavits, L. M., Daley, D. C., et al. (2007). A randomized trial of integrated group therapy versus group drug counseling for patients with bipolar disorder and substance dependence. *American Journal of Psychiatry, 174,* 100–107.

Weiss, R. D., Jaffee, W. B., de Menil, V. P., & Cogley, C. B. (2004). Group therapy for substance use disorders: What do we know? *Harvard Review of Psychiatry, 12,* 339–350.

Whelton, W. J. (2004). Emotional processes in psychotherapy: Evidence across therapeutic modalities. *Clinical Psychology and Psychotherapy, 11,* 58–71.

Wildschut, T., Pinter, B., Vevea, J. L., Insko, C. A., & Schopler, J. (2003). Beyond the group mind: A quantitative review of the interindividual–intergroup discontinuity effect. *Psychological Bulletin, 129,* 698–722.

Yalom, I., & Leszcz, M. (2005). *The theory and practice of group psychotherapy* (5th ed.). New York: Basic Books.

CHAPTER 3

Overview of
Motivational Interviewing

Motivational interviewing helps by increasing interest and energy for change, easing reluctance, and sidestepping natural defenses that hinder change. MI practitioners provide an accepting and supportive atmosphere and structure conversations in ways that evoke clients' desires and plans for living in more fulfilling ways.

Although MI integrates findings from research in social and cognitive psychology with concepts from humanistic, cognitive, and behavioral therapies, it has been developed more out of practical experience than a specific theoretical conviction. MI pragmatically focuses on motivation as a linchpin for change. Lacking motivation to change, people may be changed by external pressures, but they are unlikely to initiate and maintain change of their own volition. MI helps people change in the directions they prefer, rather than be pressed or pulled by external influences—MI helps them to change rather than be changed.

Ambivalence

Unresolved ambivalence is a common obstacle to change. Ambivalence pulls people from argument to counterargument about continuing to live as they have been versus trying something new. Cognitively, people become stuck, unable to reach a decision. Behaviorally, some people make halting steps forward, unsure of moving at all and backtracking at the first sign of potential failure. Others rush forward, only to discover that they weren't prepared for challenges in their desire to change things as quickly

31

as possible, then give up in frustration. Emotionally, people run the gamut from experiencing excitement, confidence, and determination about the possibilities in front of them to feeling dread, anger, and grief about the challenges ahead and the comforts they must leave behind. They may struggle to decide whether change is worth the effort and losses involved, and to find the will to succeed. They open themselves to the frightening possibility of failure. They have to consider details, weigh options, take chances, and risk embarrassment. When change starts, they can lose their sense of familiarity and comfort with their current way of living. Even initial success may not bring much relief, because it increases awareness of the significance of the venture they are attempting and the fact that true relief often requires permanent change. There is no diet; only permanent change in eating habits. The need for exercise never ends. Certain pleasures may need to be surrendered forever.

Making intentional changes in lifestyles, perspectives, and habits can be overwhelming. People often have to learn to value things that may bring less immediate reward than their old comforts. They may have to grasp abstract concepts to guide them through risky situations rather than follow momentary impulses and familiar habits. They may have to learn to trust others and themselves.

In MI, we stand beside those who want to change, need to change, or simply can't go on as before. Clients experience our warmth, respect, and support for creating healthier, more fulfilling lives. They discover that we strive to understand them, truly accept them, and help them envision a different future and find ways to bring it about. We carefully listen to clients' language, watch nonverbal communications, and feel the emotions that may be pulling clients forward toward change or pushing them back toward the status quo or worse. Positive movement is elicited and highlighted, while inertia and backtracking are accepted but usually not actively explored. As we work collaboratively with them, expressing support for their control over the choices they make, clients develop a greater sense of autonomy, of ownership of their lives, and of their ability to shape their own destinies.

Change

MI helps clients focus on positive changes they can make to improve their lives. Although the active ingredients of MI are not well understood at this time, several elements appear to contribute to its effectiveness. One of these is the concept (drawing from Daryl Bem's (1972) self-perception theory) that people's beliefs and attitudes are shaped by discussing them, particularly by the arguments they themselves make about them. So people who talk about the importance of exercising are more likely to remember later that they think exercising is important. While MI is not about manipulating people into doing what we want, it *is* about helping people explore their motivations to move away from patterns that are causing problems toward more satisfying lives. A key strategy for doing this is helping clients explore their thoughts, feelings, and impulses about change.

Change talk is language used by clients as they discuss forward momentum toward change. An early description of the components of change talk (Rollnick, 1998) suggested that motivation is a

> *MI helps clients focus on positive changes they can make to improve their lives.*

combination of sensing the importance of making changes and experiencing confidence that change is possible. Another summary found wisdom in the colloquial phrase "ready, willing, and able" (Rollnick, Mason, & Butler, 1999) Following the psycholinguistics studies of Amrhein, Miller, Yahne, Palmer, and Fulcher (2003), there are as many as seven types of change talk:

- Desire for change
- Ability to change
- Reasons for change
- Need for change
- Commitment to change
- Activation
- Taking steps

The acronym DARN-CAT summarizes these categories. The DARN elements are considered *preparatory change talk,* things we listen for while clients decide whether they want to make changes, and hone in on what specifically they want to change. The CAT elements, thought of as *mobilizing change talk,* include how clients want to go about changing and the elements involved in getting started.

Miller and Rose (2009) suggested a linear model of how change talk may be related to change in MI. Specific counselor behaviors elicit preparatory change talk (DARN) that then helps clients commit (C) to change, which in turn leads to activation and taking steps toward change. There has been some initial support for this model (Moyers & Martin, 2006; Moyers et al., 2007; Moyers, Martin, Houck, Christopher, & Tonigan, 2009; Walters, Vader, Harris, Field, & Jouriles, 2009) although how complete or accurate the model is, or what specific mechanisms of action are involved in the process, remain unresolved.

MI uses several strategies to elicit change talk and momentum toward change. It balances empathy and direction, specifies a collaborative and eliciting therapeutic stance, incorporates specific communication elements and general processes, and includes several broad strategies for guiding therapeutic conversations to build momentum. We review these here and in later chapters, and recommend that helpers who wish to become proficient in this approach read the general MI book (Miller & Rollnick, 2013), as well as books that target specific audiences in areas including health care (Rollnick, Miller, & Butler, 2008), mental health (Arkowitz, Westra, Miller, & Rollnick, 2008), anxiety (Westra, 2012), youth therapy (Naar-King & Suarez, 2011), social work (Hohman, 2012), and corrections (Walters, Clark, Gingerich, & Meltzer, 2007) A recent practitioner learning workbook is also available (Rosengren, 2009).

Status Quo

There is another side to ambivalence, the side that leans toward keeping things the same due to attachments to one's current lifestyle and reluctance to change. Change is hard. It involves giving up valued parts of one's life and even of oneself, and implementing new habits that feel awkward, and that may not pay off in the short term. Sometimes unanticipated challenges or disadvantages appear along the pathway to change. Old habits may also compensate for other difficulties that do not fully reveal themselves until change is attempted. How we handle this side as we help clients change is a matter of some skill, sensitivity, and timing.

Reactance theory (Brehm, 1966) is relevant here. *Reactance* is the concept that people defend their freedom whenever they perceive that others are attempting to constrain them in some way. Sometimes clients need to talk about their hesitation about changing, and if we focus only on change, they may perceive us as "taking sides" in their own internal debate and attempting to reduce their autonomy and choice, and pressure them into change. There is value in exploring the status quo side of ambivalence in some instances (referred to as *sustain talk* in the MI model), and at times it may be necessary if we are to foster change that is lasting. At the same time, there remains the obvious risk of focusing too much on problems, risks, and losses, and squashing motivation for change, if we focus too much on status quo concerns.

Balancing Both Sides of Ambivalence
(with a Tilt toward Change)

Because the goal of MI is to evoke change, it focuses mostly on clients' thoughts, feelings, and behaviors that favor positive change, giving less attention to the status quo side of ambivalence, unless it appears important to do so to help clients get unstuck. This is accomplished by actively exploring change talk, accepting and acknowledging status quo concerns as they arise, and at transitional moments, inviting clients back to actively exploring the possibilities and advantages of change.

The overall strategy is to maintain a focus on forward momentum. You may, however, incorporate nondirective moments within a larger directional strategy in order to help clients let go of attachments to the status quo. Change talk can seem elusive when you feel that you are under pressure to produce results or convince members to change. Chasing it too hard may simply chase it away.

It is easy to fall into a "uniformity myth" (Kiesler, 1966)—the idea that one correct approach is applicable across situations and clients. One size does not fit all, and there are times when it may be useful to explore the status quo, especially when group members differ in ambivalence and in what they need to help them move forward with change. There are several reasons that it may be valuable to give some attention to the status quo side of ambivalence:

- to increase trust and alliances with clients
- to allow clients to "vent," so that they can then think more clearly
- to help to reduce clients' reactance to feelings of pressure to change
- to help clients better understand some of the benefits of status quo behaviors in order to brainstorm better ways to achieve those benefits
- to help clients identify obstacles to change and strategies to overcome them

In later chapters, we discuss how you can balance both sides of ambivalence when working with challenging client styles and group dynamics. As a general principle, though, it is helpful to remember that the goal is to tip the balance toward change, while not going so far as to make clients feel they need to make arguments against change in order to defend themselves against coercion.

Empathy and Direction

MI combines Rogers's (1951) core component of empathy with a focus on providing adequate direction. Although Rogers often presented client-centered therapy as nondirective, some research indicates that Rogers was actually selective about what he reflected and what he ignored, and that clients responded directionally to what Rogers reinforced (Truax, 1966).

MI is more narrowly focused than client-centered therapy. While incorporating a client-centered stance, MI helps clients identify specific changes they can make to improve their lives. MI has a bias toward change, with an assumption that clients generally present for therapeutic services when things are not working well for them. Despite this bias toward change, MI practitioners remain client-centered, respecting and supporting client autonomy. MI works from the inside-out to elicit clients' ideas and momentum for change rather than from the outside-in, trying to install knowledge or your own preferred choices for clients.

Thus, MI incorporates therapeutic direction. It is useful to differentiate therapeutic direction from *directiveness,* which involves taking a dominant interpersonal stance, making decisions on behalf of our interactional partners, and attempting to influence them to do what we want them to do. You can be directive in a positive way, such as selectively approving the choices they make and advising them to choose in your preferred direction, or in a more negative manner by disagreeing with them, expressing disapproval of their choices, warning or confronting them, or directing them outright to do as they are told. None of these forms of directiveness is characteristic of the concept of direction in MI, which is more generally oriented toward change in a positive direction. In MI, direction involves focusing conversations on the change issue(s) being faced by clients, and interacting in a way that helps clients leverage their own motivation to change unhelpful patterns in their lives. Although there is a role for giving advice or making recommendations, it is a minimal aspect of MI, and is always done in a manner that emphasizes client autonomy and choice.

The Spirit of MI

The spirit of MI involves a *partnership* based on respectful collaboration. Clients have expertise about themselves that can be used to make healthy changes. MI practitioners have expertise in facilitating conversations that support change. MI is more a dance between partners than a wrestling match between opponents.

MI practitioners hold an attitude of deep *acceptance* of clients, which in turn facilitates change. Miller and Rollnick (2013) suggest that acceptance includes several components. The first is to recognize the *absolute worth* of clients as human beings. We don't communicate our understanding and acceptance of clients when we agree with them, then discount them when we see things differently. This kind of conditional stance is common in social interactions, yet it does not appear to be very effective in eliciting change. As Rogers (1961) explained, "The curious paradox is that when I accept myself just as I am, then I can change" (p. 17). While we may sometimes provide additional information or share a different perspective, we do so in the spirit of wondering whether clients might find these additional

ideas or perceptions useful, and never
in the spirit of being unaccepting of   *Acceptance facilitates change.*
clients.

Accurate empathy is another element of acceptance. Drawing from person-centered therapy, the goal of accurate empathy is to perceive clients' inner worlds—experiences, perspectives, emotions, meaning—and to use those perceptions to better understand their lived experience and help them become more aware, and consider the possibility of changing "inside." Rogers and colleagues describe this process as helping clients "get close" to themselves (Rogers, Gendlin, Kiesler, & Truax, 1967, p. 105). Highly accurate empathy involves perceiving experiences and meanings of which clients may not even be fully aware. This differs from interpretation, in that the practitioner is only opening up what is already inside clients, not providing an external frame of reference for clients to consider, and clients should experience this as "new, but . . . not alien" (p. 106). In addition to direct benefits, Rogers and colleagues perceived even the attempt at developing an accurate empathic understanding as beneficial, as clients experience the value the practitioner places on trying to understand them, which itself is rewarding and increases clients' motivation to understand and relate their own experiences more clearly and thoroughly.

In addition, the spirit of MI includes a fundamental *support for clients' autonomy*—for their ability and authority to make choices, consider options, and take actions. Clients' lives are their own, not ours. Supporting autonomy involves the simple recognition that we can't make clients do anything, and it reflects the belief that rather than install motivation in people, we need to help them shake free of constraining perspectives, emotions, and habits that keep them from having the kind of life they want.

Affirmation is discussed in detail later as a communication skill. *Affirmation* is not merely approving or praising those client choices with which we agree. It puts the focus on clients' strengths, effort, and vision rather than on perceived weaknesses, hesitancies, and past problems. Momentum is better achieved by building upon what is working well than by fixing what is not.

Next, MI is meant to be a *compassionate* approach to helping. We prioritize helping clients in whatever ways are best for them over ways that benefit others. MI remains focused on clients' growth needs, even while finding ways these coincide with the needs of society, their families, and so on. MI should never be used against clients' own best interests, even if there are occasions when we may choose not to help clients pursue potentially damaging self-interests due to ethical concerns.

Finally, the spirit of MI is *evocative*. MI practitioners elicit clients' perspectives on defining which behaviors might be problems, explore their own concerns, and elicit their intention to change or their optimism about change.

Miller (1999) has conceptualized the practitioner's role as providing *agape,* a selfless form of love intended to enhance others' well-being and growth. *Agape* may enhance clients' acceptance of themselves, distinct from any of the choices they have made. This acceptance may provide inspiration to actualize their potential. When you provide *agape,* you figuratively embrace clients' ambivalence and struggles. They then experiences a feeling of safety in which potential resolutions of ambivalence can emerge without arousing their defenses. A likely sign that you are operating in the spirit of MI is finding yourself in awe of your clients' strengths and humanity, regardless of any problems or negative habits they may have.

Communication Style

MI practice builds upon this collaborative relationship by incorporating a specific communication style. The style is summarized with the acronym OARS: Open questions that encourage further elaboration and consideration; Affirmations that foster positive feelings in the client; Reflections that show the helper has accurately understood and that give back to clients a particular image of themselves; and Summaries that extend the basic reflections to include a sense of momentum or build interest in changing direction. We use these techniques to build rapport and gain understanding of clients' issues, to facilitate discussion, to mend rifts in the therapeutic relationship, to redirect clients to more useful areas of consideration, and to solidify commitment to change in an established relationship where therapeutic alliance is strong. We consider each of these communication techniques in detail, discussing not only what they are but what purposes we believe they serve.

Open questions allow for open-ended answers instead of limiting respondents to specific responses. Open questions tend to invite clients to explore possibilities, to frame things for themselves, to imagine different perspectives. However, open questions can also provide significant structure that helps to focus the conversation, as in "Tell me more about how drinking fits into your everyday life," or "How might you like things to be different?" This last question elicits several things—the client's perspective, a focus on the future, and change talk about the future. Open questions stand in contrast to closed questions, such as "When did this happen?"; "How many times?"; "Where?"; "Did you . . .?" Closed questions generally ask clients to provide practitioners with specific information instead of encouraging clients to explore the topic further.

More broadly, the question is whether we are trying to open people up or close them down. One direction invites people to creatively explore options and take ownership of solutions, while the other presses people to defer to others' influence in setting the direction of their lives. Closed questions can give the message "Follow me, listen to the question, give an answer, and wait for the next question." Over time, closed questions can introduce an implicit hierarchy, in which the person asking them becomes more powerful and in control of the discussion, as the person answering them becomes ever more passive, more constrained, and more of a follower. Heavy use of closed questioning casts us as the experts, and clients as people who, somewhat helpless to solve their own problems, need expert guidance.

This is the opposite of the direction pursued in MI. MI works by eliciting perspectives, desires, and hopes; by helping people open to new possibilities rather than adhere to a plan given to them by others. It helps clients envision a new way of being, become creative, and seek it out. The goal is to help people be more in control of their own destinies—to experience greater ownership of their own lives. We want them to get excited—"This is my life, this is what I want to do with it, and this is who I want to be." When they open up to the possibilities of change and what it can bring, they focus less on what will be lost, difficult, unfamiliar, and uncomfortable. So opening up helps them think about these possibilities more concretely, in order to give them more "pull"—more power to pull themselves toward them.

Closed questions aren't taboo, of course. Sometimes, gathering specific information is helpful in focusing the conversation, and open questions are an inefficient way to gather specific information. Closed questions are appropriate when we are trying to clarify some details to guide the conversation toward a productive end. They help to lay the foundation for more open-ended exploration of a topic by first gathering some basic facts that set parameters for discussion. They may be most appropriate at pivotal points in conversations, or when a bit of specific information is needed to understand the client's more open exploration of an issue.

One last caution: Sometimes closed questions are really suggestions masquerading as questions, as in "Can you see how making that choice was harmful to you in the end?"; "Don't you think you got a bit out of hand?"; "Could you try to do X next time?" While these are technically questions, it is easy to recognize that they are really suggestions, subtle criticisms, or mild confrontations. There is a place for direction in MI, but these "leading" closed questions are instead a kind of misdirection. Open questions don't lend themselves to these kinds of tactics that are at odds with the spirit of MI, and thus are less likely to get us off track or invite resistance.

Affirmations are used to increase positive energy and mood. They often take the form of noticing something we appreciate about the client, a success of the client, or the effort invested toward a goal. Affirmations are like seasoning. Too little and the meal can seem bland and uninspiring, but too much and it becomes overwhelming or even repulsive. The amount, timing and nature of affirmations may need to vary by setting, culture, and individual client.

Affirmations increase positive energy and mood.

Affirming can be differentiated from agreeing or approving, which are more practitioner-centered than affirmations. Affirming a client strength or appreciating a characteristic does involve some opinion, but the focus remains primarily on the client. When expressing agreement with clients, you share the spotlight equally and risk that their motivations become tied to your agreement with them rather than occurring for primarily intrinsic reasons. Agreeing also puts you in a difficult position if the client then says something with which you disagree. Once you have agreed with something, you may feel more compelled to note your disagreement when the client then says something you believe is incorrect or counter to your preferences or values. Approving client choices or actions is even more practitioner-centered, potentially placing you in a more hierarchical role in relation to the client. Given the power imbalance in therapeutic relationships and clients' vulnerabilities, approving client choices or actions can sometimes further reinforce clients doing things because you think they are good ideas rather than acting on their own chosen direction.

So, generally, find things that affirm who clients are as people and what is special about them: their strengths, their determination to make some changes, their willingness to work toward goals, and how important it is for them to raise their children well, to be good to other people, or to be honest in sharing their perspective. Tread lightly when communicating approval of specific plans or agreement with specific opinions and just notice what shines about them. Ideally, look at clients with respect and a kind of awe, admiring them for their talents, energy, and attributes. You don't have to make a show of it; just casually notice these things and be appreciative of getting to know them. Avoid coming across as seeing clients as people in need of assistance, and instead look at them eye-to-eye as equals or even look up to them, noticing things to admire about them and ways you might like to be more like them yourself.

To be affirming is more than making specific affirmations. You can affirm people nonverbally by meeting them at the time you say you'll meet them, giving them your full attention and your best effort to be helpful, and your openness. It is affirming to lend them your hope, your confidence that they can make things better for themselves, your sense of excitement about possibilities, and your appreciation for who they are as people.

Affirming can be calibrated to the specific need of the moment. On the one hand, it may be especially important to be affirming when someone feels stuck, frustrated, angry, demoralized, hopeless, or bitter. When people feel affirmed at these times, when they experience your willingness to connect with them while they're in these negative states, they can develop greater positive energy. They can become more interested in change and be more willing to go out on a limb, take risks, and try harder. On the other hand, when people feel positive and focused on change, when their sense of self-esteem and self-efficacy is high, affirmations may distract them, drawing their attention away from efforts to change and back onto themselves more generally. And too much affirmation at any time can come across as patronizing or insincere cheerleading. But genuine, modest affirmation at times when people feel demoralized can lend them the energy to continue toward difficult change. It is a way of bridging over the negatives and connecting to their deeper sense of self, helping them to feel more secure and less defended, and to help stay on task.

Reflecting involves mirroring back part or all of what the client communicates (verbally and nonverbally). Reflections are used in multiple ways in MI. The simplest use of reflections is to confirm hearing what clients say. This serves not only to let clients know you are listening but it also allows them to gauge the extent to which you understand them. It facilitates further exploration by giving them a chance to hear their thoughts from the outside, which sometimes is helpful, because often people are not really listening to themselves while they speak—their focus is often on trying to communicate rather than on what they're communicating. This is essentially a nondirective use of reflection.

In descriptions of MI, reflections have typically been divided into two forms, *simple reflections,* which rephrase clients' comments to verify accurate understanding and facilitate further exploration, and *complex reflections,* which add something (e.g., a reflection of underlying meaning or feelings, tying client statements to their values, or reframing their comments into images or metaphors). Various types of content-based reflections have also been described, such as double-sided reflections (reflecting both sides of clients' ambivalence), continuing the paragraph reflections (guessing at the next thing clients might say), and so on. In this book, we organize reflections (along with the other OARS and MI strategies) into the purposes we are attempting to achieve in conversations. Chapter 8 casts these as "shaping group conversations," although we believe this framework can apply to individual interactions as well. We focus on shaping discussions with regard to breadth, depth, and momentum—how broad or narrow the focus is, how deep or superficial, and how much it focuses on review of past and present elements versus exploring momentum toward future change.

As with affirmations, there is a broader purpose to using reflections. Reflections serve as a kind of ratchet, allowing clients to continue to explore while "locking in" progress toward a more complete under-standing or plan. As with affirmations, you can reflect nonverbally as well by accommodating clients' preferred pace and style, so that their focus can remain fully on their issues, and not on how they are talking to you. You can also adjust to clients' mode of discussion, whether they approach issues in an analytical, problem-solving manner, through stories or meta-phors, with humor, etc.

Summaries are somewhat longer communications, often combining several reflections made earlier in conversation and re-presenting them to the client with a cohesive theme. Summaries help clients stand back and look at the big picture, pulling together their interests and concerns about different patterns and possibilities—seeing the forest, not just the trees. As the general focus in MI is on change, this provides a model for constructing a summary. A good MI summary might include a restatement of the out-come goals or direction in which the client is heading, clients' thoughts and feelings about change, and their current momentum toward implementing the changes they've decided upon. Generally, try to find a balance that emphasizes clients' positive thoughts and feelings about change, without ignoring the challenges involved and leaving clients feeling only partially heard, or as if you are discounting realistic concerns that they then need to explain further to you. The message you want to convey is not "Everything will be fine once you change" but "Here is what I understand about why you want to change and how you plan to go about it."

MI uses a few different types of summaries. The *collecting summary* brings together various client statements, often ending with an open ques-tion that has some momentum or direction built in, such as an invitation for clients to add more to the list or comment on what they want to do next. A *linking summary* connects a current conversation with a previ-ous conversation, perhaps on a different topic, often highlighting a shared theme, feeling, or dilemma. A *transitional summary,* used to wrap up a topic and shift to a new focus, communicates that the current topic has reached a point of diminishing returns, or that a different focus might be more productive. This allows for a sense of temporary closure on a topic, so that another can be explored. Summaries can also be used to end sessions, leaving the client with an easily recalled synopsis of an entire conversation.

MI Processes and Therapeutic Strategies

While the OARS microcommunications focus on momentary interactions, MI incorporates broader conversational strategies into the context of four general therapeutic processes—engaging, focusing, evoking, and planning (Miller & Rollnick, 2013). While the strategies may serve more than one purpose (e.g., engaging and focusing at the same time), we describe them in relation to the process that provides the best fit for each.

Engaging

The first key process is *engaging*. Therapeutic engagement is a common process across therapies, and is essential to MI as an approach that relies on deep client involvement. Clients who are deeply engaged are more able to think creatively and brainstorm new ideas and solutions. In general, a good way to start is to expect a fairly natural process of opening up, connecting, developing trust, and deepening engagement. As in the Will Rogers quote "A stranger is just a friend I haven't met yet," start with the presumption that whatever burdens clients may currently carry, however emotionally dysregulated or interpersonally insensitive they may seem, you will soon move past those surface patterns and develop a meaningful connection and working relationship. Thus, engaging has two essential functions—to enlist clients in the process of opening up and discussing personal issues, and to involve them in a meaningful relationship that provides understanding and acceptance.

Clients often have a range of interests and concerns when beginning treatment: "How helpful will counseling be?"; "How trustworthy is this counselor?"; "Will the counselor respect me and my perspective or criticize and pressure me?"; "How much of the truth should I tell, and how much should I keep to myself?" Clients may be embarrassed about things they've done, critical of themselves for having to talk to a counselor, or fearful about their ability to gain enough self-control to manage their lives more productively. As long as they have these concerns in mind, their ability to explore and reveal themselves is limited, as is their ability to envision a better future and make progress toward enacting it. Engaging helps to reduce these distractions, increasing trust and positive energy to consider change, in a trusting relationship and empathic, supportive atmosphere.

Engagement is a fairly natural process that develops as you interact with clients. However, *natural* doesn't mean automatic or assured. There are missteps that may discourage engagement as you begin this new relationship. Thus, attempt to avoid a few early traps, such as a *premature focus* on deeply exploring sensitivities or vulnerabilities before trust has developed. Another trap is taking an *expert stance,* communicating implicitly that the client's role is to answer questions, provide information, pose problems, and so forth, for you, the professional, to sort out, solve, and render advice on.

An essential part of engagement is helping clients begin to share their stories, values, and feelings. Early on, this can be accomplished through a mix of open questions and reflections directed toward developing an empathic understanding of clients' perspectives and experiences. Open questions not only inform clients that the practitioner is interested in their perspectives and experiences, but also, by their very structure, prompt clients to elaborate, which is an essential part of engaging. Reflections are used for different purposes at different times. While engaging clients, use frequent, simple reflections of key words or ideas demonstrating that you understand the key elements of their messages. Given that many clients enter services in a defensive posture, these regular, simple reflections may be more important than they seem upon first glance. They are less threatening than reflecting on deeper themes.

Reflections can sometimes be confused with closed questions. The surface difference between the two is sometimes only a matter of voice inflection. Sometimes counselors believe it is more respectful to ask a question than to make a statement about clients' experiences or perspectives. However, clients generally seem quite willing to correct off-target reflections, and they appreciate your effort to understand. To the contrary, clients who are feeling defensive or unsure may easily hear closed questions as veiled judgments or accusations.

Imagine the following two practitioner comments:

"You don't see your cocaine use as a problem?"
"You don't see your cocaine use as a problem."

The first, a closed question, demands that the client answer the practitioner's inquiry and could be interpreted as judgment or confrontation. The second example, a reflection (delivered in an accepting manner, without any hint of sarcasm), is more likely to come across as a respectful reflection of the client's current perspective, and communicates a nonjudgmental and nonhierarchical stance on the practitioner's part.

As practitioners, it is easy to miss the importance of such microcommunications. Clients, however, can be hypervigilant about such communications and react to them at a feelings or intuition level, especially if they are concerned about defending their integrity to someone with potential power over them. Such small interactions can greatly influence the direction the engagement takes—toward either an open, mutually respectful and deepening relationship, or a guarded, defensive, and superficial relationship.

Throughout MI, a goal is to average two to three reflections for every question (using other forms of communication much less frequently). This helps avoid a *question–answer trap*, in which you rely too much on asking questions (especially closed questions), essentially training clients to become more passive, to answer the questions asked, to avoid doing their own creative brainstorming, and to wait for you to provide expert advice.

This is contrary to the process we are trying to develop in MI to help clients move through lingering ambivalence about change.

Although the process of engaging clients should be established before turning attention to the process of focusing, engaging is never fully finished. At any point throughout the process, returning to an engagement focus can help reestablish the bond and clear mental clutter that competes for clients' focus or threatens their sense of well-being. Engaging can be the focus at the start of each session, when opening up new issues or discussing vulnerable matters, and anytime clients intellectualize or become overwhelmed, defensive, or detached.

Focusing

The second key process is *focusing*. Once clients are sufficiently engaged in therapeutic conversation, the focus narrows to the issue of client change. "What do you not like about your life?"; "What might be different, better?"; "What might you like to keep while moving forward, and what can be left behind?" MI focuses little on history or problems. However, the substitute is not unfocused chatting, but focusing on the future that clients would like to bring into being.

Focus is developed collaboratively rather than prescribed by the counselor or referral source. At the same time, MI is never intended to hold clients back in order to progress through a fixed treatment protocol, so when clients present with a clear view of concerns or interests, focusing may simply involve clarifying your understanding of these, then moving on to the process of evoking change possibilities and setting goals.

Often, however, clients who enter treatment experience ambivalence, wanting things to be different yet somehow still the same. They may blame themselves or others for their situation and feel pulled to focus on how things got the way they are. They may feel defensive about being put in a spotlight, being labeled or pressured to change. They may feel hopeless or afraid, or angry, and just want to escape. It can take effort to focus their attention away from these things and choose a direction, goal, or outcome to aim toward, and get moving. MI uses a number of focusing strategies to help clients focus their attention productively on the most useful issues. The goal is to join clients wherever they are, and focus conversations from there.

Many clients present with a number of concerns that compete for their focus. It can be unclear which areas are most important or urgent, or which could be most easily resolved in order to reduce distraction and build momentum toward change. One way to approach this dilemma is *agenda setting* (or mapping), which involves developing a list of topics to consider, fleshing out any that are unclear, then returning to a bird's-eye view to see how they fit together and begin to lay out a plan for the journey ahead. The plan is not fixed, of course, but it can help refocus conversation when topics seem to diverge from the plan, or when discussion seems to get bogged down and progress forward on the journey seems too slow.

At times, clients may only report that they are unhappy, or express a number of dissatisfactions. Problematic behaviors may exist alongside these complaints, but the connection isn't clear, and they do not seem to respond to invitations to explore. Rather than battling clients over focus, momentum can be established by working on issues that interest them. An alternative is to start with a general focus on greater happiness or life satisfaction, then work on narrowing focus toward specific improvements, and eventually to habits or patterns that serve as obstacles to making those improvements. Developing goals collaboratively over time allows for more thorough grounding of goals in changes that clients are already motivated to make.

There may be times when a client has different ideas than you about what to focus on. The MI model describes a *righting reflex* that practitioners can fall into, wanting to fix things that are not going well, and being drawn to shift the focus there rather than working from the inside of the client's perspective outward. During such moments, it can be helpful to take a long view and avoid sacrificing any positive engagement that has developed. This can be done by backing up, taking a broader focus to find connections between the areas, then working forward from there in such a way that integrates both focus areas.

An option is to provide information using an *elicit–provide–elicit strategy*. In this strategy, you first *elicit* clients' current awareness, knowledge, or perspective on a topic. Then you fill in the blanks and correct any mistaken beliefs, tailoring the information you *provide* to that which they truly are missing and can use. This also cues them to be ready to take in information that they might otherwise miss because they may be thinking about other things at the time. Finally, you then *elicit* their reactions to the information you shared, and whether/how they might want to use it in relation to their situation.

MI occasionally incorporates *advice-giving,* but only when clients give you permission to offer it. This can be done directly, by asking for permission (and not giving the advice if permission is refused), or indirectly, by giving the suggestion then asking them to consider how it fits for them. We have found that advice giving is rarely needed if we are engaged with clients and focused on evoking their own ideas.

Evoking

The third central MI process is evoking client perspectives and ideas about change rather than providing them our own ideas and perspectives on why and how they should change. At its core, MI is based on the idea that people motivate themselves to change, and that an effective way to elicit client change is to structure conversations such that clients identify and discuss their reasons, desires, and needs to make changes, then set their own goals for going about it. If ambivalence is a kind of internal, back-and-forth argument about making changes versus holding to a course that involves self-defeating behaviors, then we don't want to risk motivating clients to defend the status quo. Given that ambivalent people have already internalized both sides of the argument, when practitioners take a strong stance for change, they leave little else for clients to do but argue the advantages of the status quo and make "Yes, but . . ." arguments regarding the benefits of change. Thus, we are careful to avoid extolling the virtues of change. Any information we may offer in support of change includes explicit recognition of clients' personal choice to act or not act on it, and we offer suggestions only with clients' prior permission (and even then only rarely and tentatively). In MI, the focus remains on evoking clients' own motivations to change.

Key evoking tasks include eliciting and responding to change talk to build momentum toward making positive changes; accepting and responding to sustain talk in ways that prevent defensiveness or inertia; enhancing hope for success; and exploring discrepancies between clients' current actions and their goals or values, in order to encourage greater convergence.

The first evoking skill is to hear change talk when clients speak it. So much professional training targets listening for problems and pathology that it can be difficult even to notice change talk in the middle of a

> *In MI, the focus remains on evoking clients' own motivations to change.*

conversation. Early change talk can be quite mild and buried in the midst of sustain talk and defensiveness—for example, "I'm sick of being lectured to. . . . People don't really even know me that well, so a lot of their advice seems pretty useless. Maybe there are a couple things I could think about, but most of it seems ridiculous. It's not like people are making it out to be." In the midst of this client's complaining, discounting others' impressions and ideas, and denying problems is the gem: "Maybe there are a couple things I could think about." Although it is mild, tentative, and focused only on "thinking about" a few things, it is still an opening. A good MI response might be "It sounds like if you could get people off your back, you might feel a little freer to explore some things you might consider changing. What are some of the things you said you might think about more?" While such an exchange may take place earlier in the counseling process, for example, while engaging or focusing, it is important to hear change talk whenever it occurs, and to steer the conversation in that direction by evoking further thoughts (and backing off anytime the client resists). Evoking strategies focus on several areas: importance of change, confidence about change, and preparation to change.

Evoking the Importance of Change

There are several strategies to evoke clients' sense of the importance of making changes. The first is to discuss the habit or situation and the things that are good or not-so-good about it. While it may not be necessary to explore the status quo side of ambivalence, we find that exploring it initially can increase our understanding of clients' perspectives, allow them to vent some about the difficulties or drawbacks of change, so that they can then refocus their energies on change and, in the process, help us learn about perceived obstacles for later reference, when we are helping them plan their change efforts.

Evocative questions, which include the earlier example, "What things might you like to think about more?," are simple, yet invite clients to consider change. You can use the categories of change talk to generate evocative questions, such as "How do you want things to be different?" (desire), "How might things be better if you did cut back on gambling?" (reasons), or "What is the most important thing you could do to prevent things getting worse?" (need).

Importance scaling is a strategy for discovering the importance of change to the client and eliciting change talk. This strategy has three parts. The first elicits the client's rating of the importance of making a change on a scale of 0–10. This is followed by an assessment of what makes the client's answer X rather than a lower score (eliciting change talk about why a change is important), and, finally, what might increase the importance rating (risks or other developments that might increase the importance of change).

Another strategy, *looking back,* explores how things were before current problems developed, as a potential reference point for improving things again. You can trace from that point to the present as a summary that helps clients gain a broader perspective and see things more clearly. *Looking forward* involves imagining how things might be if no changes were made, and its counterpart, *envisioning,* asks clients to imagine a better life ahead, how it would look, what would be different, and how they would feel.

Typically there are discrepancies between clients' values or goals and the current behavioral choices they make. One strategy is to *explore clients' values* in this light. Because people can easily become defensive about such discrepancies, we prefer to focus on the positive, eliciting and exploring their values or goals, then exploring how they could live even more closely in line with them. We emphasize how all of us do some things we probably don't consider ideal, and we invite clients to focus on what they are moving toward rather than any current shortcomings.

Evoking Confidence for Change

Once clients are interested in making specific changes, we help them gain momentum by building their confidence that they can succeed. Once again, we use *evocative questions* that reflect and explore their perspectives to elicit change talk in this regard: "What's something you'd feel pretty confident about trying now?" or "What would help you feel more confident about getting started?" We also use *confidence scaling,* again reflecting the client's score on a scale from 0 to 10, and ask what makes it X and not zero (thus eliciting change talk regarding the client's ability to meet goals), and what would boost client confidence 2 points or so (which helps build a change plan).

You can help clients generalize from past experiences by *reviewing past successes.* Have them describe previous accomplishments, what strategies they used, what obstacles they faced and how they worked around them. It can also help to *reframe failures* as steps along the way to eventual change.

More generally, clients can talk about personal strengths and any potential external supports provided by others. Even if not directly applicable to the current change topic, building people's sense that they are competent and worthwhile, with strengths and accomplishments, no matter how minor, can help them make difficult changes.

A last strategy to increase confidence about change is *brainstorming hypothetical change.* People seem to find it easier to imagine "What if . . . " scenarios without the pressure of committing, and they are less likely to get caught up in a crisis of confidence. You can guide them to imagine their thoughts and feelings *if* they were ready to change, which can feel less threatening.

Planning

At some point, the focus of attention shifts from whether to change and why to how to accomplish change. The shift may be sudden, such as with clients who declare, "I've got to change" or "I can't go on like this anymore." Other times, the shift may be gradual, almost unnoticeable, as clients go back and forth between changing one way or another versus staying the same, considering hypothetical possibilities, then talking about how each possibility might work and what they could do toward that end. However it happens, at some point the focus of conversation is on how to go about implementing changes. At that time, shift to helping clients develop change plans and move into action.

When people have mostly resolved their ambivalence, planning strategies help them prepare for and initiate change. You can provide a *recapitulation,* or summary of the issues clients focused on and their sense of importance and confidence about making changes. Follow this with a question such as "What now?" or "Where does this leave you?"—without asking for commitment to a specific plan, leaving it open. Next, *clarify the goals* of changing, then explore clients' *options for change.* What choices might they make? Which option seems easier to try or more likely to succeed?

As you talk, listen for mobilizing change talk, and reflect and explore it. Mobilizing change talk, which relates to beginning to do something, might sound like "I'm thinking about trying . . .," "I might," or "I could." As always, take the dance one step at a time and don't press for firm commitment if clients are still tentative—keep building momentum instead and do not risk turning clients away from change.

Another strategy is to *plan the steps toward change.* What should happen in what sequence? What supports can be rallied? What rewards do clients imagine will result? What are some challenges that might interfere with the plan? Some clients like to develop written change plans, while others prefer just talking.

It can be helpful to set interim action goals rather than longer-term outcome goals. Eating healthier and exercising are interim action goals (that still need to be fleshed out), whereas being in shape and weighing 20 pounds less are outcome goals. Adopting new habits is often the key to long-term change. The new habits bring the outcome along with them.

Finally, you can help clients get started by exploring their confidence in the specific plan they are considering, and *evoking commitment* to making the change. It is helpful to modify a plan if clients express doubt that it can work as it is. Similarly, if they report low commitment, even if the plan seems solid, it is possible that their rating of the importance of change has decreased and might usefully be revisited.

As clients move into action, continue to provide support and guidance, helping them self-monitor their progress or find a supportive mutual monitoring situation. Part of moving into action may involve learning new skills, and other therapies, classes, or practice opportunities can be useful at this point. Additionally, there may be other, nonmotivational issues that can be addressed in other therapies, such as posttraumatic stress, relational difficulties, or specific issues (e.g., sleep dysfunction or phobias) that may not be directly related to the change focused on in MI but are clearly useful to clients and perhaps support the MI goal by reducing stress, and so forth.

In Chapter 4, we turn to integrating MI strategies and group therapy principles to lay a foundation for MI groups.

References

Amrhein, P. C., Miller, W. R., Yahne, C. E., Palmer, M., & Fulcher, L. (2003). Client commitment language during motivational interviewing predicts drug use outcomes. *Journal of Consulting and Clinical Psychology, 71*, 862–878.

Arkowitz, H., Westra, H. A., Miller, W. R., & Rollnick, S. (Eds.). (2008). *Motivational interviewing in the treatment of psychological problems.* New York: Guilford Press.

Bem, D. J. (1972). Self-perception theory. In Berkowitz, L. (Ed.), *Advances in experimental social psychology* (Vol. 6, pp. 1–62). New York: Academic Press.

Brehm, J. W. (1966). *A theory of psychological reactance.* New York: Academic Press.

Hohman, M. (2012). *Motivational interviewing in social work practice.* New York: Guilford Press.

Kiesler, D. J. (1966). Some myths of psychotherapy research and the search for a paradigm. *Psychological Bulletin, 65*, 100–136.

Miller, W. R. (1999). Toward a theory of motivational interviewing. *Motivational Interviewing Newsletter: Updates, Education and Training, 6*, 2–4.

Miller, W. R., & Rollnick, S. (2013). *Motivational interviewing: Helping people change* (3rd ed.). New York: Guilford Press.

Miller, W. R., & Rose, G. S. (2009). Toward a theory of motivational interviewing. *American Psychologist, 64*, 527–537.

Moyers, T. B., & Martin, T. (2006). Therapist influence on client language during motivational interviewing sessions. *Journal of Substance Abuse Treatment, 30*, 245–251.

Moyers, T. B., Martin, T., Christopher, P. J., Houck, J. M., Tonigan, J. S., & Amrhein, P. C. (2007). Client language as a mediator of motivational interviewing efficacy: Where is the evidence? *Alcoholism: Clinical and Experimental Research, 31*(Suppl. 10), 40s–47s.

Moyers, T. B., Martin, T., Houck, J. M., Christopher, P. J., & Tonigan, J. S. (2009). From in-session behaviors to drinking outcomes: A causal chain for motivational interviewing. *Journal of Consulting and Clinical Psychology, 77*, 1113–1124.

Naar-King, S., & Suarez, M. (2011). *Motivational interviewing with adolescents and young adults.* New York: Guilford Press.

Rogers, C. (1951). *Client-centered therapy.* Cambridge, MA: Riverside Press.

Rogers, C. (1961). *On becoming a person.* New York: Houghton Mifflin.

Rogers, C., Gendlin, E. R., Kiesler, D. J., & Truax, C. B. (1967). *The therapeutic relationship and its impact: A study of psychotherapy with schizophrenics.* Madison: University of Wisconsin Press.

Rollnick, S. (1998). Readiness, importance, and confidence: Critical conditions of change in treatment. In W. R. Miller & N. Heather (Eds.), *Treating addictive behaviors: Processes of change* (2nd ed., pp. 49–60). New York: Plenum.

Rollnick, S., Mason, P., & Butler, C. (1999). *Health behavior change.* London: Churchill Livingstone.

Rollnick, S., Miller, W. R., & Butler, C. (2008). *Motivational interviewing in health care*. New York: Guilford Press.

Rosengren, D. B. (2009). *Building motivational interviewing skills: A practitioner workbook*. New York: Guilford Press.

Truax, C. B. (1966). Reinforcement and nonreinforcement in Rogerian psychotherapy. *Journal of Abnormal Psychology, 71,* 1–9.

Walters, S. T., Clark, M. D., Gingerich, R., & Meltzer, M. L. (2007). *Motivating offenders to change: A guide for probation and parole*. Washington DC: National Institute of Corrections, U.S. Department of Justice.

Walters, S. T., Vader, A. M., Harris, T. R., Field, C. A., & Jouriles, E. N. (2009). Dismantling motivational interviewing and feedback for college drinkers: A randomized clinical trial. *Journal of Consulting and Clinical Psychology, 77,* 64–73.

Westra, H. A. (2012). *Motivational interviewing in the treatment of anxiety*. New York: Guilford Press.

CHAPTER 4

Blending Motivational Interviewing and Group Practice

Adapting MI to a group format requires modifying concepts, strategies, and techniques developed for individual interactions to groups with members who have different interests and perspectives. Some aspects of individual MI are directly applicable to group services, while others are ill-fitting or even inadvisable in the group context. Similarly, some aspects of group MI are not present in individual MI.

MI is a general therapeutic approach with a variety of strategies and techniques. Individual MI services are adapted for setting, context, and target issue. Strategies emphasized in outpatient addiction services may be of little use in inpatient psychiatric services. For example, outpatient MI services may focus on longer-term planning and support for moving into action, while that focus may be too removed from inpatients' current needs for crisis resolution or stabilization.

A goal of MI groups is to help people regain a sense of balance in their lives, countering the lifestyle narrowing that occurs when psychosocial or health problems dominate people's lives. Groups help members regain perspective and broaden the way they think about their lives' possibilities. Groups can help them connect with others in positive ways, often in the shadow of isolating trauma or shame. As members' perspectives expand, their challenges and struggles begin to appear relatively smaller and more manageable in context. As they successfully make changes, they gain a greater sense of owning their lives, rather than merely being along for the ride.

MI groups help people regain balance in their lives.

53

Lessons from Group Therapy
Research for MI Group Leaders

The group therapy research reviewed in Chapter 2 suggests several guiding principles for MI group leaders:

- Maximize group members' participation
- Encourage members to take ownership of change
- Explore both positive and negative experiences
- Facilitate group cohesion and collaboration
- Tailor the content to broadly address clients' experiences and interests
- Focus on potential solutions

Adapting these principles to MI groups requires multiple strategies to increase participation (e.g., OARS): eliciting member perspectives, linking members' themes and experiences, and limiting our own talking. Emphasizing personal choice and control, avoiding taking an expert stance, and showing a collaborative spirit are MI strategies that may encourage members to take more responsibility and engage with the group. Discussing the pros and cons of changing and eliciting realistic plans from group members may elicit both positive and negative emotions, and help members achieve balance, neither getting stuck in sadness or anger about the past nor pursuing significant life changes without adequate preparation. Strategies such as coaching members to use OARS with each other may enhance interactions and build a culture of positive interpersonal behavior, thus encouraging more engagement and attraction to the group. Explicitly discussing expectations about group members' roles (encouraging members to respect and support each others' choices, while remaining responsible for their own changes) may enhance group cohesion and interaction. Structuring group content to fit the needs of participants seems obvious, yet requires us to consider members' needs even before the group convenes. MI strategies such as developing discrepancy, building self-efficacy, and eliciting change talk may keep the focus on solutions and avoid excessive focus on past problems. Some of these group elements are addressed in the growing literature on MI groups reviewed in Chapter 5, while others await further study.

Therapeutic Factors in MI Groups

In Chapter 2, we reviewed the key therapeutic factors in groups. Some of these factors are fundamental to MI groups. *Acceptance* of members by both leaders and other members is a central therapeutic factor in MI groups.

Guidance also plays a role, especially in situations that involve adapting to an illness or new circumstance. However, although informational components can be woven into MI groups, MI groups are not primarily educational in nature. *Instilling hope,* a key part of MI, happens through envisioning a better future, reviewing past successes and personal strengths, and considering available supports. Hope also comes from hearing others' success stories and witnessing their change, experiencing others' support, and experiencing the general optimism that develops in a positive group climate. *Self-disclosure* is an important factor in MI groups, especially when group members feel defensive about the challenges they face (e.g., in mandated groups). Gaining greater self-understanding is the essence of the broadening perspectives phase, because it provides the foundation for taking new action toward a more fulfilling life for members in the final phase of MI groups.

Some factors that are not relevant in individual MI are important in MI groups. *Altruism* plays an important role in MI groups, especially in later phases, as members see that the support and help they provide result in benefits to other members. *Universality* also has no equivalent in individual MI, yet it is a powerful force for change in MI groups and can increase disclosure, bonding, and mutual support among members. *Vicarious learning* is not a part of individual MI, but it is another essential element of MI groups, in which leaders have less time to evoke change talk from each individual client. Instead, leaders foster vicarious learning by keeping members engaged while the focus is on others, and link members together in the process of making changes, even when their presenting issues and change targets are different.

Some group therapeutic factors are not intentionally fostered in MI groups, although they may play a role in individual members' experiences. Of these, *catharsis* is perhaps the most obvious. While experiencing strong emotions that have been held back may free members to change, MI does not focus on eliciting cathartic experiences. *Learning from interpersonal interactions* can play a role in change facilitated through MI groups, yet MI groups usually do not focus explicitly on fostering interpersonal learning through exchanging feedback about interpersonal styles or impacts, except when they are combined with a process-oriented group approach (e.g., Malat, Morrow, & Stewart, 2011).

We review the role of specific therapeutic factors, as well as leader functions and group processes, in Chapters 9–12, which are devoted to the four phases of MI groups.

MI Group Development

MI draws considerably from Carl Rogers's client-centered therapy. Rogers (1970) conceptualized a general developmental path for client-centered groups. He suggested that groups are initially unfocused, unsure of what to discuss or how to become involved or productive, and concerned with past events and experiences. As members perceive greater safety, discussion moves toward current experiences, feelings, and concerns. This fosters greater engagement among members, transforming the separate, isolated individuals into a group with a sense of togetherness. Group members shed their protective defenses to be more genuine with one another, less constrained by restrictive social norms. As members come to see the group as a source of new experiences, their sense of openness and genuineness deepens, sometimes allowing greater access to their true thoughts and feelings than ever before. Eventually, based on a sense of trust in others and belief in the growth processes they experienced, group members open to new ways of being relative to their own identity, as well as their relationships outside the group.

Rogers's process-oriented view of group development dovetails nicely with the four-phase approach we present in this book. During the *engagement* phase, leaders help members become comfortable with participating in the group, and focus as much on facilitating early group processes as on the content of members' issues and concerns. As the group moves into the *exploring perspectives* phase, leaders help to deepen members' interactions as they explore their individual viewpoints and situations together. During the *broadening perspectives* phase, interactions continue to deepen and broaden as leaders help members to consider new possibilities, allow buried hopes to reemerge, and take in others' perspectives for consideration. During the *moving into action* phase, leaders help members to get practical, take strides toward their goals, and try new ways of being, both in the group and in their daily lives.

Empathy and Direction

MI group leadership balances remaining empathic with helping members implement changes that will improve their lives. This balance can be difficult to maintain with one client, let alone 10. Some members may feel stuck and want suggestions. Others may feel pressured by other people's advice and expectations, and further suggestions may increase their defensiveness, perhaps even poisoning them against helpful ideas that they would have embraced had they not felt pressured. Some members like to talk things out in detail as they arise, while others prefer to think things through on their own before discussing them with others. Some may revel in the group's support and develop close attachments to other members. Others may see the group primarily as a source of ideas, not social or emotional connections.

In individual MI, you can watch clients' reactions as you elicit forward movement, then shift to a more purely empathic focus when a reaction suggests you are moving too quickly. In groups, it is impossible to watch everyone's reactions at the same time. Even if it were possible, you still couldn't tailor your focus specifically to individual members' reactions, because different members react to the same event in different ways.

So you are faced with a challenge. How can you follow client cues when different members have different needs, and their cues point in different directions? If you shift toward supportive, empathic exploration when a few members are not ready to move forward, the group process may bog down. However, if you press ahead when some aren't yet ready, you might leave them behind or foster discontent that can spread and eventually result in group conflict, temporarily halting group progress altogether. So you need to have different strategies for leading groups than those you use when working with individual clients.

In individual work, then, you can easily follow client cues to change focus, pick up the pace or slow it down, deepen or lighten the mood, or even pause while the client thinks in silence. You can focus on increasing the client's interest in change or easily switch to a focus on confidence, if that seems more helpful in the moment. With the client who is ready, you can switch to consider change planning, without even commenting on the shift.

Groups can be run in a similar, unstructured fashion that follows the momentary interests and readiness of group members, but it is considerably more difficult to do well. For that reason, many group leaders prefer to have at least a tentative plan for the session. How much you should structure sessions depends on members' needs, as well as your own comfort level. You can be completely unstructured and work with what emerges as the session unfolds, or you can work in a semistructured way, introducing a topic while allowing divergences that you later tie back in with that theme. Or you can use a structured approach, following an agenda and carefully managing time throughout.

Even structured groups rarely proceed in a straight line, however. One member's opinions or revelations inevitably spur other members' reactions in directions that you don't intend or even foresee. One person's momentum brings another person's reluctance to the surface. Or a moment of silence might make an uncomfortable member jump off in a different direction. Your attempts to bring the group back to focus may be overrun by members' desires to pursue the new direction. Sometimes things become uncomfortable enough that eliciting discussion at all feels like pulling teeth.

Good group leadership takes patience, flexibility, creativity, and the ability to hold many ideas and perceptions in mind at the same time. Leadership involves guiding the group forward in a way that gains traction and bringing the group back on task when it strays. As with individual MI, the guiding principle is to look for openings to move forward whenever possible, but to avoid continuing to press forward when doing so elicits defensiveness. Defensiveness is not something about which you should be overly sensitive, because there is usually some reluctance to move forward on the part of at least one member at any given time. The trick is to find the balance between providing too much direction or too little, between going so fast that you bring up strong defenses or so slow that the group loses interest or becomes frustrated.

Velasquez, Stephens, and Drenner (Chapter 14, p. 281) use a metaphor for facilitating groups:

> While the MI approach with individuals has been described as waltzing, we think that using MI in groups is more like conducting a symphony. Each member plays an individual instrument and contributes to the collective melody of the group, and at the same time responds to the conductor. The conductor, in turn, gently guides the instrumental interactions, as well as the overall orchestral composition.

If well-functioning groups are like a symphony guided by an able conductor, getting groups started can sometimes feel like directing an improvisational band of adolescents playing their instruments together for the first time, off-key, and seemingly playing different songs. Handled well, the noise eventually resembles music. The band members learn to harmonize and take turns playing lead parts, building on what came previously. They transform from individuals playing on their own to a group playing music together. The focus required of the school band teacher to hear the musical themes through the noise, and the patience to motivate the players to keep improving at times when it seems hopeless, are similar to the focus and patience sometimes required of group leaders working with new groups.

Facilitating MI Groups

A key practice for the leader is to keep moving forward as a group, neither running ahead with the fastest member nor holding back with the slowest. Avoid conducting consecutive individual mini-sessions, instead interweaving moments that focus on individuals with those that focus on the group as a whole. This builds connections between members regarding their interests, themes, or readiness to change. They listen to and learn from one another, sometimes learning what not to do. And in finding ways to support one another, they often discover their own paths forward as well, gaining greater confidence in the process.

Compared to clients in individual MI, group members' progress may depend less on overt change talk. As they listen to one another deal with challenges and make progress, members often think about their own situations and make progress even when others are doing the talking. Group MI is different from individual MI, in which the client is the only one generating change talk. Leaders who can find common themes, struggles, or hopes among members help shape the group experience so that progress is not linear, step-by-step, but exponential: slow initially, but picking up speed, like a snowball rolling down the side of a mountain.

We start by sharing some general principles for leading MI groups. Later, we present variations that are specific to each of the four phases in our model, described in Chapters 9–12:

- Focus on positives
- Bring group members into the moment
- Explore perspectives and focus on the present
- Hear complaints but do not elicit grievances
- Broaden perspectives and focus on the future
- Reflect and explore a positive focus on desires, needs, plans, and self
- Support self-efficacy
- Counteract any negative reactions before sessions end

Focus on Positives

MI groups focus more on positive growth than on resolving psychopathology or working through past injuries or traumas. Helping members become more positive may be even more productive than helping them resolve problems (Seligman, Steen, Park, & Peterson, 2005). Focusing on positives is key for successful MI groups and serves as a guide for what to emphasize, and what to ignore. It is riskier to focus on negative emotions or dissatisfactions in groups than in individual sessions. With individual clients, you can tread lightly as they discuss dissatisfactions, but in a group context it is difficult to control other members' reactions, unless you discourage them from speaking at all. When members focus on their dissatisfactions or negative emotions, other members may provide not only support but also unwanted advice or criticism.

Similarly, MI groups are not intended to bring about a catharsis of negative emotions, use "tough love" and other forms of confrontation. Furthermore, while other kinds of groups may promote the development

MI groups focus more on positive growth than on resolving psychopathology.

and resolution of conflict as important elements of experiential learning in group work, this also is not part of MI groups. Instead, the focus is on building members' energy and confidence about change. Building momentum toward change in a group setting is facilitated by focusing on positive elements—members' sense of importance about living in line with their values and goals, their sense of connection and support for one another, and their confidence that with effort they can transform their lives in satisfying and meaningful ways. For that reason, as leaders you elicit hopes more than dissatisfactions, focus on progress more than struggles, and explore solutions more than problems.

MI group leaders elicit hopes more than dissatisfactions, focus on progress more than struggles, and explore solutions more than problems.

Bring Group Members into the Moment

Clients often feel vulnerable when discussing their lives with professional helpers. They can be hesitant to reveal something embarrassing or that they feel ashamed about, and they fear being judged or patronized. Coming into a room full of strangers in a group can further amplify fears and concerns. If you start by discussing things that are "out there"—past events, current issues, and future goals—you can inadvertently extend members' feelings of being alone in a room of strangers, and it can take longer for the group to begin to coalesce. So it is useful to bring the group into the moment, communicating empathically around current thoughts and feelings. You can orient members to the group, talking a little about what the group is intended to be and helping members get a feel for each other and begin opening up to one another. In Chapter 8, we focus on engagement strategies that can help members adjust from "out there" to "in here."

Explore Perspectives and Focus on the Present

Once they are engaged, the task turns to exploring members' perspectives on their lives, values, situations and experiences. In doing this, gently steer the conversation away from recitation of past events and experiences toward members' current lives. In general, MI focuses mostly on the future. However, because people are rarely in the habit of focusing on the future, start with the present, helping members become oriented to the kinds of discussions preferred in MI. This gives you time to affirm members, underscoring positive elements that you see in their strivings and efforts and appreciating the perspectives that various members offer.

This focus helps lower defenses, as members experience support through being heard and appreciated. Group cohesion is also built in this way. All of these elements—a sense of being understood and accepted, a decreased need to keep defenses up, and an experience of bonding with others in the group—help to fortify members for the struggles and challenges they may face as they move forward.

Hear Complaints but Do Not Elicit Grievances

As part of exploring, members likely share some frustrations, complaints, and grievances. It is useful to accept and "roll with" these, neither ignoring or rejecting nor encouraging or amplifying them. Allowing members to "vent" a little and experience being heard and understood can help them shift to focusing more productively on goals, tasks, and hopes. Because these frustrations often represent some part of the problem, they can become a part of motivation to change.

Accepting defensiveness and "rolling with it" in groups can be challenging. You must roll with not only the defensiveness of members around exploring their own situations, society, and the treatment system, but also with defensiveness that takes the form of competing for perceived roles in the group (see Chapter 8), challenging you about the content and format of groups, or even challenging your ability to lead the group.

Downey and Johnson (Chapter 13) encourage leaders to embrace defensiveness (or resistance), and we agree. Embracing defensiveness is not merely ignoring unpleasant or negative interactions; it harnesses the energy present in discord and channels it into a more productive direction. This often takes a bit of time, because trying to turn discord into momentum too quickly can make you seem dismissive with regard to the concerns being expressed. Instead, try to accept negative comments but find something positive in them to focus on. The important thing is to remain nondefensive in the face of criticism.

Broaden Perspectives and Focus on the Future

It isn't necessary (or desirable) to review members' current lives in great detail. Instead, once members have shared their current situations and perspectives, help them develop new perspectives and shake free from self-limiting perspectives. You can explore some past success and present interests, but mostly focus the attention of the group on the future. The purpose of helping members develop broadened perspectives is to expand the range of perceived choices and support members as they make choices that lead toward more satisfying futures.

Reflect and Explore a Positive Focus on Desires, Needs, Plans, and Self

There are many options to choose from when reflecting change talk. Group members often have powerful reasons to change. Help them view losses and failures in ways that help to increase motivation to make changes rather than remain bogged down. Ongoing angst, rumination, and self-blame often reduce motivation rather than increase it. Furthermore, such emotional moments often elicit other members' agreement ("Yes, you screwed up"), judgment ("You were being selfish"), rescuing ("Everyone does it, it's no big deal"), or advice giving ("Just buck up and get back on track"). While these responses may be motivating, they can also backfire and elicit further self-recrimination or pessimistic thinking. This can drain the group's spirit.

Thus, while there is no need to fear moments of painful self-discovery or truthful acknowledgment to others, focus the group mostly toward the positive aspects of change. Among the types of preparatory change talk (desires, needs, reasons, ability), listen for the desire to change (how members see their lives as getting better) or steer the focus toward positive aspects of reasons and needs. Regarding expressions of need to change ("If I keep going like this, I might lose it all, and then there wouldn't be much point in going on at all"), acknowledge the reality, then pivot toward the possibilities ("So things are getting scary and you're trying to hold on to what you still have that makes it worthwhile. What are the things you want to hold onto in your life, or get back again?").

Similarly, when members focus on the difficulties posed by their choices, acknowledge the reality of the difficulties, then shift focus toward the resources available to make their plans reality ("This really does sound challenging. . . . What can you do to increase the chance of success? And how can the rest of us help?").

Sometimes, members reflect negatively on themselves, their weaknesses, and so on. Avoid directly challenging members' self-judgment or self-condemnation ("You're not a failure"), because such reassurance can elicit a defense of the negative self-judgment ("Then why am I alone now, with nothing to my name, and don't have any real friends?"). Instead, take an affirming stance that focuses on expanding members' thinking about themselves ("I'm not saying you haven't made mistakes. But I see you working hard to be honest and to do what's necessary to turn things around. Someone who cares about others, even if he's lost that focus for a while. Someone who's trying to put the pieces back together. And it seems to me that there's a lot of integrity in that").

There is a risk of overdoing it and coming across as insincere, or that members may not fully be able to take in such a response in the moment.

But the goal is to avoid debating what will probably be a losing argument and instead shift the focus elsewhere, toward more positive territory, without being naively optimistic or dismissive of members' concerns about themselves. Whether you focus on conscientiousness, honesty, autonomy, grit, or other strengths, the goal is to see the positives that members have trouble recognizing in a self-deprecating moment. Refocusing on the positives can help members experience some relief from negative self-judgment and find strengths they can build upon instead.

Support Self-Efficacy

Self-efficacy is the belief that you can accomplish the goals you set for yourself. Although many therapeutic tasks are more challenging in groups than in individual therapy, supporting self-efficacy in groups is actually easier than it is with individual clients. By virtue of "going through it together," members can support one another and help build confidence in ways that have less impact when coming from a therapist. They can share their experiences and model for each other trying new experiences or actions. Members can commiserate with one another over setbacks, bolstering determination to try again. They can brainstorm together, practice together, and share tips they've learned from their ongoing change attempts. You can reflect common experiences and themes, noting progress made and strength gained as members free themselves from the constraints of their past. There is a risk that members adopt each others' goals rather than focusing on those most important to their own growth, but you address this by reminding members that making things better means something different for each person.

Counteract Negative Reactions before Sessions End

Moments of tension and conflict are inevitable if you lead groups long enough (and they may even happen within minutes of opening the first group!), so it is important to be prepared to deal with them. While MI groups do not intentionally allow conflict to unfold in order to provide the experience of successful conflict resolution, conflict still happens at times, and facilitating positive resolution is important. Whether you help members find consensus or agree to disagree, try to prevent sessions from ending with members feeling shamed, attacked, humiliated, intimidated, isolated from the rest of the group, or resentful toward others. Members who leave feeling shamed or attacked may ruminate later and not come back (e.g., Malat et al., 2011). And although it is crucial to protect members from any ongoing attacks, it is also important that critics not get emotionally shut out of being part of the group. Although you should manage members' critical behavior, the group experience is intended to be therapeutic for all, not just for those who are friendly and supportive.

The Spirit of MI Groups

As described in Chapter 3, the formal components of spirit in the MI model are partnership, acceptance, compassion, and evocation (Miller & Rollnick, 2013). Conveying profound respect for your clients and optimism about their possibilities provides the foundation of the spirit of MI in groups. Group members may make unproductive choices, act in self-destructive ways, be neglectful of responsibilities and possibilities, behave offensively, or even hurt others at times. Still, the ideal state is to be in awe of them as fellow humans with value, strengths, and unique capabilities. You cannot know what possibilities lie within or in front of them, and the goal is to help them draw forth their best selves as they try to improve their lives. Your respect of members as individuals of worth influences the spirit of their interactions with one another. Similarly, you can explicitly encourage members to look for the best in each other and help one another build hope. Members who are optimistic that they can make things better don't wait for obstacles to be removed before they start, and getting started builds momentum toward substantive change. Optimism might even be considered the most central feature of MI groups.

Optimism might be considered the central feature of MI groups.

One way to enhance this spirit is to monitor the use of language. Avoiding the use of labels is a good way to start. Labels such as "schizophrenic," "alcoholic," or "offender" diminish people and narrow the focus to certain negative attributes, while ignoring positive elements. This is unlikely to help members broaden their thinking and increase self-acceptance. It is true that some people find clarity in these self-definitions ("Being an alcoholic means I can never take a drink without risking a relapse," "Being a schizophrenic means that I need to keep taking my medications, even when it seems like I don't need them"). However, people finding clarity in their own self-definitions is different from their being boxed in by others' labels. Thus, even if you find it valuable to incorporate a self-defining label in your reflections, remain client-centered and emphasize the person's perception ("Seeing yourself as an alcoholic helps you . . . ") rather than confirm some kind of reality of the label ("As an alcoholic, you . . . "). Keep the focus on dealing with the obstacles put in members' path by the conditions with which they struggle, not on members as examples of the condition itself. See through the pathology to the person, and avoid reducing the person to a label.

Emphasizing autonomy is another important part of the spirit of MI groups, and can enhance members' opportunities for growth by taking greater ownership of their lives, and is another important part of the spirit of MI groups. Jasiura, Hunt, and Urquhart (Chapter 15, p 289) recommend that leaders "affirm helpful group behaviors, include the group in all possible decisions and responsibilities, and seize every opportunity to elicit and make visible each member's innate desire to be well, responsible, and compassionate." Emphasizing (members') autonomy also "encourages them to take control of their lives at a time when they're feeling relatively powerless. It demonstrates nonjudgmental respect for their perspectives at a time when they're feeling discounted and misjudged. And it establishes a nonthreatening environment in which change is more likely to occur over time" (Carden & Farrall, Chapter 19, p. 358).

Emphasizing autonomy involves redirecting members when they engage in excessive advice-giving. Advice-giving is typically well-intentioned, given by a person with a real interest in helping another member. The advice given may be sound, and met with interest by the person receiving it. However, advice giving that communicates an expectation that the receiver implement the suggestion offered (beyond simply considering it) tends to move the group away from evoking a strong sense of autonomy in members. MI is intended to encourage individuals to sort through conflicting ideas, feelings, and values to achieve an owned, if fallible, plan. Instead, advice poses the risk that members halfheartedly try ideas that may not be well-suited to their situations or styles (or resist the advice altogether). It is often by carefully considering options and deciding what to do that people come to well-suited plans, secondary options to fall back on, and a deep commitment to change based on a clear vision of what they are trying to do and why.

One way of handling unsolicited advice-giving is to guide the member to ask permission to give advice:

Carmen, it seems like you want to help Mary prevent what happened to you from happening to her. That's really supportive. However, telling Mary what she needs to do, when she hasn't asked for advice, may make it less likely that Mary will hear what you have to say. Would you be willing to ask her if she's up for hearing suggestions at this time? And if she is, would you then make your suggestions without telling Mary what decision she should make? (Martino & Santa Ana, Chapter 16, p. 309)

Here the leader acknowledges the advice-giving member's altruistic intent, shares a concern with her action, asks her to consider getting permission from the receiver first, then guides her to offer her ideas as possibilities to consider rather than directions to follow.

Another approach to handling unsolicited advice is to ask members to defer any advice until after the person of focus has developed a tentative plan, then frame their comments as what has worked for them or what they have seen work (vs. making a direct suggestion). Framing suggestions into a menu of options from which the member can choose (or not) also supports autonomy. Of course, you should also avoid unsolicited advice-giving, because members are more likely to follow your actions than your directions.

In summary, MI is about helping people initiate positive changes in their lives. However, the spirit of MI is about accepting people as they are. This helps take the pressure to change off them, which can lower defenses and help them feel freer to consider making changes. As horse trainer Monty Roberts (1999) suggests, "Act like you've only got fifteen minutes, it'll take all day; act like you've got all day, it might take fifteen minutes" (p. 108). Showing acceptance can also help people better accept themselves, which in turn helps them relax, become more creative, and approach change with an eye toward what it may offer rather than as an unpleasant chore that needs to be done.

Using MI Processes

In Chapter 3, we shared the four processes of the individual MI model—engaging, focusing, evoking, and planning (Miller & Rollnick, 2013). These four processes and the four phases of MI groups presented in this book are overlapping and complementary. Miller and Rollnick make the point that while the processes in individual MI are essentially sequential, they are not meant to be stages or phases, because at any point it may be most useful to focus on a different process than the one on which you have been focusing. For example, while evoking client change talk, you may run into defensiveness that threatens the alliance, and return to a focus on engaging. Similarly, while planning, it may become clear that the goal was not ideally defined, and that it is important to return to a focus on developing a better-fitting goal. Let's consider how the individual MI processes fit with the MI group phases.

The process of engaging is obviously most applicable to the first MI group phase: *engaging the group*. Discussed in Chapter 9, the engaging process is more involved with groups than with a single individual. Not only must we engage a person in talking with us and begin to develop a one-on-one relationship, we must get a room of people to open up to each other, begin to develop mutual norms, and provide each other support within an MI-consistent style, all while tending to their different preferences, values, and interpersonal styles. In MI groups, we often begin the engagement process prior to the first group meeting, in a pregroup orientation (or screening) meeting with potential members. We also focus on keeping the group engaged regularly throughout the four phases, in order to keep members engaged simultaneously in their own exploration and in group processes that support change.

The process of focusing is most relevant to the second group phase: *exploring perspectives*. Focusing involves clarifying the goals toward which clients are moving. In individual work, it is challenging enough to help clients define goals that achieve the end of making things better—often, all clients know is that they don't like things as they are. However, you can use MI strategies on the fly—looking back, then forward; exploring values and strengths, then weave it all together in development of a promising and achievable goal. It is more difficult to weave in and out of client topics as quickly in groups, especially early on, when you (and other members) are less familiar with one another's stories. To compensate, spend more time in group laying the foundation for change by exploring lifestyles and typical days in members' lives, and exploring ambivalence about their current situation and the possibilities for change, as well as their values.

Focusing in groups involves more explicit shaping of conversations than in individual work. We must be more clear when establishing, holding, or shifting topical focus, and shape conversations in productive directions when they move too slowly or quickly, become too narrowly focused or too vague, or are too superficial or heavy to be maximally productive (discussed in Chapter 8).

The process of evoking is most applicable during the third phase: *broadening client perspectives*. Evoking involves eliciting and strengthening clients' thoughts, feelings, and motivations toward change. The process of evoking client perspectives sets MI apart from other therapeutic approaches, which focus more on providing expert input, such as instructing, advising, suggesting, or framing client symptoms with a theoretical model (Wagner, Ingersoll, & Rollnick, 2013). In using the process of evoking in MI groups, we are again challenged to do so efficiently in a group of people versus interacting with a single individual. Because floor time for individual clients is limited in the group setting, we cannot rely solely on explicitly evoking client change talk as the method of building motivation to change. Instead, we must lead groups so that clients are moving toward change even while they are silent, listening to others and processing their own reactions. Thus, we work somewhat more generally toward helping clients broaden their perspectives on their situation, challenges, and possible futures, incorporating ideas from Frederickson's (2004) broaden-and-build model of positive emotions, which focuses on the role of positive emotions in helping people use time when they are not under threat to increase physical, social, cognitive, and emotional resources upon which they may later draw to improve their situations.

The final individual MI process—planning—is used mostly during the fourth phase of MI groups: *moving into action*. In individual MI, planning involves developing and committing to a change plan. MI groups typically extend beyond planning into taking action to change. It makes little sense to us to think of MI groups as strictly preparatory, ending once members have committed to making changes. Instead, since productive groups are a strong force for change, we think it is better to use them to provide ongoing support, encouragement, and guidance, as well as a safety net when early change attempts fall short. The strength of momentum gained as a group is behind the changes individual members make in their "outside" lives. While not all MI groups extend into action depending on the setting in which they are conducted (cf. Martino & Santa Ana, Chapter 16), we think of this as an important part of the MI groups model.

Using the OARS Communication Style

As MI group leaders, we use the techniques and strategies described in Chapter 2, while adapting them for use in groups. OARS (open questions, affirmations, reflections, summaries) is the base communication style, although it is used in groups to build cohesion, and to help the group focus, in addition to helping members focus on their individual change goals. Our colleagues Velasquez, Stephens, and Drenner (Chapter 14) suggest that group conversations can be usefully facilitated by first reflecting individual members' statements, then asking an open question to the group that builds toward a shared theme.

Although they highlight reflections and open questions, you can use affirmations and summaries in a similar way. It is important that your affirmations are genuine and low-key; if you feel clever or like a cheer-leader, you may want to pass on providing an affirmation at that moment, because clients in groups may be especially primed to interpret complex comments as having implied criticism and may lose faith in you if affirmations seem over-the-top or disingenuous. As noted by Velasquez and colleagues (Chapter 14):

> We believe that the most useful affirming statements are judicious, genuine, and specific. We convey affirmations in a warm and sincere manner, because those that are rushed, tossed out casually, or delivered without eye contact come across as superficial. This "style" aspect of an affirmation is especially important when working with members whose life experiences may have made them especially sensitive to perceived hypocrisy and empty praise. (p. 274)

Affirmations are distinct from praise, and the underlying goal is to build motivation to change, rather than simply provide an experience that feels good to members. Regarding reflections, they add these recommendations:

> When reflecting client statements, we have found that less is often more. Instead of maintaining an empathic focus on a member's concerns, longer reflections tend to make instructional points or dominate the

discourse. In contrast, shorter reflections convey a real understanding of the member's remarks and have greater impact. Thus, at times, the power of a reflection is increased by using only a word or two that intensify the meaning and impact of a member's statement. In groups, reflections crystallize key points raised by members and strategically serve as punctuation marks that help clarify and draw attention to selective member responses, such as change and commitment talk. (p. 275)

Summaries can be used in group as they are used in individual therapy—to link to previous content, to provide interim ratchet points (advance the topic, then clamp down on key points during a conversation to provide a basis for advancing forward again), to transition to new topics, and to close out a session by summarizing issues discussed and members' progress toward change. In groups, you are also more likely to use *process summaries* (summaries that focus on how members worked together such as supporting each other and building off of one another's comments). This not only reinforces a sense of community but it also helps members to transition out of the group environment, back to their daily lives.

This chapter has provided an overview of integrating MI components into a group setting. We next review the evidence for MI groups, then focus on designing and implementing MI groups before returning to the practices involved in conducting MI groups in Chapter 8.

References

Fredrickson, B. L. (2004). The broaden-and-build theory of positive emotions. *Philosophical Transactions of the Royal Society of London B: Biological Sciences, 359*(1449), 1367–1378.

Malat, J., Morrow, S., & Stewart, P. (2011). Applying motivational interviewing principles in a modified interpersonal group for comorbid addiction. *International Journal of Group Psychotherapy, 61,* 557–575.

Miller, W. R., & Rollnick, S. (2013). *Motivational interviewing: Helping people change.* New York: Guilford Press.

Roberts, M. (1999). *Shy boy: The horse that came in from the wild.* New York: Harper Collins Publishing.

Rogers, C. (1970). *Encounter groups.* New York: Harper & Row.

Seligman, M. E. P., Steen, T. A., Park, N., & Peterson, C. (2005). Positive psychology progress: Empirical validation of interventions. *American Psychologist, 60,* 410–421.

Wagner, C. C., Ingersoll, K. S., & Rollnick, S. (2013). Motivational interviewing: A cousin to contextual cognitive behavior therapies. In S. C. Hayes & M. Levin (Eds.), *Acceptance, mindfulness, and values in addictive behaviors* (pp. 153–186). Oakland, CA: New Harbinger Books.

CHAPTER 5

The Evidence Base
for Motivational
Interviewing Groups

What does good MI group practice look like, and to what extent does it resemble individual MI, group therapy, or common therapeutic factors? Which models of MI groups should be considered best practices? What is the impact of these groups in different settings and populations? Which elements of MI groups are most related to improvements for individuals, and which are most related to the cohesive functioning of the group? In this chapter, we review the evidence for MI groups by examining the kinds of MI groups that have been described and the data generated in research studies. Overall, the evidence about MI groups is promising but remains limited at this time, and is at a similar stage of development as the evidence about individual MI when Miller and Rollnick (1991) wrote their first book on it.

Defining MI Groups

We define MI groups as groups that (1) use MI spirit, processes, and techniques to increase motivation for change, (2) foster healthy interaction among members and leaders to promote change, and (3) include two or more group members and one or more leaders who meet in a shared physical space. MI groups may rely on MI strategies alone. More commonly, studies combine MI and other approaches already established in clinical practice, such as CBT groups. MI groups differ from educational classes in their reliance on group interactions as the match that sparks change, and on minimal information provision as fuel to build and maintain interest in change. In our review of evidence, we do not include studies that had an individual MI session prior to another kind of group (e.g., CBT group) or Internet-based discussion groups.

What Is the Evidence on MI Group Outcomes?

Individual MI produces behavior change and symptom improvement across diverse problem areas and has a large literature of well-designed clinical trials that support its efficacy (Burke, Arkowitz, & Menchola, 2003; Hettema, Steele, & Miller, 2005; Lundahl, Kunz, Brownell, Tollefson, & Burke, 2010; Rubak, Sandbaek, Lauritzen, & Christensen, 2005). In contrast, MI groups have emerged more recently, and the research so far focuses mostly on substance use as the target behavior. Additionally, studies of MI groups as a stand-alone treatment are uncommon; more often, MI groups are a prelude to other treatment, limiting conclusions about the efficacy of MI groups specifically. Despite these limitations, studies to date suggest that MI groups are promising.

This review focuses on both MI groups and MI combination groups. *MI groups* are those that solely use the spirit, strategies, and processes of MI within a group treatment context. *MI combination groups* combine elements of MI with elements of other, distinct interventions, such as CBT.

Studies of MI Groups

Twelve published studies and one dissertation describe MI groups as distinct interventions; all target substance use behaviors among adults or adolescents, and one additionally targets posttraumatic stress disorder (PTSD). Two of these studies were randomized clinical trials (LaChance, Feldstein Ewing, Bryan, & Hutchison, 2009; Noonan, 2000). LaChance and colleagues (2009) demonstrated the greater effectiveness of a single-session, 3-hour MI group on reducing college drinking than a time-matched alcohol information group and another group that focused on alcohol concerns for two 3-hour sessions. Noonan (2000) compared a single-session MI group to an educational session as preludes to extensive substance abuse treatment among 54 men within the Veterans Administration system. No differences were found between groups, although it seems unlikely that the effects of a single group session in the context of extensive treatment in this small sample would be detectable. Five other studies were nonrandomized trials comparing MI groups to another condition, usually treatment-as-usual or assessment-only controls, that provided some information on outcomes of the MI groups (Brown et al., 2006; Foote et al., 1999; Lincourt, Kuettel, & Bombardier, 2002; Michael, Curtin, Kirkley, Jones, & Harris, 2006; Santa Ana, Wulfert, & Nietert, 2007). The remainder of studies in this category used noncomparison or pilot designs.

Taken together, these MI group studies provide preliminary evidence that MI groups affect some predicted processes of change, are equal to other active interventions in reducing substance use, and can increase the quality of subsequent participation in treatment and aftercare. These effects are similar to those identified for individual MI (Burke et al., 2003), although MI groups require more extensive study in designs of higher methodological quality. An important gap in the literature is the near-absence of targets other than substance use.

Studies of MI Combination Groups

Published studies of MI combination groups include 13 randomized trials, seven nonrandomized comparison studies, and seven case studies in which researchers observed people over time. One to four sessions of MI combination groups or MI groups preceding other treatments were common in these studies. The randomized trials focused mostly on substance abuse (Bailey, Baker, Webster, & Lewin, 2004; Hayes, 2007; John, Veltrup, Driessen, Wetterling, & Dilling, 2003; LaBrie, Pedersen, Lamb, & Quinlan, 2007; LaBrie et al., 2008; LaBrie, Thompson, Huchting, Lac, & Buckley, 2007; Marlatt, Baer, & Latimer, 1995; Norman, Maley, Li, & Skinner, 2008; Rosenblum, Foote, et al., 2005; Rosenblum, Magura, Kayman, & Fong, 2005). These studies included adolescent, college-age, and adult drinking and other substance abuse among outpatient, homeless, and psychiatric samples, and adolescent smoking. Three studies included additional target behaviors such as women's HIV risk (Carey et al., 2000), sexual HIV/ sexually transmitted disease (STD) risk (Schmiege, Broaddus, Levin, & Bryan, 2009), and college social phobia (Hayes, 2007).

These studies suggest that one- to four-session MI combination groups are superior to no treatment or treatment as usual, and equivalent to other active interventions, with a few exceptions. These results are similar to those found for individual MI when compared to other active treatments. However, MI groups in these studies were generally part of a more comprehensive treatment, and the effects of combined elements cannot be disentangled.

Other studies of MI combination groups developed long-term models of MI/CBT groups for chronically mentally ill substance abusers (Bradley, Baker, & Lewin, 2007); tested adaptation of content to mentally ill substance abusers' interests (August & Flynn, 2007); added MI strategies to address substance abuse within a family violence curriculum for domestic violence (Easton, Swan, & Sinha, 2000); combined MI with a stages-of-change (SOC) education model targeting intimate partner violence (Alexander, Morris, Tracy, & Frye, 2010); addressed problematic Internet use in a 16-week closed group combining MI, CBT, and SOC content (Orzack, Voluse, Wolf, & Hennen, 2006); integrated MI and CBT for problem gambling (Oei, Raylu, & Casey, 2010); used MI/CBT single-session groups for college alcohol violations (LaBrie, Lamb, Pedersen, & Quinlan, 2006); and used MI principles to deliver assessment plus feedback and information to reduce the risk of driving while drinking (Beadnell, Nason, Stafford, Rosengren, & Daugherty, 2012). While these diverse studies do not permit robust conclusions about efficacy, their creative use of MI in combination groups merits further testing.

Descriptive Studies

Carter, Wilber, and Sahl (2005) described an MI group for substance-using adolescents in short-term psychiatric care. The group addressed member-generated issues to increase adolescents' sense of empowerment to make changes. Specific techniques included emphasizing personal choice and control, discussing the use of substances among group members, fostering bonding to the group and group leader through reflective listening, providing affirmation and support, encouraging peer support, exploring adolescents' motivations for change, and guiding them to set small goals. Velasquez, Stephens, and Ingersoll (2005) described semistructured, MI-infused SOC groups for cocaine use, with the therapist presenting a topic followed by group discussion. Leaders linked themes and built momentum for change across members' varying levels of readiness for change, achieving high ratings of MI spirit and empathy on the Motivational Interviewing Treatment Integrity Scale (MITI-2; Moyers, Martin, Manuel, Hendrickson, & Miller, 2005).

A few descriptive studies combined elements to address the needs of specific populations. One combined MI and relational therapy in a 12-session "contemplation" group for women with eating disorders (Tantillo, Bitter, & Adams, 2001). Another combined MI with psychodrama to help psychiatric inpatients attend to group processes and participate in role playing that explored ambivalence about drug use (Van Horn & Bux, 2001).

Threshold Concerns and Embedded Designs

Some studies did not include enough of an MI intervention to be likely to produce an effect, or included an MI group as a small part of more extensive treatment. In either case, we cannot conclude much about MI groups from the results. The least intensive MI combination group intervention was a 10-minute MI group session as part of a multicomponent, Web-based smoking intervention in Canadian schools (Norman et al., 2008). Therapists leading the 10-minute MI group were rated for protocol adherence; however, MI fidelity was not evaluated. The intervention was equivalent to a Web-based attention control condition on overall smoking rates, but the intervention reduced heavy smoking more than the control condition. John and colleagues (2003) used a single MI group session embedded in a nine-session multicomponent group treatment and compared it to three sessions of individual MI in a randomized study of adults with alcohol dependence. They found that the multicomponent group intervention increased attendance at self-help groups relative to the individual MI intervention, even after controlling for confounders. Rosenblum, Magura, and colleagues (2005) compared four sessions of MI group plus 16 sessions of CBT group to 20 sessions of CBT group for adult substance abusers in a randomized trial. Both groups achieved similar rates of group attendance, days abstinent, and scores on an addiction severity measure. Hayes (2007) paired a single MI group session with CBT group sessions and compared this combination to a CBT group to address social anxiety, social phobia, and drinking among college students. These active interventions yielded similar outcomes, including reductions in social anxiety, drinking, and negative drinking consequences.

Oei and colleagues (2010) compared a group versus individual 6-week CBT plus MI intervention for problem gambling. Although they found that both formats led to greater decreases in frequency of gambling, gambling cognitions, and urges, and life satisfaction than a wait-list condition, the intervention was not described adequately enough to determine what MI or CBT elements were used.

Alexander and colleagues (2010) compared a 26-week MI plus SOC group to a 26-week CBT plus gender reeducation (GR) group in a large sample of male batterers, and found that the MI/SOC group led to a greater reduction in women's reports of violent behavior from their partners than did the CBT/GR group, especially among men who were initially less ready to change. Schmiege and colleagues (2009) treated sexually experienced adolescent offenders by adding an MI group session with personalized drinking risk feedback in the context of sexual situations following a group HIV/STD risk reduction intervention using group activities, videos, and condom use demonstrations. While their study lacked a condition with the MI group components alone, results suggested that adding the MI component to the HIV/STD risk reduction intervention was crucial to achieving sexual risk reduction in this high-risk group (described in the next section on process and outcomes).

Overall, these studies of brief MI groups or MI group elements embedded in other treatment provide examples of how to integrate MI group elements, and evidence that group interaction should exceed a minimum threshold to produce effects.

What Effects Do MI Groups Have on Treatment Processes?

The emerging literature on MI groups is diverse in both clinical and research methods. Despite the small number of controlled studies, the emerging evidence suggests that MI groups may improve the recognition of ambivalence, support autonomy, increase commitment to change, and increase treatment engagement and participation. MI groups can be adapted to prevent some of the negative iatrogenic effects that have been concerns of group researchers.

> *MI groups can improve recognition of ambivalence, support autonomy, increase commitment to change, and increase treatment engagement and participation.*

MI Groups Can Increase Perceived Autonomy and Promote Recognition of Ambivalence

Foote and colleagues (1999) found that adding an open-admission, four-session MI group as a prelude to outpatient substance abuse treatment increased members' ratings of autonomy, their perceptions of support, and recognition of ambivalence more than did standard care alone. They intentionally reshaped problematic interactions using MI-adherent communication strategies.

MI Groups Can Increase Self-Efficacy, Behavioral Intentions, and Readiness to Change

A randomized clinical trial found that a single 3-hour MI + personalized feedback group session with college students in mandated treatment for drinking violations increased members' self-efficacy and perceived risk of drinking, and decreased positive drinking expectancies compared to a two-session (6-hour) alcohol education and values exploration group (LaChance et al., 2009). The MI group reduced hazardous drinking by increasing self-efficacy to refuse drinks in three high-risk situations: social pressure, emotional stress, and opportunistic drinking. Subsequently, self-efficacy mediated drinking outcomes at 3 and 6 months. Schmiege and colleagues (2009) found that adding the LaChance model components to a 3-hour psychosocial HIV/STD risk reduction group intervention significantly improved positive attitudes, perceived norms, and intentions to practice safer sexual behavior among high-risk adolescents, and increased self-efficacy, and safer sex intentions and behavior at 3-month follow-up. In a noncomparison study, adults with learning disabilities classified as precontemplative or contemplative in regard to their drinking problems showed increased readiness to change, self-efficacy, and commitment to change drinking behavior after a three-session MI group (Mendel & Hipkins, 2002).

MI Groups Can Increase Treatment Engagement, Attendance, and Completion

A nonrandomized study of a six-session MI group intervention as a prelude to outpatient substance abuse treatment for court-mandated men who did not endorse any treatment goals produced promising outcomes (Lincourt et al., 2002). The investigators integrated OARS, MI spirit and principles; and MI strategies, such as importance and readiness scaling, eliciting change talk, and change planning, as well as related strategies (e.g., decisional balance and personalized feedback). MI group participants were more likely than those in standard care alone to complete treatment (56% vs. 32%), missed fewer appointments, and were rated by subsequent therapists as more successful at completing treatment goals.

MI Groups Can Increase Participation in Aftercare

In a nonrandomized study comparing a two-session MI group as a prelude to inpatient dual-diagnosis treatment with a control group that discussed life problems (Santa Ana et al., 2007), MI group participants attended more than twice as many aftercare sessions as those in the discussion group. The investigators integrated MI spirit, OARS communication techniques, and MI strategies (e.g., exploring and normalizing ambivalence; importance scaling; and exploring confidence, values, and strengths). Related methods included decisional balance exercises and personalized feedback. They also developed guidelines to encourage member participation and discourage arguing.

MI Groups Can Promote Recognition of Problems

Murphy, Rosen, Cameron, and Thompson (2002) piloted a seven-session, inpatient MI group targeting anger, hypervigilance, weapon possession, depression, and substance use among veterans participating in treatment for PTSD. The group was designed to increase recognition of problem behaviors and motivation to change. It emphasized a nonconfrontational personal style, reflective listening, and promotion of group interaction by encouraging members' sense of ownership of the group. The first session provided a group rationale of helping members prevent being "blindsided" by unanticipated problems posttreatment. Subsequent sessions helped them to build self-awareness by rating symptoms and problems, and comparing themselves to "the average guy." Following the group, participants had come to recognize whether they had 40% of the PTSD symptoms or problem behaviors that were initially unclear to them.

Beadnell and colleagues (2012) tested a 16-hour group motivational enhancement approach, PRIME for Life, for its impact on intentions to drink, recognition of risks, and recognition of problems. In a nonrandomized comparison group design, group members assigned to PRIME for Life were compared to participants in intervention as usual, which comprised classes. Interventions were delivered to small groups of participants mandated to Alcohol Drug Education Traffic School, usually in two 8-hour sessions. PRIME for Life emphasizes collaboration with participants, diffusion of resistance, and clear intervention directions to deliver program elements such as personalized feedback of risk and education about avoiding future alcohol-related problems. The study revealed that the motivational enhancement group showed more positive outcomes that are precursors of change, including problem recognition, greater perception of risk, and more positive ratings of their assigned intervention.

Guidance by Leaders Can Reduce Negative Group Processes in MI Groups

Group therapy researchers have expressed concerns about iatrogenic effects that can occur in groups, or about ways that the group itself may discourage positive growth or even influence clients in negative ways (e.g., Weiss et al., 2005). More recent MI group development has benefited from some of the pioneering work on MI groups that inadvertently may have elicited some of these iatrogenic effects. Some early studies used an assessment-plus-feedback approach to reshape social norms among college drinkers, delivered to groups using a primarily educational approach that did not emphasize group cohesion, or using the group experience to foster change (Walters, Bennett, & Miller, 2000; Walters, Gruenewald, Miller, & Bennett, 2001). These researchers found no advantage to the class delivery format; indeed, providing personalized feedback by mail was more helpful to change students' subsequent drinking. While not successful in obtaining the outcomes they sought, the way these early studies helped to raise questions about how best to go about conducting MI groups (Walters, Ogle, & Martin, 2002; Faris & Brown, 2003) has played an important role in the ongoing evolution of MI group models. One lesson learned from these studies is that providing personalized feedback in a group is challenging, because participants may not be able to absorb the full range of information about stigmatizing issues in the presence of others (Lincourt et al., 2002). In addition, some group members may remain defensive due to their expectations of confrontational interactions, even when they don't occur.

Faris and Brown (2003), noting the null or negative results of studies investigating MI concepts delivered in group educational format, hypothesized that negative group processes may be reducing effectiveness. They assigned college student binge drinkers to either standard or enhanced single-session MI groups with personalized feedback. The enhanced MI group that received instructions on overcoming negative group processes that reduce participation and information processing, such as focusing excessively on others and avoiding productive conversational foci, had better participation, fewer negative group processes, and increased contemplation of substance use effects among members.

What Effects Do MI Groups Have on Treatment Outcomes?

MI group outcome studies show that they may reduce problematic alcohol and drug use, and smoking, and increase risk management and disease coping.

MI Groups Can Reduce Alcohol Use and Binge Drinking

Santa Ana and colleagues (2007) found that a two-session MI group reduced drinking consumption by nearly 75%, and binge-drinking episodes by more than 50% compared to a therapist-led attention group. Michael and colleagues (2006) compared a single-session MI group incorporating MI spirit and principles, evocative questions, and MI-consistent strategies (e.g., exploring ambivalence, importance scaling, decisional balance, goal setting and change planning, and building rapport between members) to assessment only among drinking college students in a nonrandomized study. MI group participants had fewer intoxication episodes and less alcohol consumption over a 2-week follow-up period.

The LaChance and colleagues' (2009) college alcohol diversion MI + personalized feedback group (described earlier) produced significantly better drinking outcomes, including reduced hazardous drinking symptoms and alcohol-related problems, and lower average drinks per drinking day. Notably, these

MI groups can reduce drug use and smoking, and increase risk management and disease coping.

effects were larger than those in a meta-analysis of individual alcohol risk reduction programs for college drinkers. The MI group leader used OARS to lead discussion of a decisional balance exercise, to provide personalized feedback of drinking risk, and to elicit change talk. During the last portion of the session, the group leader encouraged members to help each other develop harm reduction plans to address their risky situations.

Brown and colleagues (2006) piloted a four-session, structured MI group for people with substance abuse or dependence who were recruited through newspaper ads. Following treatment, participants reported more substance-free days and less severe substance-related consequences. Marlatt and colleagues (1995) randomly assigned participants to a two-session group that integrated MI spirit and principles with personalized feedback; goal setting; and information about alcohol tolerance, laws, and social norms. The two-session group significantly decreased alcohol use compared to a no-treatment control condition. Outcomes were better for group members who had higher baseline readiness to change and for those whose attendance was voluntary (vs. mandated). Professional leaders had greater protocol adherence and overall quality of leadership compared to peer leaders, resulting in greater member participation and group cohesion.

LaBrie and colleagues (2008, 2009) have tested variations of 60- to 120-minute single-session MI combination groups for college drinkers, integrating MI spirit and strategies, such as eliciting change talk, exploring ambivalence, and goal setting, with CBT and social norms techniques. Two randomized trials comparing the groups to no-treatment or assessment-only conditions among women drinkers showed reductions in the MI group members' drinks per week, peak alcohol consumption, and alcohol-related consequences. Women with higher social motives for drinking were more likely to benefit from the MI group.

Finally, a randomized trial showed that a four-session combination MI/CBT group increased readiness to change and reduced drinking frequency compared to a no-treatment control for adolescent drinkers (Bailey et al., 2004). The group incorporated MI spirit, OARS, decisional balance, and an emphasis on participants as experts. Groups included icebreaker activities, exploration of alcohol knowledge and attitudes, alcohol education, and role play for development of alcohol refusal skills.

MI Groups Can Reduce Drug Use Frequency and Consequences

Breslin, Li, Sdao-Jarvie, Tupker, and Ittig-Deland (2002) pilot-tested a four-session MI + feedback outpatient substance abuse group for adolescents. They incorporated MI spirit, OARS, importance scaling, decisional balance and goal setting with personalized feedback, and identifying high-risk situations. They used session checklists and other measures of fidelity, and reported that members had decreased drug-using days and drug-related consequences, and increased self-efficacy.

MI Groups Can Increase Smoking Cessation

Kisely and Preston (2006) tested a 10-session MI/CBT combination group supplemented with nicotine replacement therapy in adult psychiatric and substance-dependent patients who smoked. They incorporated MI principles, pros and cons of smoking, and a menu of options for changing with CBT principles and techniques such as a focus on coping with urges. Participants assigned to the MI group achieved a high rate of smoking cessation (24%). A six-session MI smoking cessation group was compared to a six-session CBT group in a nonrandomized study of patients who did not respond to physician advice to quit (Smith et al., 2001). The MI group included the OARS communication style, MI principles, provision of information, confidence scaling, goal setting, and change planning. Of those who did not initially respond to physician advice to quit, 13% of MI group participants were biochemically confirmed as abstinent at 1-year follow-up, compared to 10% of the CBT group.

MI Groups Can Improve Risk Reduction and Disease Coping

A randomized trial compared a four-session MI + HIV risk reduction group to a health promotion group for urban women at high risk of HIV (Carey et al., 2000). Investigators used MI spirit and OARS to deliver HIV risk reduction education with personalized feedback, exploration of personal risks and ambivalence, skills building, and action planning. Compared to the health promotion group, the MI group achieved greater risk reduction knowledge and intentions overall, and better condom use, more partner discussions, and more refusal of unprotected sex among those who were ambivalent about condom use.

In a randomized clinical trial focused on safer sex behavior among high-risk adolescents in the juvenile justice system, people in an MI + feedback group targeting hazardous drinking in sexual situations paired with psychosocial sexual risk reduction strategies achieved greater reductions in sexual risk behavior 3 months later than did those in a group focused on psychosocial risk reduction alone (Schmiege et al., 2009). The investigators attributed the strong additive effect on sexual behavior to a good fit between the needs of this high-risk group and the collaborative, nonjudgmental approach of MI, as well as the provision of personalized feedback on drinking risk information in a neutral manner.

Knight and colleagues (2003) paired MI principles and OARS with an externalizing conversations strategy in an MI combination group for adolescents with type 1 diabetes. Over six sessions, they attempted to increase disease coping by encouraging group members to engage in dialogue that cast their diabetic symptoms as "the other" in conversations. Later, treatment providers rated MI group members as less threatened and more in control of their diabetes, with greater shifts to adaptive coping, than individuals who did not volunteer for the group (Knight et al., 2003).

Reflections on MI Group Research

In an evolving clinical area such as MI groups, creative therapeutic practice is often ahead of research and provides researchers with ideas and approaches to investigate. However, positive evidence about MI groups is emerging across pilot projects, nonrandomized trials, and several randomized clinical trials. The best evidence is that MI groups reduce drinking and its effects. These findings are consistent across studies by several research groups and show that MI groups can reduce drinking frequency and quantity. The evidence supporting MI groups in other areas is more preliminary but promising.

Researchers are already investigating some group processes that lead to change in MI groups. Despite having a robust body of outcomes research on individual MI, including hundreds of clinical trials, process research in that area is only now emerging. Thus, process research on MI groups is ahead of the usual curve, and a few things are already clear. First, there is a wide range of possible approaches to MI groups. Second, skillful management of group processes relates to engagement, participation, and cohesion. Third, MI groups can produce sustained improvements in self-efficacy that relate to better outcomes, perhaps by improving behavioral intentions, a concept similar to commitment.

Group therapy studies are more difficult to conduct than studies of individual therapy, due to difficulties in designing and evaluating group treatment, logistical challenges in recruiting and maintaining cohorts of participants, and managing a high number of variables requiring large sample sizes (e.g., Morgan-Lopez & Fals-Stewart, 2006, 2008). Although some aspects of MI groups may be difficult to investigate, we hope that future MI group research designs are not unduly limited by logistical inconvenience and that researchers draw broadly from study designs in the extant group counseling and therapy literature. Future studies should attempt to avoid some of the weaknesses of early studies, such as the threshold problem, embedding MI so that its unique contribution cannot be assessed, and not using effective group processes such as fostering group interaction and cohesion. Finally, the study of group education should not be confused with the study of MI groups. If future studies attend to these concerns, the evidence base for MI groups could grow substantially over the next decade.

The range of MI groups research has broadened considerably over recent years. Early innovators first tried using MI groups in a semididactic manner, pairing personalized feedback with information provision, sometimes without key elements of MI spirit and strategies. More engaging psychoeducational approaches emerged over time, with MI topics personalized to group members' experiences. More recent MI group studies incorporate more group psychotherapy strategies and nearly all MI techniques and strategies, while actively maximizing group processes to promote change. In Chapter 6 we consider these approaches to group designs, along with an array of issues that arise in adapting MI groups to specific settings.

References

Alexander, P. C., Morris, E., Tracy, A., & Frye, A. (2010). Stages of change and the group treatment of batterers: A randomized clinical trial. *Violence and Victims, 25,* 571–587.

August, J. L., & Flynn, A. (2007). Applying stage-wise treatment to a mixed-stage co-occurring disorders group. *American Journal of Psychiatric Rehabilitation, 10,* 53–63.

Bailey, K. A., Baker, A. L., Webster, R. A., & Lewin, T. J. (2004). Pilot randomized controlled trial of a brief alcohol intervention group for adolescents. *Drug and Alcohol Review, 23,* 157–166.

Beadnell, B., Nason, M., Stafford, P. A., Rosengren, D. B., & Daugherty, R. (2012). Short-term outcomes of a motivation-enhancing approach to DUI intervention. *Accident Analysis and Prevention, 45,* 792–801.

Bradley, A. C., Baker, A., & Lewin, T. J. (2007). Group intervention for coexisting psychosis and substance use disorders in rural Australia: Outcomes over 3 years. *Australian and New Zealand Journal of Psychiatry, 41,* 501–508.

Breslin, C., Li, S., Sdao-Jarvie, K., Tupker, E., & Ittig-Deland, V. (2002). Brief treatment for young substance abusers: A pilot study in an addiction treatment setting. *Psychology of Addictive Behaviors, 16,* 10–16.

Brown, T. G., Dongier, M., Latimer, E., Legault, L., Seraganian, P., Kokin, M., et al. (2006). Group-delivered brief intervention versus standard care for mixed alcohol/other drug problems: A preliminary study. *Alcoholism Treatment Quarterly, 24,* 23–40.

Burke, B. L., Arkowitz, H., & Menchola, M. (2003). The efficacy of motivational interviewing: A meta-analysis of controlled clinical trials. *Journal of Consulting and Clinical Psychology, 71,* 843–861.

Carey, M. P., Braaten, L. S., Maisto, S. A., Gleason, J. R., Forsyth, A. D., Durant, L. E., et al. (2000). Using information, motivational enhancement, and skills training to reduce the risk of HIV infection for low-income urban women: A second randomized clinical trial. *Health Psychology, 19,* 3–11.

Carter, A. L., Wilber, C., & Sahl, R. (2005). Motivational interviewing techniques and the harm-reduction model in a short-term substance-abuse group for adolescents with psychiatric problems. *Connecticut Medicine, 69,* 519–524.

Easton, C., Swan, S., & Sinha, R. (2000). Motivation to change substance use among offenders of domestic violence. *Journal of Substance Abuse Treatment, 19,* 1–5.

Faris, A. S., & Brown, J. M. (2003). Addressing group dynamics in a brief motivational intervention for college student drinkers. *Journal of Drug Education, 33,* 289–306.

Foote, J., DeLuca, A., Magura, S., Warner, A., Grand, A., Rosenblum, A., et al. (1999). A group motivational treatment for chemical dependency. *Journal of Substance Abuse Treatment, 17,* 181–192.

Hayes, B. B. (2007). Comparing the effectiveness of cognitive-behavioral group therapy with and without motivational interviewing at reducing the social anxiety, alcohol consumption, and negative consequences of socially anxious college students. *Dissertation Abstracts International B: The Sciences and Engineering, 67,* 5405.

Hettema, J., Steele, J., & Miller, W. R. (2005). Motivational interviewing. *Annual Review of Clinical Psychology, 1,* 91–111.

John, U., Veltrup, C., Driessen, M., Wetterling, T., & Dilling, H. (2003). Motivational intervention: An individual counselling vs a group treatment approach for alcohol-dependent in-patients. *Alcohol and Alcoholism (Oxford, Oxfordshire), 38,* 263–269.

Kisely, S. R., & Preston, N. J. (2006). A group intervention which assists patients with dual diagnosis reduce their tobacco use. In M. E. Abelian (Ed.), *Trends in psychotherapy research* (pp. 141–159). Hauppauge, NY: Nova Science.

Knight, K. M., Bundy, C., Morris, R., Higgs, J. F., Jameson, R. A., Unsworth, P., et al. (2003). The effects of group motivational interviewing and externalizing conversations for adolescents with type-1 diabetes. *Psychology, Health and Medicine, 6,* 149–157.

LaBrie, J. W., Huchting, K. K., Lac, A., Tawalbeh, S., Thompson, A. D., & Larimer, M. E. (2009). Preventing risky drinking in first-year college women: Further validation of a female-specific motivational enhancement group intervention. *Journal of Studies on Alcohol and Drugs Supplement, 16,* 77–85.

LaBrie, J. W., Huchting, K., Tawalbeh, S., Pedersen, E. R., Thompson, A. D., Shelesky, K., et al. (2008). A randomized motivational enhancement prevention group reduces drinking and alcohol consequences in first-year college women. *Psychology of Addictive Behaviors, 22,* 149–155.

LaBrie, J. W., Lamb, T. F., Pedersen, E. R., & Quinlan, T. (2006). A group motivational interviewing intervention reduces drinking and alcohol-related consequences in adjudicated college students. *Journal of College Student Development, 47,* 267–280.

LaBrie, J. W., Pedersen, E. R., Lamb, T. F., & Quinlan, T. (2007). A campus-based motivational enhancement group intervention reduces problematic drinking in freshmen male college students. *Addictive Behaviors, 32,* 889–901.

LaBrie, J. W., Thompson, A. D., Huchting, K., Lac, A., & Buckley, K. (2007). A group motivational interviewing intervention reduces drinking and alcohol-related negative consequences in adjudicated college women. *Addictive Behaviors, 32,* 2549–2562.

LaChance, H., Feldstein Ewing, S. W., Bryan, A. D., & Hutchison, K. E. (2009). What makes group MET work?: A randomized controlled trial of college student drinkers in mandated alcohol diversion. *Psychology of Addictive Behaviors, 23,* 598–612.

Lincourt, P., Kuettel, T. J., & Bombardier, C. H. (2002). Motivational interviewing in a group setting with mandated clients: A pilot study. *Addictive Behaviors, 27,* 381–391.

Lundahl, B. W., Kunz, C., Brownell, C., Tollefson, D., & Burke, B. (2010). A meta-analysis of motivational interviewing: Twenty-five years of empirical studies. *Research on Social Work Practice, 20,* 137–160.

Marlatt, G. A., Baer, J. S., & Latimer, M. (1995). Preventing alcohol abuse in college students: A harm reduction approach. In G. M. Boyd, J. Howard, & R. A. Zucker (Eds.), *Alcohol problems among adolescents: Current directions in prevention research* (pp. 147–172). Hillsdale, NJ: Erlbaum.

Mendel, E., & Hipkins, J. (2002). Motivating learning disabled offenders with alcohol-related problems: A pilot study. *British Journal of Learning Disabilities, 30,* 153–158.

Michael, K. D., Curtin, L., Kirkley, D. E., Jones, D. L., & Harris, R. J. (2006). Group-based motivational interviewing for alcohol use among college students: An exploratory study. *Professional Psychology: Research and Practice, 37,* 629–634.

Miller, W. R., & Rollnick, S. (1991). *Motivational interviewing: Preparing people to change addictive behavior* (1st ed.). New York: Guilford Press.

Morgan-Lopez, A. A., & Fals-Stewart, W. (2006). Analytic complexities associated with group therapy in substance abuse treatment research: Problems, recommendations, and future directions. *Experimental and Clinical Psychopharmacology, 14,* 265–273.

Morgan-Lopez, A. A., & Fals-Stewart, W. (2008). Analyzing data from open enrollment groups: Current considerations and future directions. *Journal of Substance Abuse Treatment, 35,* 36–40.

Moyers, T. B., Martin, T., Manuel, J. K., Hendrickson, S. M., & Miller, W. R. (2005). Assessing competence in the use of motivational interviewing. *Journal of Substance Abuse Treatment, 28,* 19–26.

Murphy, R. T., Rosen, C. S., Cameron, R. P., & Thompson, K. E. (2002). Development of a group treatment for enhancing motivation to change PTSD symptoms. *Cognitive and Behavioral Practice, 9,* 308–316.

Noonan, W. C. (2000). Group motivational interviewing as an enhancement to outpatient alcohol treatment. *ProQuest Digital Dissertations Database,* Publication No. AAT 9998849.

Norman, C. D., Maley, O., Li, X., & Skinner, H. A. (2008). Using the Internet to assist smoking prevention and cessation in schools: A randomized, controlled trial. *Health Psychology, 27,* 799–810.

Oei, T. P., Raylu, N., & Casey, L. M. (2010). Effectiveness of group and individual formats of a combined motivational interviewing and cognitive behavioral treatment program for problem gambling: A randomized controlled trial. *Behavioural and Cognitive Psychotherapy, 38,* 233–238.

Orzack, M. H., Voluse, A. C., Wolf, D., & Hennen, J. (2006). An ongoing study of group treatment for men involved in problematic Internet-enabled sexual behavior. *Cyberpsychology and Behavior: The Impact of the Internet, Multimedia and Virtual Reality on Behavior and Society, 9,* 348–360.

Rosenblum, A., Foote, J., Cleland, C., Magura, S., Mahmood, D., & Kosanke, N. (2005). Moderators of effects of motivational enhancements to cognitive behavioral therapy. *American Journal of Drug and Alcohol Abuse, 31,* 35–58.

Rosenblum, A., Magura, S., Kayman, D. J., & Fong, C. (2005). Motivationally enhanced group counseling for substance users in a soup kitchen: A randomized clinical trial. *Drug and Alcohol Dependence, 80,* 91–103.

Rubak, S., Sandbaek, A., Lauritzen, T., & Christensen, B. (2005). Motivational interviewing: A systematic review and meta-analysis. *British Journal of General Practice, 55,* 305–312.

Santa Ana, E. J., Wulfert, E., & Nietert, P. J. (2007). Efficacy of group motivational interviewing (GMI) for psychiatric inpatients with chemical dependence. *Journal of Consulting and Clinical Psychology, 75,* 816–822.

Schmiege, S. J., Broaddus, M. R., Levin, M., & Bryan, A. D. (2009). Randomized trial of group interventions to reduce HIV/STD risk and change theoretical mediators among detained adolescents. *Journal of Consulting and Clinical Psychology, 77,* 38–50.

Smith, S. S., Jorenby, D. E., Fiore, M. C., Anderson, J. E., Mielke, M. M., Beach, K. E., et al. (2001). Strike while the iron is hot: Can stepped-care treatments resurrect relapsing smokers? *Journal of Consulting and Clinical Psychology, 69,* 429–439.

Tantillo, M., Bitter, C. N., & Adams, B. (2001). Enhancing readiness for eating disorder treatment: A relational/motivational group model for change. *Eating Disorders, 9,* 203–216.

Van Horn, D. H., & Bux, D. A. (2001). A pilot test of motivational interviewing groups for dually diagnosed inpatients. *Journal of Substance Abuse Treatment, 20,* 191–195.

Velasquez, M. M., Stephens, N. S., & Ingersoll, K. S. (2005). Motivational interviewing in groups. *Journal of Groups in Addiction and Recovery, 1,* 27–50.

Walters, S. T., Bennett, M. E., & Miller, J. H. (2000). Reducing alcohol use in college students: A controlled trial of two brief interventions. *Journal of Drug Education, 30,* 361–372.

Walters, S. T., Gruenewald, D. A., Miller, J. H., & Bennett, M. E. (2001). Early findings from a disciplinary program to reduce problem drinking by college students. *Journal of Substance Abuse Treatment, 20*(1), 89–91.

Walters, S. T., Ogle, R., & Martin, J. E. (2002). Perils and possibilities of group-based motivational interviewing. In W. R. Miller & S. Rollnick, *Motivational interviewing: Preparing people for change* (2nd ed., pp. 377–390). New York: Guilford Press.

Weiss, B., Caron, A., Ball, S., Tapp, J., Johnson, M. & Weisz, J.R. (2005). Iatrogenic effects of group treatment for antisocial youth. *Journal of Consulting and Clinical Psychology, 73,* 1036–1044.

PART II

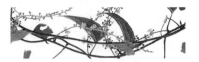

Motivational Interviewing Groups in Practice

In this part of the book, we focus on practical matters in designing, implementing, and conducting MI groups.

Chapters 6 and 7 focus on designing and implementing MI groups, training and supervising MI group practitioners, and developing a continual quality improvement program intended to enhance the effectiveness of services offered.

We turn in Chapter 8 to issues related to conducting MI groups. We first focus on shaping group conversations toward MI-consistent communications and establishing the therapeutic focus. We then focus on the advanced conversational shaping skills of optimizing pace, depth, and breadth of conversations.

In Chapters 9–12, we present a four-phase sequential model of motivational tasks to include in group sessions. This sequential model first focuses on *engaging the group* by facilitating group development through linking members, working with challenging interpersonal styles and roles, and structuring sessions to promote maximum benefit. With these general principles in place, we focus on facilitating the first group session.

The second phase, *exploring perspectives,* involves developing mutual understanding of members' perspectives on their current life situations and challenges. We help members take a step back, look at their situations, and identify ways that they are currently stuck, reflecting upon past experiences when it might help them move forward, but otherwise focusing on the present. As the group becomes more cohesive, members further explore and define their values, perspectives, and identity.

In the third phase, *broadening perspectives,* MI groups help members gain new perspectives on their situations and challenges, envision a more satisfying future, and build confidence to implement changes in their lives.

In the final phase, group members *move into action*—defining, planning, implementing, and maintaining changes that they believe will improve their lives, in collaboration with the other members.

We view these phases as generally sequential but not fixed. Not all groups will cover all phases or engage in all of the topics or exercises we present, and very brief or single-session approaches may only borrow a few exercises that are most relevant to their purposes. Each chapter focuses on group dynamics, therapeutic factors, and leader functions before presenting MI strategies. These are especially relevant to leaders who conduct MI groups in unstructured ways.

CHAPTER 6

Designing Motivational Interviewing Groups

We believe that MI groups have a valuable role to play in the array of group services that help people who are stuck or suffering. We think of MI groups as time-limited, focused mostly on facilitating change for those who are stuck due to unresolved ambivalence or demoralization. We believe there is more value in this approach to groups than is currently appreciated. On the other hand, MI groups are no panacea, and we are not suggesting that they replace other group services. Rather, we believe they could be added to a continuum of care services to enhance the potential for good outcomes.

Tailoring the group approach to fit the needs of your clients helps them succeed. In this chapter, we discuss the considerations involved in designing MI groups, and outline some steps to help design and customize an MI group for your situation.

Why Offer MI Groups?

When clients remain ambivalent about change and unclear about how services can help them achieve their goals, they are less likely to engage and more likely to develop conflicts with staff and other participants. MI helps to increase engagement and reduce dropout, leading to improved outcomes (Hettema, Steele, & Miller, 2005). MI helps clients resolve their ambivalence about change, develop specific goals, and implement plans to pursue these goals. Once clients have clearer goals, they may see participating in services as a way to help them move toward those goals.

MI groups can provide other benefits as well. Group members often benefit from the support and experience of others in similar situations, potentially developing connections that will exist beyond the life of the group. MI groups can help to increase the efficiency of services for clients with poorer attendance rates, by preventing holes in scheduling that are common in individual services. MI groups can also serve as alternatives to wait lists, keeping clients engaged and priming them to participate in other services as they become available.

MI groups are well-suited for these purposes, because they often focus on the content issues that predict group therapy dropout, such as substance problems and somatic complaints, while using a therapeutic style that overcomes some of the interpersonal issues leading to group therapy dropout, such as hostility and introversion (MacNair & Corazzini, 1994; Project MATCH Research Group, 1997).

Skills Involved in Designing MI Groups

Several experiences and skills are useful for developing MI groups. Ideally, you should have experience working with the target population, preferably in groups, and be comfortable using MI techniques, strategies, and spirit. You should also be aware of your locality's service needs. Given the diversity of skills needed, it may be useful to take a team approach to designing your MI group. For example, a practitioner skilled in individual MI may collaborate with another skilled in group processes, and with a program manager who understands the clients and the expectations of referral sources and payers. These three people, each with a different area of expertise, could collaborate to consider the issues outlined in this chapter. By tailoring the design of MI groups to your needs, you maximize their effectiveness and efficiency. Once you develop your initial plan, then pilot test it, trying different approaches, observing the effects upon group members, and gathering their input and feedback. You can refine your plans based on the input of all involved, along with the data you collected during pilot testing.

Take a team approach to designing your MI group.

Group Objectives

The first step is to consider your objectives for the group. Defining the desired outcomes will help you make decisions about the group format, composition, and structure.

Enhancing Engagement and Participation in Other Services

MI groups may foster *engagement in an array of services*. MI groups can help clients become interested in available services, and comfortable participating in them. MI groups may be especially useful for those who are reluctant to participate in services. During the group sessions, members learn that they gain most from active participation, partly by observing peers who are already involved in services. Some who initially may be reluctant to commit to change due to past failed attempts may gain realistic hope for change by hearing from members who have overcome similar challenges. This increase in optimism or confidence can lead them to participate more fully, often improving their retention and outcomes (Katz et al., 2007; Walitzer, Dermen, & Conners, 1999).

MI groups also promote another type of engagement process: *preparing members for a change in services*. For example, it is common for people enrolled in substance abuse treatment to transfer to a less intensive service upon achieving certain goals. In a medical setting, patients in a physical rehabilitation unit who regain enough strength to be discharged from the hospital setting may continue to need in-home services. In this situation, an MI group approach can help people currently in one type of service consider what comes next, and what they'd like to achieve. The MI group may focus on familiarizing members with a different treatment approach that requires a shift in self-definition. For example, engaging in optimal health behaviors may require one to shift from considering oneself a medical patient being cared for to a person actively managing one's health with the support of community resources.

In some cases, the group involves cohort members who will participate together in a subsequent experience. For example, a group of patients currently hospitalized for heart attack might participate in an MI group that helps them start a group cardiac rehabilitation program together after discharge. Students adjudicated within the same month for underage drinking might attend a single-session MI group that prepares them to engage in an alcohol awareness program together. In these cases, the MI group can be designed to encourage a group of at-risk people to consider making changes they previously had not thought were relevant.

Engaging group members early is important. Having members drop out damages group cohesion, which is critical to treatment success (Fieldsteel, 1996). MI groups can be designed from the outset to generate active participation rather than passive attendance. We recommend including strategies that foster immediate engagement, such as those that elicit members' ambivalent feelings, evoke their primary concerns, and enable them to identify and set key goals.

Fostering Motivation and Change among Group Members

Often the MI group is a stand-alone intervention (as we describe in Chapters 9–12), intended to build motivation and facilitate change. While broad improvements are often desired, MI groups typically focus on making a few specific changes. Desired outcomes for each group member often include a combination of *behavior initiation, behavior reduction,* and *behavior cessation.* For example, medical patients are often advised by their healthcare practitioners to initiate behaviors such as exercise, regular medication use, or blood glucose monitoring. They may be guided to reduce other behaviors such as eating high-sugar foods or drinking alcohol excessively. They may be advised to cease some behaviors, such as smoking. Clients with addictions may be expected by the courts to stop using all substances and initiate alternative behaviors, such as attending mutual support groups.

> *While broad improvements are often desired, MI groups typically focus on making only a few specific changes.*

When MI groups are intended to help people maintain goals they have already achieved, such as regular exercise, good medication adherence, or abstinence from substances, there may be less need to focus on ambivalence about the presenting issue. Instead, these groups can help members identify current challenges that threaten to undo gains, monitor any increase in ambivalence about maintaining changes, or address temptations to return to the old behaviors.

Multiple objectives are common for MI groups. You may design a group that you hope will engage and retain participants, help them to make decisions about change, and implement change. You should consider all possible objectives, yet focus on a few primary objectives to help you choose formats, time frame, and other design elements.

Group Format

Once the group's objectives are clarified, the next step is selecting a group format. We consider three common group formats—support groups, psychoeducational groups, and psychotherapeutic groups. Although we present these separately, they are more prototypes falling along a continuum rather than distinct formats. Many groups combine elements of each.

Support groups typically include members who share a specific condition, such as cancer, or have a new status in life, such as being unemployed and seeking a job, or becoming the caregiver of a relative with Alzheimer's disease. The goal of support groups is to facilitate acceptance and adjustment to the new situation. Support groups sometimes have a scheduled topic or guest speaker, followed by group discussion. They are often facilitated by leaders without extensive training in group therapy. Using an MI approach, support groups can focus on making changes that help members adjust to new circumstances or behaviors, such as medication adherence or healthy eating. Support group leaders who have relatively less training and experience can use basic MI techniques and strategies to encourage members to change (e.g., the OARS communication style) and strategies such as exploring values, envisioning the future, reviewing successes and personal strengths, and developing some initial plans for change. These strategies themselves have elicitation of change "built in," so groups can still be helpful even with leaders who are less experienced at responding strategically to change talk or using other advanced MI skills.

Psychoeducational groups provide personalized information and skills building to help people adjust to a new situation, as well as change some aspect of their functioning. In most psychoeducational groups, leaders provide information about clinical conditions and challenging life transitions, along with common coping strategies that can help members improve their lives. Leaders help group members personalize the concepts presented, integrate them into their lives, and practice specific skills. The group may focus on enhancing motivation, knowledge, or skills and rely on theoretical models such as behavioral theory or social learning theory. For example, many addiction treatment programs provide psychoeducational groups that review symptoms of addiction, signs of relapse, treatment options, and social and psychological support, and practice skills such as drug refusal. HIV risk reduction groups, assertiveness training groups, or gamblers' coping skills groups are all examples of psychoeducational groups. MI psychoeducational groups may include a semistructured focus on topics such as exploring a typical day, envisioning a better future, sharing change success stories, exploring importance and confidence about change, and change planning (Ingersoll, Wagner, & Gharib, 1999). These groups may also integrate strategies from related approaches, such as identifying stages of change or conducting a decisional balance.

One psychoeducational group variation includes assessment feedback and discussion among group members about that feedback and their experiences. Such assessment feedback groups are often used to raise awareness of problem behaviors in people not seeking treatment. For example, assessment feedback groups are offered to help college students evaluate their drinking compared to real rather than perceived social norms, and to encourage them to consider change based on related risks. To date, evidence on this format is mixed (LaBrie et al., 2009; LaBrie, Pedersen, Lamb,

& Quinlan, 2007; LaChance, Feldstein Ewing, Bryan, & Hutchison, 2009; Walters, Bennett, & Miller, 2000). One concern is that processing assessment feedback in the presence of others may induce embarrassment or shame. Another concern is that feedback discussed in the group could result in a negative renorming process. For example, a drinker whose blood alcohol content reaches risky levels may perceive his or her drinking to be normal if several members of the group drink more than that. Some groups attempt to prevent this inadvertent normalizing of harmful behavior by using a feedback process designed to discourage sharing of personal results. Rather, they use the group time to focus on goals for change, thus reducing the risk of pathological renorming. This is an example of adapting the group design to fit the needs of the group.

The third common format is *psychotherapeutic groups,* in which process-oriented therapy is conducted in a group setting (e.g., Malat, Morrow, & Stewart, 2011). These groups are usually facilitated by experienced group leaders, are typically unstructured, and are based on a specific theory about the origin of distress and its resolution. For example, in a university counseling service, while students with a variety of adjustment challenges may discuss their situations and reactions, the leader may use group processes to illuminate patterns of interpersonal dynamics and conflicts related to the presenting problem that may stem from their early life experiences with significant others, as suggested in object relations theory. One advantage of unstructured MI groups is greater freedom to use members' interests and energy as a catalyst to move toward change (as in individual sessions). This allows you to be more creative, rather than following a semistructured or structured curriculum. However, it requires greater skill in guiding the group to focus productively in the moment, as well as managing unexpected events that can arise in these groups.

Matching the Format to Your Objectives and Setting

Let's consider how these formats may fit with some possible objectives for your group. If your primary objective is *engagement,* then a format that intrigues members may make them want to come back. A support group may invite ongoing participation by helping members bond around experiencing similar struggles. A psychoeducational group that provides some personalized feedback in the first session might leave members wanting more. A psychotherapeutic group in which members experience the power of a highly involved, cohesive group might increase their interest in returning to gain new ideas. If a primary objective is *behavior change,* you might design a psychoeducational or psychotherapeutic group that focuses on resolving ambivalence and increasing motivation to change, to help members feel more empowered. At times, mixing the formats may be beneficial. When your objective is *behavior initiation,* you might mix a support group format to increase members' motivation to make a habit change together with a psychoeducational format to practice new skills. MI groups can be conducted in any of these formats, and we encourage you to consider formats that vary from your typical approach, to ensure that you don't overlook a promising possibility.

Group Structure

The degree of structure you use is influenced by clients' needs, abilities, and preferences; the amount of time available; and the demands and norms of your setting. Using an *unstructured* approach may include simply opening the group in a neutral way and using MI strategies to work with what emerges in conversation. Another approach is to open the session by inviting discussion of a specific issue, then elicit and explore client reactions. Alternately, sessions can be *semistructured,* focusing on an identified topic, while remaining flexible to member interests and desires, and deviating from the agenda when useful. Finally, sessions may be *structured,* managing group time with an agenda that includes subtopics and planned exercises.

A number of factors can influence which approach you adopt. Psychologically minded clients, particularly those who are voluntary, may respond well to unstructured groups. Leaders trained to lead process-oriented groups, who may be most familiar with unstructured work, thrive with this approach after becoming familiar with MI concepts and strategies. Semistructured and structured approaches may work better initially with mandated or reluctant clients, and with clients whose situations, culture, or experiences lead them to be less open to sharing personal matters. These approaches are also a good fit for leaders who have experience with more structured therapies, such as cognitive-behavioral therapy. Leaders who work in medical, corrections, or addiction fields also may be comfortable using more structured approaches, as may leaders who are new to leading groups.

You can also combine these approaches. You may sequence sessions to flow from an initial, structured format while participants are first getting to know one another, to a semistructured format as they become more comfortable, and finally to an unstructured format when they are able to openly share vulnerabilities or personal matters. Alternatively, you may design the group so that some sessions are more structured and others are less structured, or you may begin by openly exploring interests, then shift to a more specific task focus.

Group Composition

Next, consider who should be in the group. MI groups balance understanding and acceptance of clients as they are with inspiration and support for change. Determining how best to promote these can guide your selection of a group composition strategy. The group should be perceived by most clients as a comfortable place to share, explore ideas, and try new behaviors, without fear of negative judgment or conflict. For some, this may best be achieved by participating in a homogeneous group.

> *MI groups provide a balance between understanding and acceptance of clients as they are, and inspiration and support for change.*

Homogeneous Groups

Homogeneous groups include members who are similar on a key variable. For example, a group may include members working on a specific change goal, such as weight loss. While members may change different habits (e.g., reduce overall food intake, limit late-night eating, or increase exercise), all share a goal of losing weight. Groups may also include individuals who share broader life challenges (e.g., those who have lost a partner or child) or clinical conditions such as depression or posttraumatic stress disorder (PTSD). In these cases, members may engage in different approaches to reaching change goals, and may not even share similar goals. However, they do share similar diagnoses, and perhaps similar histories, struggles, and treatment experiences are common among them.

Homogeneous groups may also focus on specific subpopulations, such as urban youth, college students, or women. Members may have different reasons for participating in these groups, different goals and strategies, and different struggles, but share an identity in common related to their demographics, gender, or role.

You can also design MI groups around the degree of client readiness to change, or specifically around the stages-of-change model. Using the stages-of-change model, for example, groups can be designed for each stage of contemplation, preparation, action, and maintenance. A contemplation group might target clients who have mandates for behavior change, as is common in criminal justice settings. These clients may not have decided whether they are committed to changing behavior that violates some legal statute, such as impaired driving or domestic violence. The group members are similar in that they face external pressures and legal constraints, and may face a choice of participating in group or being jailed, or fined. Such groups are also common in medical settings, where patients who have been advised to make a number of health changes are as yet uncertain which specific changes they want to make. In these situations, if and when clients decide upon specific changes they want to make, they may transfer to a preparation group, where they share with others this commitment to change but have not yet developed a specific plan to do so. Another possibility is to combine stages, such as a predecision group and a planning/action group. Either way, dividing groups in this manner allows clients to work with those at a similar level of readiness. This can protect those who have made the decision to change from being pulled back into ambivalence about change by being around people who are as yet undecided, and protect those who are undecided from feeling pressured by those already in action.

There are several advantages in offering homogeneous groups, however one defines homogeneity. Bonding may happen more readily among members who share a common status or similar difficulty. The focus of group discussions may revolve around a limited number of related issues, making resolution of ambivalence about specific issues more likely. When group members see clearly how their difficulties relate to those of other members, they may share more of their concerns and develop trust with less fear of being stigmatized. Thus, there can be high engagement, participation, and cohesion, all of which facilitate better outcomes.

There are also disadvantages with homogeneous groups. One challenge is logistical. There may not be enough similar members to make such groups feasible. Another disadvantage is that clients with similar difficulties sometimes feed off each other's fears, resentment, and pessimistic attitudes about change, leading to a spiral of negativity. While they sometimes can inspire one another by conquering shared challenges together, at other times they lack the creativity and multiple perspectives that come from mixing clients with different issues or backgrounds. In mandated treatment, facilitating a homogeneous group can at times feel like facing an angry mob with a grudge against you for representing "the system" forcing them to be there. We consider issues related to subgrouping in Chapter 9. One important subgrouping split to avoid is having your clients all in one subgroup, yourself in another, and tension between the two!

Heterogeneous Groups

The other option is to initiate a heterogeneous group composed of members who differ in significant ways. This type of group is easiest to run from a logistical perspective, because separate groups are not required for different backgrounds, diagnoses, change targets, or levels of readiness to change. Time spent on screening is reduced as well, as there is no need to verify that clients fit the designated homogeneous grouping, only that they are reasonable candidates for group services. Having members who differ in important ways may also provide the greatest potential for growth, as the range of perspectives and experiences is broadened, and members may avoid the trap of seeing themselves with potentially limiting identities centered on their diagnoses or problems. This increases the likelihood that members experience the therapeutic factor of universality.

Heterogeneous groups, however, can be more difficult to facilitate. It may require extra effort to elicit commonalities and link members who have a wide range of backgrounds and challenges. Stronger group facilitation skills may be required to help groups develop cohesion around change process issues such as envisioning or goal setting than developing cohesion around problem or subcultural similarity. Therefore, design the group so that it affirms each member's participation and personal explorations in a way that helps bring members together. Because it is the similarity clients perceive with one another that is most important, not demographics or diagnoses, a heterogeneous group that helps people find deeper connections despite surface differences may be the most powerful experience of all MI group possibilities.

Group Size

How many members should be included for the most effective group composition? Group sizes of five to 15 members may be feasible, although group sizes toward the upper end risk seeming like classes or meetings rather than group sessions. It can be difficult to explore vulnerabilities in a room with six or eight other people, and many members simply won't even try in a room with over 12 people. If your focus is on information provision as part of a psychoeducational group, or basic support in a support group, group sizes of 10–12 members may be workable. For psychotherapeutic groups or groups focused on complex or sensitive issues, we believe that eight to 10 members are ideal for two co-leaders, and five to seven if there is a single leader. Note that there is some evidence that a single therapeutic group of 10 clients with two leaders is more effective than two smaller groups with individual leaders (Kivlighan, London, & Miles, 2012). At the other end of the spectrum, when groups fall below five or so members, they can devolve into sequential individual work rather than group work, unless leaders reinforce deeper connections between members. If the numbers are that low, brief individual MI sessions may be better than group.

Some clients feel safer in smaller groups. You may also find that no matter how many members you try to include in a group, your groups typically end up around a certain size after a while. In this case, members are voting with their feet. Accept the wisdom or at least the reality in these reactions and adjust plans accordingly. Contact clients who don't return, and offer them individual services or the opportunity to participate in a smaller group.

Overall, the best size of any specific group is affected by a number of factors: the number of leaders and their experience and skill levels; the length and frequency of group sessions; the severity of client problems; and the reliability, social skills, and openness to participation of clients, as well as the goals of the group. Be realistic about the potential limitations of the design you develop for your MI group. Group members with severe difficulties and unreliable attendance habits, limited social skills, and hostility to the group endeavor are unlikely to achieve major changes such as recovery from addictions, significant weight loss, or perfect adherence to medical recommendations from a large, 50-minute group that meets every other week and is led by one less experienced leader. While resources everywhere are stretched, MI groups will not achieve the impossible. On the other hand, designing your MI group to fit the needs and abilities of clients in your setting could increase the chance of having a significant impact by using resources efficiently.

Group Duration

MI groups can be scheduled for a specific number of sessions or a specific time period. Psychoeducational groups typically have a set number of sessions and a specific sequence of topics and activities. Generally, MI groups are *time-limited,* and can be a single-session, very brief (two to four sessions), short term (four to 12 sessions) or longer term (12 to 20 or more sessions). Group duration may be based on its purpose, as well as its function. For example, if engagement is the goal, and the function is to provide a holding zone while members wait for more extensive services, a briefer duration would fit. If there are multiple objectives, and the group is to stand alone, a longer duration could be better. In a setting with high client turnover, a single-session group can stand on its own, because it is unlikely that members will be together more than once.

MI groups can also be *open-ended,* continuing indefinitely. Members leave as their goals are met, and new members replace them. An open-ended, unstructured psychotherapeutic group might incorporate MI strategies but avoid a predetermined progression of topics. Open-ended structure can also be used in wait-list groups or groups intended to prepare clients for other services, particularly if the typical period of enrollment in the group is fairly brief. Using a semistructured approach, you could rotate perhaps four topics continuously, allowing members to join in any given session and stay as long as is appropriate for them.

An advantage of open-ended groups is that clients can progress forward and exit the group at their own pace. Clients who are eager and ready to move forward are not constrained by a group that has a time line commitment or that has members who move forward at a slower pace. Clients who progress more slowly can remain in the group without the pressure of having to end at the scheduled time along with everyone else. These might include clients who are highly ambivalent; clients for whom each step forward poses new challenges, with an increase in reluctance, difficulty, or other barriers to change; or clients who simply prefer a slower pace. A potential disadvantage of open-ended groups is that momentum for change can be slower to develop without a defined ending to the group that presses for forward movement.

Session Length

Another consideration is session length. The length of sessions ideally should relate to group size and format. You might consider 1 hour for small groups of six or fewer members, 90 minutes for groups of six to 10, and 2 hours for groups of 10 or more. This should allow time for discussion with the group as a whole, time to focus on each member individually, and time for wrapping up at the end. Sessions that last 2 hours or longer are challenging for logistical reasons, such as the need for breaks. More importantly, a 2-hour session is a long time to keep the group engaged. We encourage you to experiment with various sizes and lengths to determine what works for your setting. Two smaller groups, each meeting for an hour, may work better in some settings, whereas one larger group meeting for 2 hours may work better in others. An additional consideration is the format. Support groups often run for about an hour, psychoeducational groups for 90 minutes, and psychotherapy groups from 90 minutes to 2 hours.

Selecting and Preparing Members for Group

It is helpful to meet with clients individually before they join the group in order to consider their readiness for group and prepare them for group participation. The pregroup meeting can screen out people who are inappropriate for an MI group, or at least identify potential challenges that may need to be managed in the group setting. In composing a group, it is important to consider that an MI group may not benefit certain clients, or that their style or issues may reduce the group's effectiveness for other members. Clients should be able to tolerate some interpersonal intimacy, stress, and conflict. They should be able to report on events and behaviors outside of the group and reflect upon how these may relate to their thoughts, feelings, and decision making. They also should be willing and able to participate regularly in group sessions, and to interact appropriately.

Members with disruptive, domineering, or hostile styles may have difficulty participating in an MI group, and may drive other members into hiding vulnerabilities or quitting due to the group's unpleasantness and the potential for harm. Similarly, members with dramatic symptoms can impair group members' ability to bond and develop trust. On the other hand, members with extreme levels of social anxiety, impaired cognitive ability, or ongoing severe crises may not be able to participate fully in group interactions and may be better candidates for individual services. You might exclude them from MI groups, or have them first work with an individual counselor to become better prepared to participate in group.

Pregroup interviews also serve to prepare clients for success in the group. They allow you to engage potential group members, learn details that they may be initially hesitant to disclose in a group, and develop a direct connection that may be useful later with members who struggle during group or if conflict emerges between group members. You can also work with clients to increase preparedness for group participation. You can elicit and respond to any concerns of potential members, convey interest in having them join the group, and communicate confidence that the group will be supportive and beneficial. Finally, it is important to inform group members of the limits of confidentiality and the possibility that emotionally difficult interactions may occasionally occur during sessions. Potential group members are more able to give truly informed consent to participate in individual pregroup meetings than in group sessions.

Chapter 9 provides more detail on conducting pregroup interviews. Although pregroup meetings may seem like a part of the process that might easily be skipped over, particularly if you are not able to screen out undesirable clients, we recommend that you skip them only in rare instances. Forming an individual connection with clients prior to and separate from group interactions can pay healthy dividends should group processes become challenging. If you absolutely cannot conduct pregroup meetings, offer to meet new members individually for 30 minutes or so before their first session, to form a connection and prepare them for their first group session.

Admission Practices

There are several ways to handle group admissions. *Closed-admission groups* enroll a cohort of members at the outset and maintain the same membership for the duration. These can be used when groups are time-limited, such as semistructured psychoeducational groups that have a set agenda over a number of sessions. Closed admission can also be used in unstructured therapeutic groups that are constrained by external schedule, such as a college group that meets for a semester, or a specialty group that may run four times a year and build up a wait list for the next run. If a member leaves during the ongoing group, this transition is usually marked by significant discussion. Some groups establish expectations that members provide notice if they plan to stop participating, so that open discussions involving the departing member can be completed and other group members can discuss the impact of the impending departure. Some groups have a formal "goodbye" ceremony for departing members.

Because closed-admission groups retain the same members throughout, intimacy is higher than in open-admission groups. Tight-knit closed groups often contain the best elements of a family or a group of close friends: Members come to know one another deeply, learn about themselves through the relationships that develop, and benefit from helping one another altruistically. On the other hand, on occasions when closed groups become toxic, the experience can be traumatizing if leaders are unable to guide the group through the crisis, to a deeper level of shared tolerance, intimacy, and trust.

In contrast, some MI groups run as *open-admission groups,* in which each session may be attended by different members, some of whom attend repeatedly and others who only come to a single session. A logistical advantage of open-admission groups is that clients can join the group immediately upon presenting for services—an advantage that is especially useful if the group is a wait-list service. You don't want clients to have to wait to get into the wait-list group! A disadvantage of open-admission groups is that members are likely to be fairly superficial among a group of strangers.

A *staggered-admission* approach admits new members at specified times, such as monthly intervals, or when a subgroup of members graduates to a different service. This approach capitalizes on the strengths of both open and closed admission groups. Incoming clients do not have to wait long to participate, and current members bond and develop trust by working together for several sessions before adding new members. When new members join, the group is better prepared to absorb the new dynamics they bring. These transitions can also prompt current members to consolidate their gains as they summarize their situation for new members, marking where they are and how it differs from where they began.

Relative Difficulty of Design Choices

A final issue to consider as you design your group is the relative difficulty of various options. Although meeting objectives should be the primary consideration, some design options may increase the difficulty of group facilitation, depending on your clients' and your own previous experiences. Figure 6.1 ranks the design choices by their relative difficulty.

You might be tempted to select the elements that, when combined, seem simplest. In general, when you select the easier elements, there is less risk of unintended negative consequences but potentially more limited positive effects. This approach can yield a manageable group and may be advisable if leaders are relatively inexperienced. In contrast, more difficult choices may be potentially more effective in eliciting deep change but require more advanced skills to do well.

When less experienced leaders facilitate groups with many of the more difficult design components, there can be greater risks. Risks that should be considered include uncovering more extensive emotional distress or psychopathology, the emergence of challenging interpersonal conflicts, and other challenging group processes. Groups leaders don't need to avoid these challenges entirely, because they improve by taking on a bit more than they can comfortably handle. Still, it is important to be realistic in matching the anticipated difficulties of a group with the current skills of the leaders. It is good to stretch beyond one's comfort zone, but the task of facilitating the group should not be so complex that it causes panic. It is important to new leaders and clients alike that the group sessions go well.

Designing MI Groups That Work

You have many choices in designing an MI group. Once you decide on objectives, you can select group format, composition, duration of both the group experience and each session, and your approach for enrolling new members. Table 6.1 shows typical design choices for support, psychoeducational, and

	Easier..More difficult
Format	Support................ Psychoeducational ....Psychotherapeutic
Structure	Structured............... Semistructured.............Unstructured
Composition	Homogeneous...Heterogeneous
Size	5...15
Session length	60 minutes...120 minutes
Admission	Staggered......................Closed...................Open

FIGURE 6.1. Relative difficulty of design choices.

TABLE 6.1. A Template for the Design of MI Groups

	Support	Psychoeducational	Psychotherapeutic
Objectives	Engagement	Any	Behavior change
Structure	Any	Semistructured	Unstructured
Composition	Homogeneous	Homogeneous	Heterogeneous
Size	Up to 15	8–12	6–10
Duration	Either	Time-limited	Open-ended
Session length	45–60 minutes	60–90 minutes	90–120 minutes
Admission	Open	Closed or open	Staggered
Counselor preparation	Low	Medium	High

psychotherapeutic MI groups. This template is meant only as a starting place—you can mix and match elements as they work for you.

For example, a support group that focuses on helping members adjust to a new medical condition helps members engage with health care providers who may recommend specific changes. In this situation, the MI group might be conducted as an unstructured discussion group, responding to the issues members face in their current situations, or it might be semistructured, balancing limited education around relevant topics with an open discussion period. Generally, this type of group would be limited to members who have the relevant medical condition. Group size may vary from session to session, with up to 15 people with open admission, so that patients become involved immediately upon diagnosis, when it is timely and they are most likely to want support and guidance. Sessions might last 45 minutes to 1 hour—long enough to yield benefits but short enough that participation isn't perceived as a major time commitment. Patients may use the sessions as informal meetings with nurses or other providers, to touch base on issues between scheduled individual appointments. The group may be set up on an ongoing, open-ended basis or a time-limited, repeating basis. Although basic training in MI and group leadership helps leaders organize the group and prepare for challenges, such as members who dominate discussion or raise sensitive or complex issues, extensive training in MI or in group therapy is probably not needed to facilitate support groups as long as one has a colleague to consult with as needed.

A psychoeducational group can meet objectives of engagement, preparation for other services, or behavior change. These groups are typically semistructured, with targeted focus and some planned activities but also time to explore issues that emerge. Psychoeducational groups may include members who are homogeneous on one or more variables. A group size of eight to 12 members allows increased efficiency of services, while preserving opportunities to function as a therapeutic experience rather than simply as a class. Admitting 12 participants may be necessary to ensure that eight to 10 members are there for any given session. Psychoeducational groups are typically time-limited, with sequential topics that fit the needs of the setting. For example, one 8-week sequence that we suggested in a manual for community-based addictions programs is (1) introduction and exploration of lifestyles, (2) stages of change, (3) good things–less good things, (4) looking forward/exploring goals, (5) decisional balance, (6) exploring ambivalence/developing discrepancy, (7) change success stories, and (8) planning for change (Ingersoll, Wagner, & Gharib, 1999). A four-session model intended to take the place of a waiting list used topics 1, 3, 5, and 6. A single-session model used a menu of options of several strategies to choose from: lifestyle, stresses, and substance use; health and substance use; typical day; good and less good things; providing information; the future and the present; exploring concerns; and helping with decision making. No fixed model is universally appropriate; brainstorm, experiment, and find a fit that works in your setting.

Sixty to 90 minutes is a good session length, although shorter lengths are possible if you adjust goals accordingly. Psychoeducational groups are typically closed if they use sequential topics, but they may be open if participation in earlier sessions is not required to benefit from subsequent topics. Counselor preparation is important to keep these groups from becoming strictly educational classes, which appears ineffective for promoting client change (Faris & Brown, 2003; Miller & Wilbourne, 2002). Psychoeducational group leaders should be well-versed and experienced in providing MI, and participate in training or mentorship in providing group services.

Psychotherapeutic groups may be the most challenging. These groups focus on clinical change and may be members' primary therapeutic service, supplemented by case management or other services. Psychotherapeutic groups may be unstructured, with the MI model implicitly guiding leaders, or a theme identified, but no session plan. Leaders address issues as they arise on clients' paths toward change rather than sequenced topics. Psychotherapeutic groups are often heterogeneous, emphasizing commonalities that members experience in making intentional changes rather than a shared condition, situation, or role. Group sizes often range from six to 10 members, with open-ended duration. Each session may last 90–120 minutes, depending on group size, complexity, sensitivity of issues, and members' psychological mindedness and assertiveness. Admission may be staggered, allowing deeper work around sensitive issues and greater use of group dynamics that come with a stable set of group members. Admitting new members at intervals can keep the group from becoming too small or stale, while also meeting service needs of new clients. Because of the usual unstructured nature of psychotherapeutic groups, the sensitivity of issues involved, the complexity of managing group dynamics in unstructured and heterogeneous groups, and the goal of achieving significant and lasting change in participants, leaders should have substantial preparation. This includes both expert MI practice skills and group leadership skills needed to lead these groups effectively.

There is no single design that leads to the best outcomes. Consider what might work best in your setting, then draft a design for your MI group. An important aspect of design is willingness to refine the original plan—experimenting and modifying it along the way until you, the group members, and organizational stakeholders are happy with the result.

References

Faris, A. S., & Brown, J. M. (2003). Addressing group dynamics in a brief motivational intervention for college student drinkers. *Journal of Drug Education, 33,* 289–306.

Fieldsteel, N. D. (1996). The process of termination in long-term psychoanalytic group therapy. *International Journal of Group Psychotherapy, 46,* 25–39.

Hettema, J., Steele, J., & Miller, W. R. (2005). Motivational interviewing. *Annual Review of Clinical Psychology, 1,* 91–111.

Ingersoll, K. S., Wagner, C. C., & Gharib, S. (1999). *Motivational groups for community substance abuse programs.* Richmond, VA: Mid-Atlantic Addiction Technology Transfer Center.

Katz, E. C., Brown, B. S., Schwartz, R. P., King, S. D., Weintraub, E., & Barksdale, W. (2007). Impact of role induction on long-term drug treatment outcomes. *Journal of Addictive Diseases, 26,* 81–90.

Kivlighan, D. M., Jr., London, K., & Miles, J. R. (2012). Are two heads better than one?: The relationship between number of group leaders and group members, and group climate and group member benefit from therapy. *Group Dynamics: Theory, Research, and Practice, 16,* 1–13.

LaBrie, J. W., Huchting, K. K., Lac, A., Tawalbeh, S., Thompson, A. D., & Larimer, M. E. (2009). Preventing risky drinking in first-year college women: Further validation of a female-specific motivational enhancement group intervention. *Journal of Studies on Alcohol and Drugs Supplement, 16,* 77–85.

LaBrie, J. W., Pedersen, E. R., Lamb, T. F., & Quinlan, T. (2007). A campus-based motivational enhancement group intervention reduces problematic drinking in freshmen male college students. *Addictive Behaviors, 32,* 889–901.

LaChance, H., Feldstein Ewing, S. W., Bryan, A. D., & Hutchison, K. E. (2009). What makes group MET work?: A randomized controlled trial of college student drinkers in mandated alcohol diversion. *Psychology of Addictive Behaviors, 23,* 598–612.

MacNair, R. R., & Corazzini, J. G. (1994). Client factors influencing group therapy dropout. *Psychotherapy, 31,* 352–362.

Malat, J., Morrow, S., & Stewart, P. (2011). Applying motivational interviewing principles in a modified interpersonal group for comorbid addiction. *International Journal of Group Psychotherapy, 61,* 557–575.

Miller, W. R., & Wilbourne, P. (2002). Mesa Grande: A methodological analysis of clinical trials of treatments for alcohol use disorders. *Addiction, 97,* 265–277.

Project MATCH Research Group. (1997). Project MATCH secondary a priori hypotheses. *Addiction, 92,* 1671–1698.

Walitzer, K. S., Dermen, K. H., & Conners, G. J. (1999). Strategies for preparing clients for treatment: A review. *Behavior Modification, 23,* 129–151.

Walters, S. T., Bennett, M. E., & Miller, J. H. (2000). Reducing alcohol use in college students: A controlled trial of two brief interventions. *Journal of Drug Education, 30,* 361–372.

CHAPTER 7

Implementing Motivational
Interviewing Groups

Once you have an initial group design, the next task is to lay the groundwork for implementing and evaluating your group. Anticipating challenges to implementing MI groups in your setting, and gathering stakeholder and participant input can help make the group a success. However, the most important factor is the skill and preparation of group leaders. Thus, we begin with ways for practitioners to become more skilled at leading MI groups, including training, supervision, and practicing facilitation skills within existing groups and with colleagues.

Preparing to Offer MI Groups

Anticipating Challenges

When beginning a new service, there are some predictable challenges. Often, many people have heard of MI but may not understand it accurately or know enough to judge its potential in groups. The first challenge is that some staff members may not be very familiar with MI. If MI is new to the setting, some preparatory MI training, especially its spirit, can help colleagues to understand the purposes and methods that are a part of MI groups. When staff members are familiar with individual MI, they often advocate for more infusion of MI throughout the continuum of care. Gaining the support of informal opinion leaders (who often are not the supervisors or directors!) helps to avoid resistance to "yet another new initiative." It can help to share the challenges that led you to design the MI group, and the desired outcomes. Continue to seek the input of opinion leaders and others as you proceed.

A second challenge is that important people outside your setting may prefer that services stay the same. Even if you perceive MI groups to be a positive step forward, some referral sources may favor how things are currently done. Again, sometimes the source of this reluctance is a lack of information about MI, MI groups, or your plans for how the change may affect other practices and procedures. Therefore, in conjunction with your efforts to gain support internally, consider how to explain new or revised services to external stakeholders. Staff members of some referral agencies may expect progress reports that are inconsistent with the MI spirit. If you are changing the format of reports, you might provide an orientation about all of the changes you are making as you implement MI groups and ask colleagues to review the proposed forms. When these professionals have an opportunity to review the information you propose to provide, they may identify specific information they require and help you to fine-tune plans.

Informing other colleagues who provide different services to your clients is also important, because it can be confusing for clients to move among several types of services smoothly without information about how service A differs from service B. Brainstorm with colleagues about clients' experiences when they participate in MI groups and other services. When the care providers in the alternative system understand and support your efforts, and you reciprocate this, it can only benefit your clients.

Finally, when planning MI groups, ask clients, past clients, or focus groups to review materials and implementation plans. This process provides important feedback that can help you to strengthen the fit between your plans and actual client needs. With all of these stakeholder groups, getting feedback fosters good communication, provides important context and content for your groups, and shapes realistic expectations for MI groups.

Preparing MI Group Leaders

Learning to master MI group facilitation may take an extended period and include several phases. Both MI practice and group leadership skills take time and effort to learn, and so does their integration in MI groups. Ideally, practitioners are competent in conducting individual MI and group facilitation before they participate in MI group training. However, some potential leaders may have relative strengths in one or the other skill set. Some may have solid MI practice skills and familiarity with the population and its issues. Others may be relatively unfamiliar with MI but have training and experience in group psychotherapy, group substance abuse treatment, or family or couple therapy. Thus, they are familiar with managing group dynamics and balancing the focus on individuals and the group as a whole, as well as managing subgroups that develop. When practitioners have a good grasp of both the empathic and directive elements, and are familiar with group dynamics and sensitive to the population, they can readily grasp MI group process concepts and use MI in groups with some training and practice.

To achieve competency in MI, practitioners typically require several concentrated days of MI training, followed by ongoing coding and coaching of their work to achieve solid MI skills. Similarly, most practitioners also require theoretical and practical training in running groups, which can require an extended period. Theoretical training should include group treatment concepts and skills such as monitoring individual behavior, interpersonal behavior, and group processes, and intervening at the group level. There is no substitute for practice to develop group facilitation skills. We favor an apprenticeship model, in which practitioners build group skills over time with a more experienced colleague as a co-leader. This apprenticeship should include using each other or peer observers to process the experience.

Sometimes practitioners who lack extensive training in either MI or group therapy want to learn to facilitate MI groups. If this is your situation, we encourage you to obtain further training in your less developed area before engaging in training of MI group practice. You may best serve your clients by first offering MI groups that are relatively less difficult in their design, as described in Chapter 6, preferably with an experienced co-leader with strengths in your less developed area. You can increase your learning by obtaining careful supervision of this practice.

When you have a good background and skills in both MI and group practice, we recommend several days of experiential training specifically in MI groups, followed by coaching and supervision as you begin to run MI groups. In addition to obtaining this background and training, you can increase your skills and confidence by practicing MI group skills both with real groups (not necessarily designed as MI groups) and with your colleagues as a practice group. You may be able to practice and build your MI group skills by sequentially trying various components of the MI groups within your current setting. Specifically, if you are working in a setting that runs groups, join as a co-leader and try some of the following MI group skills.

First, we recommend practicing the appropriate MI group facilitation skills for each phase of treatment using selected MI group techniques in your group. For example, when your group first meets, members should engage with one another and explore perspectives on lifestyles, values, and ambivalence. During this phase, practice being empathic, using an eliciting rather than a providing style, and using OARS strategically to link participants' perspectives, interests, and experiences. These experiences give you a feel for starting the group, shaping early conversation, and demonstrating empathic understanding of individual member issues and their relation to those of other group members. In addition, notice when members give each other advice rather than listening, and when they reduce others' motivation by supporting the status quo rather than supporting change. Practice reframing or briefly coaching participants to paraphrase what they hear in an exchange, before reacting to each other.

Later, try out some of the *broadening perspectives* strategies such as envisioning, exploring importance and confidence, changing success stories, and evoking strengths. Practice handling issues pertinent to this phase of MI group work, such as working with a co-leader, understanding the group on both content (what is discussed) and process (how the discussion unfolds) levels, and managing silence or tension within a heterogeneous group. You and your co-leader might try specific roles that help to build these skills. For example, you might observe the group as a whole and make reflections or ask questions that draw group members into the discussion. Your co-leader can then focus on strategies rather than using OARS skills. If you have observers or the opportunity to record your groups, get feedback about your use of specific skills or strategies. Try different elements that include emphasizing choice and control, avoiding MI traps, and using reflections and open questions with more difficult members.

If you are practicing MI group skills in a group focused on change planning and taking steps, try techniques that are useful for the *moving into action* phase. Here you can try different ways to manage unresolved ambivalence, or improve your skills in managing incongruence as some members plan and implement changes, while others remain inactive. Here, you can gain skills in keeping a positive momentum flowing by inviting members to look toward the future rather than the past. You and your co-leader can also try different roles, such as content facilitator and process facilitator. The *content facilitator* focuses on eliciting change talk and commitment talk during a change planning discussion, using key questions, such as "What do you hope to gain from making this change?"; "How will you do it?"; "How will you know it is working?"; "How will you know if it's not working?"; "How can the group (and others) help?" This type of discussion can be guided by a worksheet, with group members writing in their responses before, during, or after discussion, with key points recorded by the content facilitator on a chart. In the meantime, the process facilitator summarizes and creates links between members' feelings about change, ambivalence, or where they are along the pathway toward change, as well as interpersonal aspects, such as how they support one another. Following the session, discuss what you learned from each role or from observing each other.

An alternative to trying out MI techniques in a real group is to help each other build skills. One or two of you can facilitate a practice group, while three to five others serve as members, ideally exploring current issues in your own lives, as well as role playing some moderately challenging client situations. This can be a safe way to build MI skills, especially in more difficult situations, such as managing discord among group members with differing levels of readiness for change, or with significant psychopathology. To foster your learning in these situations, your colleagues should display varied levels of challenging or withdrawn behavior to help you build confidence using MI skills. Practice exploring importance and confidence using several different methods (e.g., open discussion vs. scaling, verbal vs. written exercises), while also observing group process and making summaries that link themes and different group members' experiences. After each mini-practice, elicit your colleagues' ideas about managing interactions within that phase of group work, and brainstorm alternative ways to facilitate group interactions. Since this is a practice group, you might "stop the action" and ask your colleagues/group members for their ideas about how to proceed. You might also use this practice group to gain skills using different methods to elicit and strengthen commitment and planning for change. Following this plan, you will have practiced six to 10 specific MI group strategies, as well as group skills, such as managing multiple clients simultaneously. You will also have practiced co-facilitation skills. This should increase your comfort level with conducting MI groups and heighten interest in developing more MI groups for your setting.

You and your colleagues might also experiment with potential MI group designs and conduct pilot groups to refine what works in your setting, and with your population. This period of experimentation may help you to develop ownership of the group and confidence in its implementation.

Implementing MI Groups

Once you've designed your group, prepared leaders, and built support with collaborators and stakeholders, it's time to start the group. The rest of this chapter describes how to support and supervise MI group practices, as well as how to evaluate these practices and the outcomes you hope to achieve. The next several chapters focus on the specific "how-to's" of running the group and strategies that are helpful in different phases of group work.

You need ongoing support in MI group practice. Supporting the leaders usually includes training in MI and group processes, followed by ongoing, clinically focused supervision. Supporting the group might mean examining clients' perceptions of benefit and, when possible, the aggregate outcomes. Ongoing quality assurance and evaluation processes can help you improve MI group services over time based on the information you gather.

Supervision of MI Group Practice

Supervision can include discussion of cases, clinical methods, and clinical decision making. Supervision also helps the leaders to facilitate group processes that elicit client change. New leaders have various concerns that can be addressed in supervision. Leaders may feel anxiety about managing the group while maintaining an MI style, especially when handling

Supporting group leaders involves training followed by ongoing supervision.

challenging members. Supervision is a productive place to brainstorm solutions to difficulties that arise. More importantly, it can help leaders view members' experiences in group through an MI lens. When leaders focus keenly on the perceptions, perspectives, concerns, and thoughts of group members, overly self-evaluative performance concerns tend to diminish. When leaders are too focused on what to do next while leading the group, their listening skills are diminished. In contrast, relaxed leaders trust fundamental listening and group facilitation skills. Supervision can guide less experienced leaders into this relaxed, trusting posture with the group, and this in turn often fosters comfort and commitment of group members to their own aspirations and movement toward them. Supervision can also help less experienced MI group leaders learn to structure the group proactively, link important content across members, and attend to members' interpersonal and intrapersonal processes that occur but are unaddressed. Leaders can then return to the group with an open ear and ideas about how to address these issues more skillfully. Whenever possible, we recommend video-recording group sessions for review in supervision (using audio recordings when video is not feasible).

Supervision can help less experienced leaders learn to structure the group proactively, link across members, and attend to processes that are unaddressed by members.

Support for MI Group Practice

Some ongoing support for MI group practice is crucial to implementing effective group services. In-service training can focus on MI concepts, strategies, skills practice, and group processes. Case conferences allow practitioners to present challenging cases or situations, sometimes by reviewing recorded segments with colleagues, followed by discussion that may include invited MI group experts. Case conferences should focus on the use and timing of specific MI skills and strategies that are pertinent to the group's phase of work, developmental level, and target behaviors.

Informal meetings can also provide valuable support. These may include informal lunch meetings in which MI group issues are discussed, or in which specific chapters, treatment manuals, or books are reviewed. Least formal is peer-to-peer discussion of MI, group processes, MI groups, or a challenging group session in which a leader talks with a peer who serves as a sounding board and brainstorming partner. When several of these options are available, leaders gravitate toward those that suit them best to foster their skills, learning, and confidence.

Quality Assurance for MI Groups

Quality assurance (QA) helps to determine whether MI groups adhere to quality standards and produce positive outcomes. QA differs from supervision, which focuses on practitioner skills and specific cases. QA has two components: (1) Treatment fidelity, which determines how well the service adheres to guidelines and principles, and (2) outcome evaluation, which focuses on the extent to which a specific service benefits participants.

Treatment Fidelity

The treatment fidelity of individual MI sessions is evaluated by rating systems that code MI global skills and specific behaviors. MI global skills include attributes such as empathy and direction. MI is characterized by specific communication patterns. MI prescribes consistent use of reflections, open questions, affirmations and summaries, and occasional use of other communication elements, such as emphasizing client choice and control. Some communication methods (e.g., such as confrontation, giving directives or warnings, or advising clients without permission) are avoided. Coding systems are used to verify practitioner adherence to these patterns. The most commonly used coding system, the Motivational Interviewing Treatment Integrity Scale (MITI-3; Moyers, Martin, Manuel, Miller, & Ernst, 2009), reliably codes the overall level of empathy, direction, MI spirit, and specific therapist MI adherent and nonadherent behaviors in individual MI sessions (Madson & Campbell, 2006; Moyers, Martin, Manuel, Hendrickson, & Miller, 2005; Moyers & Martin, 2006). Patterns of behavior are also important; for example, adherent MI practice involves twice as many reflections as questions, twice as many open questions as closed, and as many complex reflections as simple ones. However, MI global patterns and behavioral skills are different in group MI, and direct assessment of treatment fidelity in MI groups awaits the development of reliable and valid MI group measures. We consider these differences and return to how current measurement systems might be useful in quality assurance.

Practice Differences between Group and Individual MI

With treatment fidelity in mind, let's consider how MI in groups differs from individual work. Group leaders strive to foster an atmosphere of empathy, direction, and MI spirit for the whole group. At first, these characteristics may come from leaders, who model these attitudes. As the group becomes more cohesive, leaders guide members to interact in MI-consistent ways, in addition to modeling MI behaviors themselves. During this phase of work, leaders may coach members to help them be more empathic and collaborative with one another. Over time, members should show increasingly collaborative attitudes, support for the autonomous choices of other members (MI spirit), and even interest in understanding others' experiences (empathy). The MI group continually moves toward MI-consistent communication. Even with coaching, some members may not communicate fully in the spirit of MI, but they may reduce hostile-sounding confrontation or advice-giving. Eliminating negative interactions among members may be more critical than fostering MI-consistent interactions.

Direction and talk time also become more MI-consistent in the MI group over time. MI groups clearly differ from classes, in which leaders may do nearly all of the talking. In MI groups, it is helpful for leaders to step back once the group members are engaged. This helps group members to be more involved and autonomous. Group members should be talking more than leaders, generating most of the conversation. However, a challenge for evaluating MI treatment fidelity arises as the leaders generate fewer utterances for coding. In addition, reflections may focus on linking emotional or experiential themes.

Obviously, both leader and member behaviors contribute to a productive and MI-consistent atmosphere, but the nature of a group complicates rating any individual's contribution. Practitioner behavior frequencies will be quite different from those observed in individual MI sessions, and definitions of some behaviors may need to be modified, as in the earlier reflection example. These differences between group and individual MI affect ratios calculated from behavior counts. A very important quality to evaluate is the "group" itself, and here the process is rated best using global codes, including those that reflect the level of member participation and benefit. For research, it may be possible to code each member's speech, or to generate some kind of aggregated rating that combines group members, but such a system is unlikely to be feasible in practice.

Adaptations to Coding Needed to Capture MI Group Characteristics

MI coding measures should be adapted for the group environment. For example, consider the MITI-3 category of "collaboration," one of the key measures of the spirit of MI. The MITI defines the ideal in this category as "Clinician actively fosters and encourages power sharing in the interaction in such a way that the client's ideas substantially influence the nature of the session." Thus, in individual MI, collaboration involves the clinician drawing out client perspectives, and not dominating the client in interactions. However, because successful group sessions include a sharing of focus across multiple members, interaction among members, and development of cohesion between members, the MITI definition of collaboration for individual MI does not capture all aspects of collaboration in a group session. A group adaptation of this definition might be "Leaders encourage group interaction and sharing, and actively balance contributions across members. Leaders guide members to give attention to whoever is speaking, not to interrupt or divert focus, to share helpful experiences and ideas, and to shape the group agenda." As the group is not intended to comprise successive, individual mini-sessions, the definition should consider not only leaders' direct interactions with clients but also how well they foster a collaborative atmosphere with the group as a whole. The opposite might be captured as "Leaders use excessive time with individual clients and discourage interactions between group members."

Adapting definitions for other MITI coding targets is also appropriate, as in *autonomy support,* when different group members may make different choices and do not need to come to similar solutions. *Direction* involves not only directing the focus of conversation toward the target behavior of an individual but also good time management, so that all members move toward change in sessions, and thematic management, so that time is spent focusing on the future more than the past or the present. Leader skills in linking motivational or change themes across participants is also an important part of direction in group sessions, because finding broad themes that combine the motivations of many members is more fruitful than approaching each member's change as an isolated phenomenon, specific to that person.

We have begun to develop some principles and methods for evaluating MI groups. In the meantime, it is useful to consider how group themes supplement individual MI themes when we attempt to coach leaders based on individual MI session measures.

Process Evaluation

A recent review documented 160 different measures in the research literature on group process components (Strauss, Burlingame, & Bormann, 2008). We recommend considering a few of the group therapy measures in the battery proposed by the American Group Psychotherapy Association (AGPA) CORE-R Task Force (2006; Strauss et al., 2008). While these instruments are not specific to MI groups, they may help you evaluate important elements. The CORE-R battery includes instruments for group selection and preparation, group process, and group outcomes. Although the full battery requires ample resources, a few instruments may be implemented to evaluate group process and outcomes, and serve as feedback tools to leaders and program administrators during the active life of groups. All of these measures assess elements of group process and outcomes from client perspectives.

Alliance

For process evaluation, the CORE-R includes the Working Alliance Inventory (WAI; Horvath & Greenberg, 1989) to assess the relationship between individual members and group leaders. Despite the other important variables involved in good group therapy, alliance with the therapist remains an important element in group services as well. This 36-item instrument takes about 10 minutes to complete and measures the bond between members and leaders, as well as members' perception of agreement on the goals of treatment and the tasks required to achieve those goals. The AGPA task force recommends this instrument as the primary measure if only one measure of process can be used. A second useful measure of leader performance is the Empathy Scale (ES; Persons & Burns, 1985), a 10-item scale measuring members' perceptions of leaders' warmth and empathy, including both positive and negative items.

Group Processes

The Group Evaluation Scale (GES; Hess, 1996), a seven-item measure, assesses members' perceptions of overall feelings about the group, ease of discussing problems within the group, feelings of being understood and supported in efforts toward greater autonomy and responsibility, and sense of helpfulness of other members. The Group Climate Questionnaire (GCQ; MacKenzie, 1983), a 12-item scale, assesses engagement (perceived closeness of members, perceived importance of the group, willingness to engage with and understand others in the group, willingness to self-disclose), avoidance (reluctance to assume responsibility for change), and conflict (perceived amount of tension, anger, distrust, and distance within the group). The Therapeutic Factors Inventory (TFI; Lese & MacNair-Semands, 2000) Cohesiveness subscale is a nine-item scale measuring perceived trust, cooperation, acceptance, and sense of belonging within the group. A final measure to consider for your groups is the Critical Incidents Questionnaire (CI; MacKenzie, 1987), a narrative open-ended questionnaire focused on perceived critical incidents in the life of the group. The CI provides information about which events members perceive as especially important in promoting change.

Outcomes Evaluation

There are many standard markers of outcomes that are beyond the scope of this chapter, such as measures of overall quality of life, overall medical outcomes, social support, and changes in specific behaviors. One could make the case that if individuals within the group change problematic behaviors, this is good evidence of progress, even if this is not a formal measure of group outcomes, since there are likely other factors influencing members' improvement. This may be sufficient for the needs of most programs. On the other hand, a more complete evaluation of outcomes would attempt some comparison of outcomes from the MI groups to a wait list or other services, to consider whether the MI group produced change and to determine its efficiency compared to other services.

Client General Outcomes

The Outcome Questionnaire 45 (OQ-45; Lambert, Lunnen, Umphress, Hansen, & Burlingame, 1994) measures symptom distress (anxiety, depression, and substance abuse), interpersonal relations (satisfaction in friendships, family life and romantic relationships) and social role performance (level of functioning across work, family, and leisure). While these issues may or may not be specific targets for change in MI groups, they may affect and vary with other behavior changes and are of importance within many clinical services (and may improve through participation in MI groups). The OQ-45 takes approximately 10 minutes for clients to complete and can be used pre- and post-service to determine change or be incorporated at regular intervals as a feedback and planning tool. There are alternative versions (30-item Short Form, Severely Mentally Ill Form, and 10-item Medical Settings Form when referral for psychological services is indicated). The OQ suite also has group readiness screening instruments, and group environment and session-tracking instruments.

Self-Acceptance

The 10-item Rosenberg Self-Esteem Scale (SES; Rosenberg, 1965) measures current degree of client self-acceptance, which is likely an important element of resolving ambivalence and proceeding toward long-term change.

Interpersonal Problems

We recommend considering the 64-item Circumplex (IIP-C; Alden, Wiggins, & Pincus, 1990) and 32-item Short-Form versions of the Inventory of Interpersonal Problems (IIP-SF; Soldz, Budman, Demby, & Merry, 1995).

Client problems in interpersonal interactions (e.g., aggressiveness or difficulties with assertiveness) can hinder behavior change, even if they are not the target behavior in MI groups. This instrument can be used for screening or pre–post comparison. Any of these measures can be useful to assess MI group service outcomes, and provide relevant, easily gathered information both pre- and postgroup.

Individualized Client Goals

The Target Complaints measure (Battle et al., 1966) assesses clients' perceived improvement on three individualized goals as well as current distress level. This brief measure can be used at the end of group to gather retrospective perceptions of progress on goals.

Individual change plans generated by clients can also be used to track progress and outcomes. While all of these group psychotherapy outcome measures provide useful information about MI groups, the most useful evaluation may be determining what goals were set and how well clients reached them.

> *The most useful evaluation may be determining what goals were set with clients and how well they reached them.*

Client Perceptions of Outcomes

It seems important to query participants directly about their perceptions of the benefits of the MI group, and to query the leaders about their perspective.

Beginning in Chapter 8 we turn to the specific skills and strategies that represent good MI group practice in different types of groups and during different group phases.

References

AGPA CORE-R Task Force. (2006). *Core Battery—Revised: An assessment toolkit for providing optimal group selection, process, and outcome* (1st ed.). New York: American Group Psychotherapy Association.

Alden, L. E., Wiggins, J. S., & Pincus, A. P. (1990). Construction of Circumplex scales for the Inventory of Interpersonal Problems. *Journal of Personality Assessment, 55*, 521–536.

Battle, C. C., Imber, S. D., Hoehn-Saric, R., Stone, A. R., Nash, E. R., & Frank, J. D. (1966). Target complaints as criteria of improvement. *American Journal of Psychotherapy, 20*, 184–192.

Hess, H. (1996). Zwei verfahren zur einschätzung der wirksamkeit von gruppenpsychotherapie [Two methods to assess the affectiveness of group psychotherapy]. In B. Strauss, J. Eckert, & V. Tschuschke (Eds.), *Methoden der empirischen gruppentherapieforschung—ein handbuch* [Methods of empirical group psychotherapy research—A user guide] (pp. 142–158). Opladen, Germany: Westdeutscher Verlag.

Horvath, A. O., & Greenberg, L. S. (1989). Development and validation of the Working Alliance Inventory. *Journal of Counseling Psychology, 36,* 223–233.

Lambert, M. J., Lunnen, K., Umphress, V., Hansen, N. B., & Burlingame, G. M. (1994). *Administration and scoring manual for the Outcome Questionnaire.* Salt Lake City, UT: IHC Center for Behavioral Healthcare Efficacy.

Lese, K. P., & MacNair-Semands, R. (2000). The Therapeutic Factors Inventory: Development of a scale. *Group, 24,* 303–317.

MacKenzie, K. R. (1983). The clinical application of a group climate measure. In R. R. Dies & K. R. MacKenzie (Eds.), *Advances in group psychotherapy: Integrating research and practice* (pp. 159–170). New York: American Group Psychotherapy Association.

MacKenzie, K. R. (1987). Therapeutic factors in group psychotherapy: A contemporary view. *Group, 11,* 26–34.

Madson, M. B., & Campbell, T. C. (2006). Measures of fidelity in motivational enhancement: A systematic review. *Journal of Substance Abuse Treatment, 31,* 67–73.

Moyers, T. B., & Martin, T. (2006). Therapist influence on client language during motivational interviewing sessions. *Journal of Substance Abuse Treatment, 30,* 245–251.

Moyers, T. B., Martin, T., Manuel, J. K., Hendrickson, S. M. L., & Miller, W. R. (2005). Assessing competence in the use of motivational interviewing. *Journal of Substance Abuse Treatment, 28,* 19–26.

Moyers, T. B., Martin, T., Manuel, J. K., Miller, W. R., & Ernst, D. (2009). *Revised global scales: Motivational Interviewing Treatment Integrity 3.1.1* (Unpublished manuscript). Retrieved May 3, 2011, from *http://casaa.unm.edu/download/mitI3_1.pdf.*

Persons, J. B., & Burns, D. D. (1985). Mechanisms of action of cognitive therapy: The relative contributions of technical and interpersonal interventions. *Cognitive Therapy and Research, 9,* 539–551.

Rosenberg, M. (1965). *Society and the adolescent self-image.* Princeton, NJ: Princeton University Press.

Soldz, S., Budman, S., Demby, A., & Merry, J. (1995). A short form of the Inventory of Interpersonal Problems Circumplex Scales. *Assessment, 2,* 53–63.

Strauss, B., Burlingame, G. M., & Bormann, B. (2008). Using the CORE-R battery in group psychotherapy. *Journal of Clinical Psychology, 64,* 1225–1237.

CHAPTER 8

Shaping Group Conversations

Groups do not spontaneously develop the cohesiveness, task focus, and mutual support that are critical to their success. For groups to be helpful, some guidance is needed to establish conversational flow, turn taking, member-to-member communication, and full-group involvement. Maximizing impact requires advanced skills in shaping conversations.

Successful therapeutic groups develop through focused exploration of members' experiences, perspectives, attitudes, hopes, and plans. Spontaneous conversation is usually more chaotic, dominated by a few individuals telling stories, making small talk, and focusing on past

> *Guidance is needed for groups to establish conversational flow, turn taking, member-to-member communication, and full-group involvement.*

events. Your work as group leader is to shape group conversations, so that they have a productive focus and flow, leading members toward ever greater clarity of their values and goals, and investment in their plans for change.

While facilitating groups, you are always engaged in one or more of the following conversational strategies:

- Establishing a topical focus
- Eliciting discussion
- Linking members and guiding their communications with each other
- Holding the focus on topic and preventing unproductive drift
- Shifting focus

121

- Guiding the conversation to move forward at a productive pace
- Guiding the group to slow down in order to consider certain issues more carefully
- Guiding members to broaden or narrow their focus
- Inviting and helping members to go deeper into feelings, values, or themes
- Helping members to return to the surface or lighten the mood
- Closing the conversation

Shaping group focus is like directing conversational traffic. Part of your job is signaling when to stop, when to go, when to change direction, and when to wait for others to proceed first. This includes initiating a topic and engaging members in discussion. Once members are engaged, it is important to maintain focus on productive conversation while building cohesion by linking members together. Eventually, it becomes time to close discussion of the topic.

> *Shaping group focus is like directing traffic—signaling when to go, when to stop, when to change direction, and when to wait for others.*

In addition to establishing and maintaining focus in order to make group conversations productive and hold the group together while moving forward, you also need to shape the conversations so that they are maximally helpful. Some conversations move too slowly or too quickly, or are superficial rather than very meaningful. At times, conversations that are too vague to promote change place the group at risk of becoming a discussion group rather than one that leads to action. Other times, conversations are too narrowly focused on story details to be broadly motivating.

In shaping conversations, it is helpful to consider depth, breadth, and momentum:

- *Depth* refers to level of meaning, ranging from a surface level, with a superficial focus on daily events, factual matters, and general interests, down into deeper conversations about more personal matters, values, identity issues, and underlying perspectives or emotions.
- *Breadth* refers to how narrowly the conversation focuses on a single event, specific issue, or idea, versus how much it broadens into more general themes.
- *Momentum* refers to the pace of forward movement in the conversation—the degree to which new ideas emerge in the conversation or how the conversation proceeds toward some conclusion or commitment to action. In contrast, a slower momentum occurs when the

conversation proceeds at a more leisurely pace, merely exploring an idea or issue, with no particular movement toward a conclusion.

Using advanced conversational shaping—accelerating or decelerating momentum, broadening or narrowing focus, deepening or lightening focus—helps members get the most out of group conversations. We first consider basic conversational shaping tasks, then the more advanced tasks.

> *Shaping the breadth, depth, and momentum of group conversations maximizes impact.*

Basic Conversational Shaping

Establishing and Maintaining Focus

Focusing therapeutic group conversations leads to improvement in members' outcomes (Barlow, Burlingame, Harding, & Behrman, 1997). Your basic tasks in facilitating conversation are to establish and develop a particular focus (on a topic, theme, person, experience, etc.). Because group conversations tend to drift, holding the group's attention on a focus is essential. Knowing when and how to change focus to keep momentum moving forward is also important. Table 8.1 summarizes these strategies, which we detail below.

Establishing Focus

The first task is to establish a focus of conversation. Whether you are opening a topic at the beginning of a session, introducing an exercise or

TABLE 8.1. Basic Conversational Shaping Strategies

Aims	When is this most appropriate?	What conversational methods?
Establishing, developing, and holding focus	• During initial session • Opening additional sessions • When conversation is productive	• Introductory framing • Evocative, open questions • Simple reflections • Emphasizing personal control
Changing focus	• When members focus on unproductive stories, details, or concepts	• Transitional summary • Shifting focus • Amplified reflection • Agreement with a twist

activity, or focusing attention on a new person or issue, it is important to keep the group from meandering in an unfocused manner. It is also important to remember that MI groups are not member-led—it is up to you, as the leader, to guide the group in a productive manner. Even when you incorporate periods of brainstorming or open exploration to find the energy or interests of the group, it is useful to guide the group into those tasks, and indicate how long you want to explore them. Often, establishing initial focus is as simple as describing in a few sentences what you'd like the group to discuss. Lengthy explanations are likely to be tuned out and inhibit exploration. If you are leading a support or psychoeducational group, you can use a handout, material on a whiteboard, or a visual cue (e.g., artwork) to introduce the focus. Using rounds or dyads (discussed below) can be helpful for new topics, especially when it would be useful for members to share some details before delving into underlying concerns or overarching themes. Some groups might even incorporate movement as part of establishing focus (e.g., having group members line up along a 0- to 10-point importance or confidence ruler on the floor or along the wall to establish visually different levels and explore them by eliciting comments from representatives along the line rather than having to explore each individual's answers).

Eliciting Discussion

Even in groups whose members are mandated to attend, most are fairly easy to engage in discussion (although their comments may not be universally positive at first!). However, not all members speak up, and some only speak up during more superficial conversations, not at times when they feel vulnerable (and would likely benefit more from participating).

Ask the Group. Often, simply asking members to comment is enough to get the conversation started. You can lay the groundwork by emphasizing first that the group is intended only to help—that members won't be pressured to make changes and will only change by personal choice. You can also emphasize the importance of hearing everyone's thoughts, even when they're similar to something another member has expressed. Explain that sometimes when multiple people make similar comments, themes that emerge across comments are important to discuss. Mention that people sometimes feel more comfortable sharing ideas and reactions when they get a response than when others stay quiet, even if the response is agreement or just a comment (e.g., "That makes sense"). Then, asking an evocative, open question encourages comments from the floor. Once a few members have spoken, asking "What else?" or "Who else?" is usually enough to encourage others to join in (avoid asking the closed questions "Anything else?" or

"Anyone else?" unless you are ready to finish the conversation, because it can seem more a courtesy than true interest). Reflecting themes and asking other members to share how they might think or feel similarly or differently carry the conversation forward. Asking members to talk with each other rather than directly to you also helps. If the conversation slows before you are ready to change focus, including the names of those who haven't yet participated, without singling anyone out, can elicit conversation ("Steve, Astrid, Stella, I'm curious about what any of you think").

Similarly, using your eyes to engage members can help. If a member discusses a theme or situation that you know is relevant to another member, simply glancing (but not staring) toward the other member while the first person is speaking, and perhaps again when the first person finishes, may be enough to invite the other member to speak. If you don't yet know whether particular members relate to specific situations or themes, regularly scanning the faces of other members (in a low-key, easy manner) will cue you to who is reacting and who is simply listening (while also helping keep all members engaged). In fact, we regularly look around the circle while a member is speaking, which helps keep everyone engaged and communicates nonverbally that even if one individual temporarily has the floor, this is still a group conversation.

Pairs. If open discussion is not sufficiently drawing people out, break the group into smaller groups or pairs for discussion, if that fits with your approach to group. This can be useful in larger groups, where some may feel uncomfortable or intimidated sharing about vulnerable issues, especially early on. If you do break into subgroups, make sure to give clear instructions for the pairings (e.g., pairs should share their perspective or experiences with each other for 10 minutes, making sure that both people share evenly). If you plan to elicit large group follow-up discussion that involves sharing of what group members discuss in pairs, be sure to let members know ahead of time and instruct them to clarify with their partner anything that is not to be shared with the larger group. When members are done with their breakout work, bring the group back together and elicit highlights of what was discussed, if you think there are important ideas to reflect upon and reinforce. Alternatively, you can skip the content and discuss something about the process ("What did it feel like to share with your partner?") or the effect of the exercise ("How does that leave you feeling now?"; "What did you learn or what thoughts has that triggered?"; "How do you want to take that forward as a group?") Often, breaking the group into pairs rejuvenates members and full-group discussion takes off again.

Rounds. You can also draw out members by using a *round*—going around the circle and having each person share a small amount ("Who is one person you find supportive in your life, and what does he or she do that you appreciate?"). Before you start the round, it is sometimes helpful to give people a few seconds to a minute to think about what they might want to say. If you use multiple rounds, start with a different person, go in a different direction, or both. Remember that people tend to pay greater attention and remember more about the beginning and the end of any sequence, so try not to start or end with a member who feels negatively about the issue being discussed, or who is confused about the question or the answer. An exception might occur when you are intentionally putting the person in the last spot for strategic reasons, such as cueing to focus more positively on something about which he or she typically is negative. Once the round is finished, focus attention on any themes that would be useful to explore further, or on specific members who may benefit from further exploration. If a member becomes emotional during the round, you might mention that you'd like to check in with him or her once the round is finished, allowing the member a little time to get composed and consider what he or she wants to explore. On rare occasions, you may think it is best to pause the round and explore a situation or issue with a specific member in the moment, particularly if you think it is a limited opportunity and the person will block further discussion if you first complete the round. In that case, indicate that you are pausing the round temporarily and will finish it after exploring this member's concerns (then make sure to do that).

Visual Aids. If appropriate for your group, use handouts or worksheets. You might ask members to read something and think about it; write answers to questions; complete sentences; draw a picture that represents some situation, feeling, or idea; or make a list. Allow sufficient time for most to complete it, then give notice that there is perhaps a minute left. You can follow this with any of the previous discussion approaches—pairs or small groups, rounds, or full-group open discussion.

Invite Rather Than Expect. Although it is important that members participate in group activities and interactions, some may be less talkative than others for various reasons—introversion, having a different background than most members, experiencing shame or anger about participating in the group, and so on. We suggest inviting members to participate in group interactions rather than pressuring them to do so. You can use processes, such as rounds, that communicate an expectation that each person will briefly participate in turn, or invite individual members to comment on a topic or respond to a question, but if a member hesitates, simply acknowledge that it's okay if he or she wishes to remain silent. By shaping interactions over time, so that talkative members listen more and quiet members talk more, things tend to even out. At the same time, try not to let anyone go without speaking for a whole session, unless extenuating circumstances make the member feel unable to participate but still want to be present and perhaps benefit from just being with the group. Generally, however, it becomes harder to speak if a person remains silent too long: Too many topics have gone by, there is too much pressure to say something important, and the person is no longer a part of the natural flow of interaction.

Considerations on the Quiet Group. If the group is generally quiet, consider more broadly what might be happening (or not happening) to inhibit conversation. It is not terribly uncommon in the beginning for a group to be on the quiet side while focus is being established, or while group members are sizing you up to see how you will interact with them, and as long as you do not pressure them and are reasonably friendly (without going overboard), any cultural or other differences between you and the majority of group members should not unduly limit conversation. However, if members are overly quiet for long periods, there is probably some general sense that the group is either unsafe or unlikely to be helpful.

Unlike psychotherapy process groups in which you may let silence continue in order to press members into assuming responsibility for their group experience, MI groups have a more practical focus. Generally, silence should not be left to linger, unless it is a particularly productive silence that occurs while members focus on some solo task. Outside of such moments, silence can be caused by many things, requiring different responses. Generally, a good place to start in addressing silence is to consider the group's focus in the session and attempt to counter it. If silence occurs because the topic has gotten too narrow and no one has much to say, broaden the focus. If members run out of things to say because the discussion remains at the surface, deepen the conversation by focusing on underlying themes, feelings, or values. If the focus has become too deep and members have become uncomfortable, lighten the mood.

If members are silent at the beginning of a session, you may not have provided sufficient guidance, or you may have prematurely attempted to explore a topic that members have not previously thought about (and so have little to say) or feel vulnerable about (and so do not want to put themselves at risk). Generally, slowing down or focusing first at surface level can help. Making small talk before sessions, transitioning gradually into the start of the session while attempting to sustain the informal mood, and beginning group with some warm-up discussion or exploration of efforts made since last session, or hopes for the current session, usually help to address silence at the beginning of the session.

One option is to use this as an opportunity to talk a bit with members about group processes (Faris & Brown, 2003). You might mention that the more people involved in a conversation, the longer it can take for everyone to feel "in sync," and for comfortable ways of interacting to develop. No one is sure whether he or she should speak; people forget their own ideas while listening to someone else, or they get caught up in a new topic and become focused on their own thoughts for a bit and tune out. Invite members to recall past group discussions in other settings where these things might have happened and share those with the group. Instruct members just to notice these normal processes in group discussions as they happen, and to take a chance by sharing their ideas, even if they only remember them later, after the topic had shifted elsewhere. Let them know that they don't need to worry about being off-topic or sharing something similar to what someone else has already said, that you'll make sure the group discussions stay productive, so they can just relax and join in.

Silence during the middle of the session can be caused by fear of vulnerability around a sensitive topic that is being discussed. In such moments, the silence is a message that the group is either not ready for the topic at hand or needs to approach it in a more structured way or at a more superficial level, at least to get started. Silence also occurs when a member has violated a group norm, whether explicit or implicit. Similarly, members who disclose too quickly and too transparently, members who have an aggressive edge to their communication, and members who feel hopeless all can elicit silence from other members. In such moments, it is helpful to take clear leadership of the group (decisive but not necessarily hierarchically strong leadership) and work to reduce the tension that is intimidating members. While it is sometimes useful to work individually with the person who is eliciting the reaction, often it is better to shift the focus off that person and the energy he or she is emitting. If you choose to shift focus, it is important to not do it in a way that it adds credence or power to the mood that has been elicited, as if you, too, are intimidated by it. Rather, try to draw a theme from the moment that connects all members, without isolating the person causing it or pathologizing his or her communications. It is often fairly simple to reflect about the negative emotions that can arise while attempting to make significant changes, and to invite others to share some of the feelings they experience that put their change attempts at risk. If needed, use this as a teaching moment to reflect on how people sometimes turn away from change because of discomfort in dealing with the negative feelings and thoughts involved.

Silence can occur at the end of a particularly heavy session, or when a substantial topic has been explored and members are hesitant to open something new. It is useful to have a few topics you can visit briefly (e.g., checking in on plans for making change efforts between sessions) that don't make it seem like you are just running the clock out. We generally don't end sessions early, because it can start expectations that ending early will become common.

Linking Members. Linking members is a crucial group leadership strategy. Cohesion is so central to group outcomes that you should nearly always look to increase it. There may be no better way than linking members' concerns, themes, feelings, attitudes, goals and motivation. While there are rare times when you might want to emphasize differences (e.g., to emphasize personal choice), generally you should look for connections, similarities, shared experiences, and so on, and drawing members' attention to them.

Usually, this can be done with reflections or summaries that emphasize underlying themes or feelings, going beyond individual details and highlighting connections between members. Even questions that implicitly include everyone can help build cohesion, as well as using terms such as *we, us, you* (plural), *the group,* and *everyone* whenever possible. You can also use your eyes to link members, noting connections whenever they exist (and often silently influencing members to notice them as well, especially at times when they may be paying less than full attention to another member's story). In MI groups, it is especially useful to link members' interest in change, confidence about change, and commitment to making change happen. And at times it is helpful simply to assume similarities, even when you are not yet sure whether they exist. In fact, anytime you are unsure what to do, finding a way to link members together will create a valuable moment for the group.

Guiding Member Communication. Because MI has a specific communication style, it is important to guide member interactions in such a way that they are generally consistent with the spirit of the MI approach to communication, even if not technically so at all moments. While some leaders explicitly teach group members to use OARS, it may not be necessary to go to these lengths or always be the best use of group time (though we're not arguing against it, either). However, we do think it is important to identify early on the general nature and spirit of the group, as we discuss in Chapter 9, to emphasize the idea of supporting one another without pressure, focusing on positives rather than negatives and on the many possibilities for change, and how the only rule about it is that all members must decide for themselves what to change, if anything. Beyond that, we generally focus on guiding members during specific interactions to express their experiences and perspectives on their own situations, and to avoid advice giving or claims of having "the" answer regarding any specific matter.

Downey and Johnson (Chapter 13, p. 259) suggest that you "invite members to use 'I statements' (e.g., 'I think,' 'I feel,' 'I prefer') when expressing their views," allowing them to speak their minds without having to justify or defend their beliefs. Other collaborators give additional suggestions about how to manage challenging interactions within the group. While all of these ideas are important, perhaps the most important thing you can do to facilitate good member communications is to model them consistently yourself, especially when opening the session or managing difficult situations, because these are times when it is easy to be too didactic or controlling.

Holding Focus

The effectiveness of MI groups depends on maintaining a focus on moving toward implementing change, and this may make them different from other approaches to group treatment. MI groups are not centered around members becoming more assertive, increasing their interpersonal sensitivity, or expressing their emotions (although all of these things can be valuable). Similarly, MI groups are not about members learning to find self-direction by taking responsibility for structuring group sessions themselves in ways that they find most useful. MI groups are client-centered, in that the focus is on members developing greater ownership of life choices and behavior patterns. However, although you should respectfully involve members as you conduct the group, it is your responsibility to manage the group process and conversational focus, so that members proceed through the broad steps of engaging, exploring and broadening perspectives, and moving into action. Moving through these steps involves exploration of the various topics involved (exploring strengths, past successes, etc.), which requires carefully monitoring and guiding the group's focus. There is value in guiding the group to deepen and broaden the focus (and so on), as described later in this chapter. Even in unstructured MI groups, however, it is important to keep the group on task, which rarely happens spontaneously, because group conversations tend to diverge onto different topics in the absence of guidance.

Generally, your own internal cues can alert you when the group is veering off focus. However, focus is looser in groups than in individual counseling, and it is more important to be able to refocus the group as needed than to prevent the group from going off-focus. Our experience with groups is that there are almost always divergences and asides as people react to one another's thoughts and stories. This is okay, and it often builds cohesion. It is important to not react with anxiety or frustration, or to come across as scolding the group about divergences (and if you do fall into this trap, be prepared to return to the work of eliciting discussion from a fairly silent or flat group). Instead, keep your sense of ease and good humor, and steer the group back to a productive conversation, ideally finding some way to link the preferred focus to the current focus.

Being on focus doesn't necessarily mean maintaining a consistent session topic. Instead, it is about remaining on a productive path toward change. Sometimes, despite your best laid plans for a topic of conversation, the group's energy is elsewhere. It can be more productive to follow that energy and make something useful of the group's momentary interests than to attempt to keep the group focused on a specific topic that members clearly are not interested in discussing. Know the MI model well, and if the group diverges and isn't responding to attempts to focus on a specific topic, work to relate the group's current interests to some other aspect of change— such as importance, confidence, readiness, envisioning, resolve, planning, or ambivalence—or to important aspects of group development—such as openness, cohesiveness, support, universality, or altruism. There are many right paths and many ways to make a productive moment out of a seeming divergence. Sometimes the group needs something other than the planned MI focus, and the best you can do is ride out the divergence as productively as possible and refocus the group on the topic you'd planned later in the session or the next time you meet.

Sometimes it is useful to hold the focus on a specific member who is discovering something new, exposing a well-guarded vulnerability, or reflecting on something he or she has avoided, even if the topic is not consistent with what you have been discussing. This is especially important if the member has been fairly quiet, superficial, or has focused more on others than on him- or herself.

Patience is also important to good group leadership. Sometimes what at first seems like a divergence becomes an unexpected deepening or broadening of focus. However, when you recognize that the group is steering toward something not only unexpected but also irrelevant or unproductive, it is important to act quickly and confidently. The longer you wait, the harder it is to bring the group back. You have many options. You can simply steer the group back with a bit of direct guidance, or offer to come back to the new topic later in exchange for the group's return to its focus on the planned topic. You can remind the group of the importance of focusing on a single topic rather than multiple topics or conversations occurring simultaneously. You can work for a time with a particular person and more directly explore the focus with that person before returning to group conversation. You can introduce a new process—change from unstructured conversation to pairs, small groups, rounds, activities, exercises, or group brainstorming. Get people on their feet temporarily. Part of the drift in group conversations can result from boredom, and changing some aspect of the focus—topic, person, or process—usually helps restore energy.

Changing Focus

While it is important to maintain the group's focus on productive topics, processes, or themes that achieve the goals of the group, at times it is important to change course. For example, you may notice that you've become so focused on one member that the rest of the group has drifted, or a member keeps on talking, without moving toward a conclusion. Sometimes, when a conversation is going around in circles, it is important to move on to a new focus to keep the group moving forward. At other times, one member may become critical of another; perhaps some hot button has been pushed by something said, or the critical member thinks it is in the other member's best interest to be challenged or confronted. In all of these cases, if you don't change focus, then your group may lose momentum and begin to fray.

Given the desire to be helpful, it may run against your natural tendencies to step in when needed. However, when the leader doesn't interrupt to stop negative processes, the group can become dull or toxic. While dull groups are not necessarily harmful, they are less likely to promote exploration and change. MI groups rely on inspiring people to look harder, consider more carefully, and overcome the challenges facing them by becoming more proactive and living with confidence and courage. Dull groups do not inspire such efforts. Energy and momentum build upon themselves, and groups generally either move toward stronger, more focused energy and greater momentum or trudge along and fade to the point that they fail. When a group dies prematurely, it is not necessarily due to outright conflict but often results from lagging energy due to the loss of critical elements such as group identification, cohesion, perceived task interdependence, instillation of hope, altruism, and so on. Some groups die because the leaders allow negative interactions to go unchecked and unrepaired, until it is too late, and the group environment becomes toxic and unsafe, and members no longer see it as a likely source of help in their lives. Groups are organic creatures that require more than starting and ending on time, and going through a scheduled set of topics to keep them alive. Thus, whatever hesitations you may have about the social discomfort of taking direct charge of interactions, we think that to be a good group leader you must sometimes interrupt members and redirect their energies and focus.

Individual MI strategies include a basic (but crucial) one called *shifting focus*. The general lesson is that when clients become more resistant as a conversation continues, it is a signal that the interaction is going in an unhelpful direction and you need to shift focus. While it is great to harness the energy of the resistance and turn it in a more productive direction, this is not always possible. Often, a simple shift in focus prevents further escalation of resistance.

Although we don't focus much on discord or resistance in this book, the basic idea is the same with groups: When things start to turn bad, do something different. It is not helpful to continue down a path that is not working. While it is possible that the group may reach a point of crisis that then resolves itself into a higher level of group functioning, it is equally likely that conflict breeds further conflict, defensiveness, distrust, closes off possibilities. Because MI groups are not intended to be psychodynamic process groups that allow group conflict to develop so that members can learn from it, once conflicts develop, the goal is to diminish them and return to a more positive atmosphere.

Changing the focus of an unraveling group requires quick, confident action. Sometimes, even stopping to explain yourself in the moment can weaken your attempt to change focus, and it is better simply to shift gears and stop the negative interaction, before it does harm. It may help to think of it as redirecting the group rather than interrupting an individual. You can always revisit and process the redirection later.

In Chapter 9, we review situations in which group momentum is highly negative or the group is being hijacked by a few members' negative interactions or problems. In these instances, shifting focus or changing direction is often quite overt and clearly in response to a negative event. However, when the level of urgency is lower, you can use the advanced conversational shaping techniques to which we now turn—shaping momentum, shaping breadth and depth of discussion, and shifting the group's focus in more subtle, gradual, seamless ways.

Advanced Conversational Shaping

Momentum: Accelerating or Decelerating Focus

The first advanced conversational strategy involves shaping group discussions to move the story line forward or to slow down and explore the current focus. Table 8.2 summarizes when and how to accelerate or decelerate the momentum of group conversations.

Accelerating

Sometimes members explore histories and current situational details longer than is needed to establish a basis for moving toward change. It is useful to know enough details of members' situations to be able help when they get stuck moving forward, but beyond that, explore details only for specific purposes (e.g., engaging members, establishing a focus, slowing the group down). Members place importance on the things on which leaders spend time. A focus on exploring histories, interpersonal conflicts, and negatives about change underscores their importance to members. It also deprives the group of time to envision a better future and move toward it, especially

TABLE 8.2. Advanced Conversational Shaping Strategies: Momentum

Aims	When is this most appropriate?	What conversational methods?
Accelerating	• After initial exploration of perspectives • When members focus on the past or "stop short" of tying ideas/values to choices or behaviors	• Open questions about change • "Continuing the paragraph" reflections • Affirmations • Group brainstorming of change possibilities
Decelerating	• When members skip or race through difficult issues • When members seem to have overconfidence about a complex, risky change	• Suggesting slowing down • Exploring a related secondary theme • Incorporating a written exercise or working in pairs or small groups • Using linking reflections • Exploring potential obstacles to change and backup plans

when unearthing situational details for every member threatens to take the entire time available.

The focus in MI groups may be unfamiliar to members, but over time, groups generally settle more into the habit of focusing forward than looking back. Waiting for people naturally to stop reviewing details and begin to consider options for change can be a long process, especially when people get stuck in conversational "loops." Accelerating involves guiding the group toward change rather than continuing to explore problems or delve into the past. So when members focus on the past or on current details to the point of becoming unproductive, or "stop short" of tying ideas/values to choices or behaviors, it is a good time to consider accelerating the conversation.

As with other conversational shaping strategies, you can address this directly by asking members how things might be better in their lives, what options they might have, and what would help them let go of their negative emotional reaction to what is bothering them or wrap up "unfinished business" that is an obstacle to moving forward. Another method is *continuing the paragraph reflections,* in which you guess the next thing members might say if they were moving toward change, and express that as a reflection of something as yet unspoken in the current conversation (note that this is not a way to "sneak in" advice giving without first gaining permission).

MEMBER: It's just so hard getting started exercising again.

LEADER: And so that's where these little rewards you mentioned come in handy to get through those first few weeks.

MEMBER: He just never really seems to hear what I'm trying to tell him about not drinking in front of me, even though I've told him a million times (*sigh*).

LEADER: So you've been reminding him as clearly as you can, then letting it go and focusing on taking care of yourself, even if it means getting out of there for a while. And so far that seems to be working.

Another way to help when members get stuck in conversational loops is to use affirmations to underscore members' strengths to change things that bother them.

MEMBER 1: It's like they're determined to get you down.

MEMBER 2: They don't really want you to change. They just like being in charge.

LEADER: And you both seem determined to do what you think is right for you, no matter how anyone else might try to stand in your way.

Another way to accelerate the conversation is to use the group to brainstorm a menu of options (i.e., several ways a member might move forward). Rather than provide advice, ask the member whether he or she would like the group to help brainstorm possibilities. Don't go forward if the member says no, but assuming that the member says yes, ask him or her to frame what input the group should provide. Be clear with everyone that the idea is first to generate a number of possibilities, then have the member react, to see whether anything he or she wants to try or think about comes up. After a few possibilities are generated, stop and ask the member to reflect upon them. If this is the first time you've done this, you might set it up so that rather than reflect on options he or she doesn't like or isn't ready for, or justify any reactions, the member simply comments on the options he or she likes most or wants to think more about. Repeat the process until the member has a few possibilities to consider further, or one definite path that he or she would like to pursue. Thank the group when the process is done.

Decelerating

There are times when instead of moving forward, you may want members to slow things down to consider more detail or choose more carefully. This can happen when groups move too quickly to strategies for change, before members have developed enough cohesion to trust one another with their more vulnerable perceptions or experiences, or have even explored options. Sometimes members race past considering issues, experiences, or possibilities that have some discomfort associated with them. This can also occur when a member seems to be overconfident about a change that seems unlikely to be as simple as he or she thinks, especially when there is substantial risk in the attempt. While it is not consistent with MI to try to pressure someone, there is a difference between pressuring and simply inviting him or her to slow down and open up, then moving on if the member doesn't respond.

If group members are racing past important topics or elements, it can be helpful to slow the forward momentum. As always, you can simply suggest that they slow down and stay on the current issue, perhaps noting explicitly that this is important. It can help to introduce a new wrinkle related to the topic to help group members consider things in a new way. If the group members seem to not trust one another enough to address a particular issue, one strategy is to put that issue on the shelf for later. Leaving it behind to focus on issues about which members feel less vulnerable allows them to build connections, trust, and cohesion. If this is not practical, you might approach the current topic in a less threatening way, by dividing into small groups or pairs, using a structured worksheet approach, or stepping out of the discussion temporarily to focus on metacommunication. *Metacommunication* involves focusing on the current processes or dynamics of group interaction and exploring how members perceive the group environment, how they feel in the room, and brainstorming ways to help them feel more comfortable and trusting. Sometimes group members have specific ideas about making the atmosphere more comfortable. Other times, it is enough simply to open the door, to show that it is not taboo to discuss their experience in the group.

If it is simply one member jumping over important issues, one way to decelerate is to use a linking reflection, one that relates the current conversation to a previous one, and invite the member to consider the connection between the two. This not only helps the member stay on topic but it allows him or her to do so without diverting attention from the content being explored.

The issue of overconfidence is a bit trickier. Generally, in MI, you avoid taking a stance that opposes the client's perspective. In judging that a person's confidence is falsely high, you stand outside and above the person. Similarly, you wouldn't want to risk potentially undermining a bold new and healthy stance, since it is impossible to know for sure whether the person's confidence is truly too high, or whether you are simply underestimating him or her. At the same time, as professionals in a position of some experience and knowledge, we don't want to contribute to clients attempting to take steps so large that they are likely to be unsuccessful. While there is no special harm in being unsuccessful at a change attempt when a person is fairly humble about the likelihood of immediate success, it can sometimes be devastating when the person has been overconfident.

Addressing this issue is nearly always a bit sensitive, and more so in a room full of peers. You don't want to approach it in a way that leaves the member feeling shamed, insulted, or challenged to prove him- or herself at any cost. And if you approach it in a way that the group perceives as embarrassing the member, even if the member doesn't see it that way, the group will retreat to a more superficial level. One way of approaching this situation is to accept the member's own perspective on the relative ease of change, and explore potential obstacles and backup plans exactly as you would with a plan that might seem more realistic. Another is to affirm the member's determination to change, and see whether he or she would like to hear other members' experiences with such a change, what went well, what they found more challenging than expected, and how they overcame those challenges. Remember that your goal is not to warn the person off an attempt to change—that, of course, is the purpose of the group in the first place—but to cushion the fall and soften any blows to ego, emotions, or perceived social status should the plan not work. You can invite the person to share in the next session how things are going and any observations or unforeseen challenges that might be helpful information to other members. The purpose is simply to provide a reset and reformulation of plans if things don't work out the first time.

Breadth: Broadening or Narrowing Focus

The second advanced shaping task is to broaden or narrow the conversational focus in order to make it more productive, as summarized in Table 8.3.

Broadening

Broadening is used when group members are too focused on details or are overwhelmed by numerous, seemingly unrelated problems. With broadening, you link behaviors or situations to establish a theme that extends across them. When this is effective, members broaden their perspective so that they make one broad change that encompasses several smaller elements, allowing them to be more planful about change and reducing their stress.

Imagine that a client has a list of things she wants to change—eat less junk food, get back to swimming, take a yoga class, be less stressed, and get more sleep. She is demoralized after several rounds over the last year of making good progress toward these goals, then "falling off the

TABLE 8.3. Advanced Conversational Shaping Strategies: Breadth

Aims	When is this most appropriate?	What conversational methods?
Broadening	• When members are too focused on details or have limited perspectives	• Linking summaries • Open questions • Double-sided reflections • Imagery or analogy reflections • Elicit–provide–elicit sequence
Narrowing	• When focusing on one aspect of a multifaceted issue will help promote progress toward change • When members speak vaguely, or talk about principles or values, without tying them to change	• Closed questions • Selective reflection

wagon." When this happens, she becomes anxious and depressed, and enters a period of binge eating, drinking wine to excess and staying up too late and missing sleep, leaving her more frustrated and less motivated. She says, "When I am on top of things, everything is in sync but then something happens—a work deadline or relationship problem or whatever—and it all comes crashing down. Then I get depressed and just say 'screw it' and I give up, become lazy again, and just go back to eating and drinking and watching TV all the time."

While addressing each of the situations separately and making individual plans for them can be valuable, there is a clear benefit to developing a connecting theme—healthier living—because if she decides to pursue this broader goal, each of these specific changes will become part of a larger whole and can be approached in a more unified manner, likely increasing her ability to maintain the changes. Instead of trying to do it all at once, and thinking of herself as "bad" or a failure when her life can't accommodate so many habit changes at one time, she can continue to work toward her general goal of healthier living by sustaining any one of these changes until it is a well-established habit, at which time she can add another specific habit change that allows her to continue to progress toward her more general change goal. She may come to believe that, even if it feels uplifting for a while, it is not actually healthy living to try to change too many things at once, only to fail, become disillusioned, berate herself and fall back into an entrenched unhealthy lifestyle. Healthier living may involve making incremental changes while gradually adjusting her lifestyle to accommodate those and consistently building toward greater overall health over the course of months or even years.

Some changes are more complex than this, and the connecting theme is not always so obvious, but the goal of broadening focus is to find more general patterns to approach as a unit, so that the person may think of it as making one general life change rather than multiple separate changes. Even when the person may benefit from breaking it down and approaching individual elements as separate changes, the presence of a broader theme that links the elements together can make changing easier, because the person is more likely to spot specific, smaller patterns that exemplify a larger theme, and borrow from the motivation for broad change to fortify his or her efforts on specific discrete elements.

Broadening is also useful in another common situation. Members often have been referred for some specific reason or perceived problem that may not be of interest to them. This presents a challenge when using a client-centered approach that is intended to focus on things of interest to the clients themselves. While there are various ways to approach this situation, one of the best is broadening in such a way that the focus includes both the client's interests and those of the referral source, whether this be the court, an employer, or a family member. For example, the court may refer a member who is mandated to abstinence. That member may not be interested in abstinence, and may be angry about the mandate. The court and the client are at odds with one another, and you may feel that you are being forced to choose which side you're on. If you side with the court, you are directly opposing the client and inviting resistance. If you side with the client, you are encouraging him or her to further a battle that he or she is not likely to win, and "winning" such a battle is often not in the client's best interests anyway. Broadening focus, trying to find a goal that meets the interests of both the client and the court, is one way to resolve such a dilemma. It may involve helping the client identify ways life could be better, such as improving career opportunities by going back to school or taking on a personal growth challenge, such as developing a new skill or interest area, and exploring how to make improvements. In pursuing broader goals, often the initial conflict becomes not worth the fight to the client if fighting gets in the way of pursuing the new goals. If the initial problematic behavior is at odds with the new goals, then the situation is even better. When a habit is seen as an obstacle to a goal in which a client is invested, the client often gives it up, without much direct focus on it at all. In any case, by broadening the focus, the initial investment in fighting against external control is usually lessened, and the client is less likely to continue the battle.

Broadening focus is most directly accomplished through open questions, since that is what such questions do naturally: "How does this fit into the bigger picture?"; "How does this relate to other things you are trying to achieve?" One way is to ask the person an open question that links two separate, defined issues: "How are eating too much junk food and staying up too late related?"; "What connection might there be between your sister always coming to you to borrow money and your coworkers giving you more than your share of the grunt work?"

Another broadening possibility is to use a *linking summary*. If you notice a connecting theme or pattern between an issue a member is currently exploring and a previous conversation you've had, you can offer a summary that links elements from both conversations for the member to consider. If you can tie this kind of content-oriented linking summary to an interpersonal linking reflection that ties together multiple members of the group, you may not only broaden the discussion beyond a specific content focus but also broaden the focus from a single individual to a shared theme across members.

In an HIV support group, for example, you might offer:

> "Cory, you mentioned how you keep meaning to tell your doctor about the increasing fatigue and nausea you've been experiencing lately. You said it's on your mind when you go to your appointments and you plan to talk with her, but then other things come up and you decide it's not that important to mention. And a few weeks ago you talked about sometimes skipping your medication because you just get tired of always having to think about having the infection. And Angelos, you mentioned how you like our group sessions but sometimes dread thinking about coming until you get here and remember how you like the group having your back. It seems like one of the ways to cope is to keep HIV out of mind, which seems better than always dwelling on it, but keeping it off your mind takes some energy, too, and might have some downsides. What do you think?"

Double-sided reflections also work well to broaden the focus. The nature of ambivalence is that people often go back and forth between two sides of a dilemma. Often people become frozen in indecision, and other times they engage in two very different patterns in alternating fashion, unable to stick with either for long. A smoker, for example, may think for months or years about quitting, yet never quite get to it, despite wanting to, at least in part. Another smoker may quit cold turkey, maintaining a smoke-free pattern for a while, until a new life stressor becomes too much, then return to smoking as a coping mechanism that ends up outlasting the new stressor to become a habit again, until the process begins all over again. While double-sided reflections do not magically resolve the ambivalence about the issue, they can help open a door to integrating the thoughts, feelings, temptations, and frustrations of both directions (or valences) and help the person explore solutions that may offer both the health benefits that come from not smoking and the stress reduction (and other benefits) that smoking provides, in such a way that eventually the balance is tipped in a more stable and lasting way. Double-sided reflections can sometimes kick off this process, along the lines of "You like a lot about the way it feels when you're not smoking, and at the same time smoking really relaxes you and helps you get through some of the rough times."

Reflections and affirmations that include imagery or analogies can also broaden focus.

- "It seems like you're juggling seven balls at once."
- "It's like whack-a-mole, just when you get one problem knocked down, another one pops up somewhere else."
- "You're like a cat, always landing on your feet."

An advantage is that these methods can refocus members—from talking about problems to talking about what they do to manage problems. For some, this can be a perceptual shift, from seeing themselves as passive victims of problems to seeing themselves as people who actively manage problems. Such shifts in perception can pay enormous dividends.

One other broadening strategy is the *elicit–provide–elicit* approach to information exchange, which can help members incorporate new information into thinking about their own perspectives and plans. This is described in more detail in Chapter 11.

Narrowing

Although some conversations begin too narrowly focused, others start at the opposite end of the spectrum: Members are clearly unhappy but have only a vague sense of what they might like to change. When asked what they might like to be different, they may answer, "Everything." Pressed a little, they may say, "I want to be happier" or "I want to stop wasting my life." Others might be somewhat more specific but still broad enough that it is difficult to link their concerns or interests to specific actions they might take: "I want to feel like I'm more in control" or "I want to procrastinate less." The strategy of *narrowing* involves shaping conversations from general, broad themes about how life could be better toward more well-defined interests and targets for change.

Narrowing is also useful with some cognitive or psychological difficulties that clients may have. People with chronic psychological disorders sometimes lose the connection between action and consequence. People with anxiety may not be aware of how avoiding anxiety-provoking situations heightens their anxiety over time by reinforcing their fears. People with chronic depression may be unaware how their pessimistic style and depressed mood may keep others at a distance, thus perpetuating their feelings of loneliness and isolation. It can be quite difficult in individual treatment to help these clients narrow their focus toward implementing changes that can affect their lives more broadly. Ideas that sound good in session lose their relevance or urgency back in everyday life, where the person's emotional reactions and interpersonal habits may automatically resume their position of priority. These issues can be addressed more directly during group sessions, because others are affected by the patterns as they occur in session, and they can be explored *in vivo* and developed into goals for change. MI groups are not interpersonal process groups that focus mostly on ingroup interactions. Still, there are still plenty of opportunities to help members discover problematic patterns and work with other members to resolve them in MI groups, which is not always possible in individual MI.

Incorporating the strategy of narrowing allows clients' interests to emerge over time. Members don't need to begin groups with specific change goals in mind, and they are not pressured to identify goals just for the sake of identifying them. As leader, you don't need to have a very specific goal in order to focus on a general direction of positive change. Having members brainstorm various ways their lives could be better is energizing, and often results in more impactful change goals than those that clients initially conceive early in process of group development. Direction is already built into MI strategies, and you can meet clients wherever they are along a pathway to change and help them take steps forward from there. Narrowing occurs naturally as you help group members define what *better* means to them, begin to figure out ways to make things better, and move toward action.

Asking clients to be more specific in their focus, to sort out what they think they should change, what they are willing to do and to give up to make it happen, and how they want to start, are all examples of narrowing. Although MI does not encourage heavy use of closed questions, they are not taboo, and they can help narrow focus at times as well. In addition, selectively reflecting aspects of client statements that narrow the focus toward specific change can help members discover goals and plans that direct questioning sometimes cannot. Like broadening, narrowing is a kind of discovery process.

Depth: Deepening or Lightening Focus

In addition to the scope of conversation (how broad or narrow), conversations can be focused at the surface of an issue or delve deeper into underlying emotions, values, or themes. Table 8.4 summarizes when it is

TABLE 8.4. Advanced Conversational Shaping Strategies: Depth

Aims	When is this most appropriate?	What conversational methods?
Deepening	• When members are ready to share more vulnerable issues • When members are too focused on surface details, intellectualizing, or are stuck in unresolvable ambivalence	• Reflections of emotions, values • Affirmations
Lightening	• When closing sessions or ending the group • When mood becomes too intense or heavy, or when conflict emerges	• Closing summary • Shifting focus • Linking reflections • Using humor

appropriate to deepen or lighten the focus, and the most common conversational methods to do so.

Deepening

MI generally has a somewhat practical focus on setting and achieving goals once ambivalence is on its way to resolution. However, that practical focus does not prevent helping clients hone their goals to be as meaningful as possible. Look for ways to safely deepen the focus once members have developed some trust in one another. Beyond making discrete behavior changes, MI groups can be powerful tools for changing people's lives, and sometimes a single pattern change at a deeper level can encompass many surface-level specific behavior changes (e.g., deciding to be more honest with significant others can change the frequency of lying, arguing, avoiding, and even motivate clients to not do things they would later have to hide from their loved ones). Deepening the focus can increase cohesion and trust as members become ready to address more vulnerable issues together. Deepening is also useful when you become aware that members are too focused on surface details, are intellectualizing, or are stuck in ambivalence.

As an example, it is good when clients with addiction problems set goals to abstain from using and to attend peer support groups. These are certainly valuable goals when substance use becomes dysfunctional and takes over clients' lives. As many who have overcome addictions indicate, however, achieving abstinence is often not all there is to making such a change. Many who successfully change from having substance use at the center of their lives to having it play a negligible role undergo deeper change. They develop increased awareness of their emotions and incorporate them more functionally in their lives, becoming more open and honest, and developing stronger purpose and commitment in life. These deeper changes often come to be defining aspects of such all-encompassing change.

While considered spiritual by some, that frame is not required for the process of becoming more grounded in one's own skin, more open, more trusting, and flexible. Rogers promoted the role of deepening in both individual and group person-centered work, and it fits nicely within MI groups, helping to increase the value of the group in members' lives regardless of the problem set or change goal on which they may be focusing. Finding opportunities to reflect emotions, values, purpose, and commitment all deepen the MI group experience. Linking members together by their deeper levels of commitment and purpose heightens awareness of how their values influence behavior choices, and helps to develop the group's sense of community.

Reflecting emotions, values, purpose, and commitment deepens the MI group experience.

Affirmations contribute to deepening when they highlight a core value underlying members' actions (e.g., altruism), particularly when those actions take place in the group session itself. Affirming positive acts highlights opportunities for members to grow through their group participation, and often increases group cohesion. The experience of helping another person in some meaningful way can be profoundly deepening. Look for these opportunities, especially as the group members travel through experiences together. Of course, do so only in a gradual and genuine way: MI groups are not meant to be like encounter groups, where immediate, explicit, intense striving for genuineness and transparency can make the whole thing somewhat artificial and sometimes abusive. Going into deeper aspects of people's personal lives is a privilege that develops over time as trust is earned.

Lightening

The complementary strategy to deepening involves lightening the mood, tone, or intensity of discussion. The purpose is to bring people back to a surface level, which is particularly important when you sense that things have gone deep too quickly for members to handle, or when time is running short toward the end of a session. Some issues that can be explored in group leave members powerfully transformed, such as transcending the consequences of past abuse. However, these require not only advanced skills on your part but also readiness on the part of individual members, a deep trust and openness among group members as a whole, and sufficient time. Without all of these elements, it is important to prevent exploration from going too deep, or allowing a member to reveal too much to the group, only to regret it later and feel that the group no longer feels like a safe place. Even when it is meaningful to work at a deeper level, it is our responsibility as leaders not to allow clients to be overly exposed and vulnerable when they leave the session. Until a group is working regularly at deep levels, take special care to return the focus to more surface-level discussion and lighter topics well before group sessions end. While deep and intense explorations can be compelling, especially when members indicate they've never talked about an experience or issue before, it is crucial never to leave such a conversation hanging because time ran out. Always leave plenty of time to return to a surface-level focus before ending group sessions, even if you have to redirect a group member as he or she starts a topic.

You can lighten by acknowledging that things may be getting too deep, without enough familiarity, trust, or time to support deeper work, and steer the group toward safer topics, while acknowledging the value of deeper exploration at a better time. Affirm members' willingness and courage to go into deeper and more vulnerable issues, and the trust that group members are developing. You can explicitly link the deeper aspects with the more everyday, surface elements involved in members' change, so that the transition feels natural. If appropriate, some lighthearted and uplifting humor can help you ease the group out of the moment (just be sensitive, as this is not a time for cynical or hardened humor). You can gradually return the group to a surface level using selective reflections that focus on more surface or action-oriented details of clients' issues, without commenting on your intention. Members will naturally follow your focus back to the surface.

Comparing Advanced Conversational Shaping Strategies

In MI groups, one of the primary strategies is managing the focus so that group conversations involve all members (and their perspectives), while remaining productive. There are various ways of managing conversational focus to achieve these goals and also shape the momentum, breadth, and depth of discussion. While these are abstract concepts and advanced skills, we think they are critical to incorporate as you continue your practice. To help you incorporate these skills into your practice, we offer Table 8.5, in which practitioner responses that attempt to shape the conversation in the ways we mention are followed by client reactions.

TABLE 8.5. Comparing Advanced Conversational Shaping Strategies

Aims	Practitioner	Client
(Initial client statement)		"Everyone keeps telling me to get my act together, more or less. And I keep thinking, you don't think I want to get better? You think I want to die?"
Accelerating	"Let's just focus on that, then. What are you already doing? What else have you thought about trying?"	"I quit smoking! That's a big deal! I'm trying to eat better and exercise more, but not doing as well on those."
Decelerating	"You seem to feel pressured, and like that only makes things worse. I don't want to do that to you, so let's just take it slow. Getting it right over the long run may be better than rushing into things just to be doing something."	"People keep acting like I'm lazy or not willing to put effort into it. But I quit smoking and have been trying to eat better and exercise more, it just isn't as easy as everyone acts like. It's like I really want to, but then I just kind of forget about it after a while."
Broadening	"It sounds like it's even more than just wanting to get past being sick, it sounds like you want to be healthier overall, happier, less stressed. You don't want to just keep your head above water, you want to really enjoy swimming."	"Right. I'm so sick of being sick. And always having to think and talk about it. I don't want to just stay out of the hospital, I want a better life. Maybe a less demanding job doing more what I want to do. Maybe relax more, spend more time with friends. Not just survive, but actually live."
Narrowing	"It sounds like this is very important to you and you're ready to focus on something specific instead of talking about it in general."	"Yes. It doesn't help to just keep hearing how I need to lose weight and have less stress. I've tried a couple diets. I've tried deep breathing. It hasn't really helped."
Deepening	"Right. You want to grow old with your wife and be a part of your granddaughter's life as she grows up."	"More than anything. I just am so afraid that I worry all the time, and it makes me want to eat, it makes me want to smoke. I can't get it off my mind and it's just making me sicker."

(continued)

TABLE 8.5. (*continued*)

Aims	Practitioner	Client
Lightening	"Whoa, back off people! (*Smiles.*) Hmm ... I guess I'm wondering what you can do so you don't get dragged down by all this. How you can let go of their comments so you can keep working on your plan this week."	"Oh, trust me, I've thought of a few things I could do to really get them off my back! (*Laughs.*) But seriously, what bothers me the most is when other people doubt me. It makes me doubt myself. So maybe if I just focus on doing what I can do and ignore them, it'll keep me on track and maybe even my wife will see that and not worry so much herself."
Changing focus	"It sounds like there is a lot for us to talk about. I appreciate you sharing what this is like for you, and I don't doubt you. Since we only have a little time right now, I wonder if we could come back to this when we can explore how this has you frustrated, and how we can all help you put this behind you."	"That would be great. I didn't mean to unload you on right now as I know this is just a check-in, but I'm really overwhelmed and just had to say something. If we could plan another time, maybe I could think a little more about why I feel so stuck and frustrated, and then we could figure out what to do."

Closing the Conversation

At some point, when session time is running out, when there are other tasks to do, or when a topic has run its course, it is time to close the discussion. Goals include summarizing key points of the conversation or exercise, clarifying whether the topic is completed or to be continued at a later time, and helping members transition out of the topic, activity, or session. If you need to close due to a time issue and sense that there is still energy that will distract members as they move to the next task or transition out of the session and back to their lives, you can address this in a number of ways. One way is to do a round with a key question or instruction, such as "Share what you got from this conversation, and whether you think it is now settled for you or if you will continue to think or work on it." Alternatively, ask the group members to develop together a summary of key points as a collaborative task. If several members are unsettled, ask whether this topic should be reopened the next session, before moving on to a new focus. Otherwise, wrap up the session with an acknowledgment that this is one more piece in the puzzle or one more step on the road to change, and thank members for their participation and support of one another.

There may be times when you prefer not to summarize, such as when members should consider issues further after leaving the session. Generally, though, summarizing in some way helps members to solidify a perspective or understanding of the issue covered, so they can more easily switch back into daily life, without forgetting the interaction.

References

Barlow, S. H., Burlingame, G. M., Harding, J. A., & Behrman, J. (1997). Therapeutic focusing in time-limited group psychotherapy. *Group Dynamics: Theory, Research, and Practice, 1,* 254–266.

Faris, A. S., & Brown, J. M. (2003). Addressing group dynamics in a brief motivational intervention for college student drinkers. *Journal of Drug Education, 33,* 289–306.

CHAPTER 9

Phase I

Engaging the Group

Our conceptualization of MI groups involves members working together as a group to make positive changes in their lives. It lies between approaches that focus heavily on group processes and those that focus on individuals. At one end of a continuum of group styles, the interpersonal process approach uses group interactions to draw out interpersonal patterns and perceptions that members developed through early experiences with significant others. These patterns and perceptions are then corrected in the here and now by examining the dynamics in the group and working to change how members approach and perceive others. At the other end is an approach in which leaders conduct sequential individual mini-sessions, while the other group members silently witness the interaction and provide summary feedback afterward. We advocate an approach in the middle that interweaves a focus on exploring individual issues with a focus on generalizing issues by linking them with others' concerns, then exploring those together. While our approach does not focus explicitly on group dynamics, we do use the group to provide support for change.

In this chapter, we focus on facilitating group development and managing challenges so that groups reach their optimal effectiveness. We discuss the advantages of having co-leaders in MI groups. We focus on general strategies for structuring sessions, then on preparing for and conducting the first MI group session, which is typically sufficient to engage the group.

Facilitating Group Development

MI was developed as an individual counseling approach. A crucial difference in MI groups is that we do not have as much time to explore each

149

person's individual situation in depth. Another difference is that while exploring a person's situation in depth can be quite engaging in individual counseling, it can deaden groups. Some early practitioners conducted group sessions as a series of individual mini-sessions, with other participants observing. The bulk of group research since that time has identified engagement in group process, group cohesiveness, and mutual task involvement as key contributors to group success. This accumulated wisdom points group leaders away from conducting one-on-one interventions within group sessions and toward promoting therapeutic interactions among members. In essence, it moves away from interviewing individuals and toward facilitating group interactions.

Figures 9.1 to 9.5 show the difference between dyadic interactions with witnesses and group interactions (figures are adopted from Farrall, 2007). Figure 9.1 shows a group leader working with a small group of five members. In this sequence of interactions, the leader communicates one-on-one with the various group members, interacting with each individually. As shown in Figure 9.1, such an approach makes it in essence a leader-centered group, with members relating only to the leader, who then by necessity has more speaking turns than group members. This leaves members somewhat isolated even in one another's presence.

Because much of the power of groups comes from members interacting and working together, it is important to link members together by similarities in experiences, challenges or attitudes about change, and so on. As members internalize the linkages, they begin to interact as a working group rather than coexisting as separate individuals in a room with a leader. The following figures show what begins to happen when the leader works to link two members who have raised individual issues. In Figure 9.2, the leader suggests/reflects a similarity between their interests, concerns, or

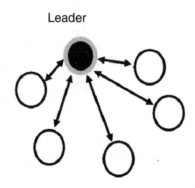

FIGURE 9.1. Leader-centered group.

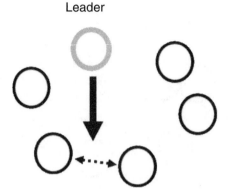

FIGURE 9.2. Linking two members.

motivation to change, facilitating a linkage between the two (e.g., "Even though you're focusing on different issues, you both are working to be more assertive with others about your needs").

As the leader highlights similarities, the two members begin to interact with each other, prompting two other members to join in. The leader reinforces this involvement with further linking reflections, affirmations, or questions directed to the group as a whole, as shown in Figure 9.3.

After the fifth member remains uninvolved for a period, the leader reaches out, maintaining a connection even if the member otherwise remains disengaged during this particular discussion (Figure 9.4).

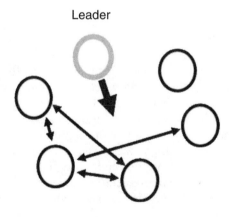

FIGURE 9.3. Connecting to the group as a whole.

Leader

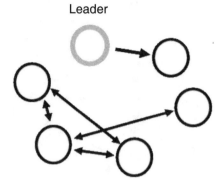

FIGURE 9.4. Connecting with an isolated member.

Over time, the goal is for the group to sustain itself without constant leader involvement, demonstrating a high level of group involvement and cohesion. Members interact with all or nearly all of the other members. While the leader still has periods of interacting directly with individual members, many comments are directed to the group as a whole. As we are developing a group, we often envision this web of connections being woven, as depicted in Figure 9.5. Once a strong web of ongoing connections exists, we have facilitated the development of a powerful working group and can shift our focus toward deeper aspects of group functioning.

Our goal is for the group to sustain itself without constant leader involvement.

It isn't necessary for every member to speak to every other member. Rather, the point is to try to develop links and interactions between members to maximize the power and efficiency of the group. Not only do cohesive groups work together better, but they also reduce the need for each individual member to discuss all of the details about his or her concerns, challenges, and motivation to change. Members who are fully engaged gain vicariously through one another, and when one person explores ambivalence, decides to change, and begins considering how to go about it, other engaged group members are brought along on the journey and often only need to explore their own key points with the group, not their full story, exploration, and decision-making process. Member-to-member interactions are encouraged in order to achieve this end. Once the group is engaged and interconnected, you can spend more sustained time on individual members, while keeping the group engaged by interweaving individual exploration with group interaction.

Leader

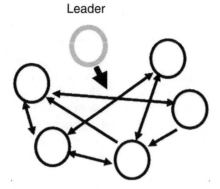

FIGURE 9.5. Web of connections.

Subgroups

One thing to watch for is the development of subgroups, in which you may struggle to communicate with the entire group and instead must interact with different groups within the group, as shown in Figure 9.6. While subgrouping is bound to happen (and may even be helpful) briefly in regard to specific topics, it is important to prevent subgroups from becoming stable, because stable subgroups reduce cohesion and group power, and either become neglectful or compete with other subgroups.

Leader

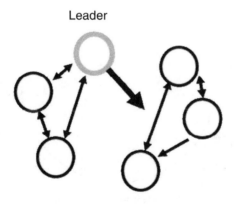

FIGURE 9.6. Subgrouping.

Engaging Members
with Challenging Interpersonal Styles

One leadership task is to manage group dynamics so that members' different interpersonal styles don't cause unnecessary friction. Another task is to allow members to take on healthy roles within the group, while steering them away from roles that interfere with group functioning. It is also important to intervene if members make insensitive or prejudicial remarks toward other members, in order to keep the group positively focused.

Interpersonal Problems

A well-researched model of interpersonal interactions describes eight problematic styles (Alden, Wiggins, & Pincus, 1990; Hopwood et al., 2011; Locke, 2000), spread in a circular fashion around the dimensions of control (from dominance to submission) and affiliation (from friendliness to hostility) as shown in Figure 9.7.

Generally, these styles are problematic (and challenging) due to rigidity and extremity. Healthy interpersonal functioning typically involves people being flexible in their approach to others. When it is best to be assertive, they can do that, and when a situation is better served by remaining silent, they can do that as well. They can lead, follow, nurture, and be

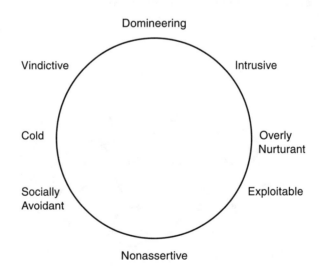

FIGURE 9.7. Interpersonal problems circumplex.

tough-minded when necessary. Healthy functioning also involves the ability to adjust one's intensity to the extremity of the situation. In two situations that both call for a friendly style, a pleasant and easygoing friendliness may be appropriate to one, whereas more intense comforting or nurturing may be needed for the other. People with interpersonal problems often have difficulty reading social cues, adjusting their style to the different needs of different individuals or situations, and moderating the intensity of their interactions (Kiesler, 1996). In groups, this can have a strong impact on the ability of the group to remain cohesive and supportive, to accomplish tasks, and to weave between a focus on individuals and the group as a whole (MacNair-Semands, 2002). People with interpersonal problems also interpret group climate and events in ways that are consistent with their own problematic style (Kivlighan & Angelone, 1992; MacNair-Semands & Lese, 2000), mediated by varying attachment insecurities that underlie the problematic interpersonal styles (Chen & Mallinckrodt, 2002). In addition, because of their often rigid and extreme styles, they can actually *experience* different group climates. For example, a vindictive group member is likely to receive less support from the group, and thus perceive the group climate as distant and unfriendly. A member of the same group who is highly nurturant, on the other hand, is more likely to elicit warmth and friendliness from other group members and come to perceive the same group as accepting and supportive (MacNair-Semands & Lese, 2000). Thus, while managing interpersonal issues is not a significant part of individual MI, it requires attention in MI groups.

Given that personality styles are usually firmly established and slow to change, even in a group specifically intended to reduce interpersonal problems (e.g., Malat, Morrow, & Stewart, 2011), it is probably better to focus on facilitating the MI group in a way that accommodates different styles, while minimizing any disturbance in group functioning that they may provoke. Since we focus on building positive energy in groups, one of our preferred ways of accommodating these styles is to look for and affirm the strengths associated with them. Table 9.1 highlights strengths that accompany the various interpersonal problems (drawn from Locke & Sadler, 2007; Sadler, Ethier, & Woody, 2011) you should watch for and verbally recognize from the outset of group. Engaging group members based on their strengths helps to bring out their best, builds your *Look for and affirm strengths associated with different personality styles.* relationship with them, and fosters group cohesion. This can provide important reserves for any moments of group conflict that may occur. In addition to affirming these strengths throughout group development, we offer strategies for addressing these styles in an MI-consistent manner that

TABLE 9.1. Interpersonal Problems, Corresponding Strengths, and MI Group Strategies

Style	Description	Strengths	Strategy
Domineering	Has problems with controlling, dominating, and trying to change others.	Ambitious, determined, decisive, persuasive, assertive	1. Elicit/reflect member's intention to be helpful. 2. Guide member to focus on his or her own experiences, interests, and concerns. 3. Ask member to invite others to share reactions in order to explore discrepancy between the member's intent (to help) and its actual impact upon others (often, to make others resistant to suggestions the member offers). 4. Affirm member's determination.
Vindictive	Is distrustful and suspicious of others and is unable to care about others' needs when they conflict with one's own.	Clever, skeptical, watchful, witty	1. Emphasize personal choice and control. 2. Elicit that member's intent is to protect self from perceived attacks or criticisms, rather than to attack others. 3. Affirm member for "keeping it real" (when appropriate).
Cold	Is unable to express affection and feel love for others; is unable to be generous to, get along with, and forgive others.	Thick-skinned, straightforward, focused, tough-minded	1. Emphasize pragmatic solution finding. 2. Invite sharing of "hard truths" learned along the way. 3. Affirm member's ability to "go it alone" when needed.
Socially avoidant	Is anxious and embarrassed around others; has difficulty initiating social interactions, expressing feelings, and socializing with others.	Private, soft-spoken, solitary, sparing	1. Invite participation during discussion of strengths. 2. In rounds, arrange for person to speak second or third to prevent too much anxiety buildup (but also so the person does not have to go first). 3. Give permission to observe silently until comfortable, then invite participation later in the session. 4. Affirm individual virtues and strengths.

(continued)

TABLE 9.1. (*continued*)

Style	Description	Strengths	Strategy
Nonassertive	Has difficulty making needs known to others; experiences discomfort in authoritative roles; is unable to be firm with and assertive toward others.	Content, a contributor, avoids getting in others' way, able to avoid arguments	1. Encourage person to share understanding and reactions to others' dilemmas. 2. Ask person to observe and comment on group dynamics or processes. 3. Emphasize personal choice/control. 4. Affirm member for being a "team player" (when appropriate).
Exploitable	Has difficulty feeling and expressing anger for fear of offending others; is gullible and readily taken advantage of by others.	Modest, humble, forgiving, gentle	1. Evoke perceptions during periods of low stress. 2. Invite to share perspective when another member describes feeling taken advantage of or being unable to express anger. 3. Emphasize personal choice/control. 4. Affirm gentle, forgiving nature.
Overly nurturant	Tries too hard to please and is too generous, trusting, caring, and permissive in dealing with others.	Considerate, warm, welcoming, likable, helpful, soothing, understanding	1. Gently guide back to focus on own needs, desires. 2. Ask the person to help other members better interact with significant others. 3. Emphasize personal choice/control. 4. Affirm attempts to understand and help others.
Intrusive	Is inappropriately self-disclosing, attention seeking; has difficulty spending time alone.	Sociable, approachable, energetic, expressive	1. Reflect themes or emotions to guide away from storytelling. 2. If in rounds, put this person at beginning, emphasizing need to hear from everyone (or at end). 3. Ask the person to observe others quietly during activity, then summarize. 4. Affirm energy, exuberance.

is intended to draw from people's strengths and minimize any negative impact on the group.

Member Roles

In addition to these challenging styles, some members seem to take on certain "roles" in the group. Often this is a just a feature of the current group, and not problematic, such as when a client seems to take on the role of "supporter" who regularly affirms others. However, certain roles can be disruptive, or at least can limit a full flowering of the group process. One problematic role is a kind of pseudotherapist, in which the member acts as he or she imagines a group leader might. This can involve analyzing, interpreting, probing, challenging, and even confronting at times. While having one member elevate him- or herself above others is generally problematic for developing cohesion and other group dynamics, these behaviors can be particularly problematic for an MI group, because they contrast the approach and threaten to undermine the effectiveness of the group.

While it is important to intervene in this situation, it is also important to avoid conveying any negativity, as it is in tense moments that the spirit of MI is crucial if the group is to carry through to its full development. In the first few occurrences, or when interactions are mild, you can simply redirect the conversation in a more productive direction, such as reminding the person of the supportive intent of the group or redirecting the member taking the negative role to reflect on how this relates to personal issues. If you need to go beyond redirecting, restate the member's comments in a more MI-consistent manner, then check with the recipient of the comment on the accuracy of your restated reflection. Closed questions can be restated as open. Interpretations can be restated as complex reflections. Challenge statements can be restated as issues of personal choice.

If the pseudotherapist behavior is more intense or ongoing, a stronger reaction than redirecting or restating may be required. Two options are exploring intent and exploring reactions. *Exploring intent* involves stopping the interaction after the member taking on a pseudotherapist role makes a challenging or demanding comment, and checking the intent of that person. Since exploring intent is riskier than redirecting or restating, it can help to "seed" positive intent (leading a bit). This might be something like "Chuck, it sounds like you care about Amy and are a little worried about her situation and so are trying to help by pointing her in a direction that seems good to you." If needed, you can add some feedback into your reflection to cue Chuck as to why you're stopping the interaction: "I'm not sure it's coming across like that to her, though, so I wanted to check with you." If the role taking continues, you can elicit feedback from the group or the recipient, possibly again emphasizing the difference between intent and impact. Of course, you can also ask him or her to avoid taking this kind of guiding role with other group members. Regardless of how you choose to approach it, take care to model the type of communication you are trying to facilitate among members.

There are other roles that members can take, such as "class clown," "guru," and so forth. While we generally dislike such labeling, it probably captures the essence of such role taking for our purposes here and can help us see it for what it likely is—a form of avoiding the feelings associated with the ambivalence that often develops when members focus on their own issues, and indirect feedback that, for at least one person (the person taking the role), the group feels a little unsafe. When this happens, your options include responding in ways that range from mild and safe, yet possibly ineffective, to stronger and possibly more effective but riskier. Whenever possible, we prefer a gentle touch when addressing such issues. It is easier to ramp up your response if it fails to redirect the interaction than it is to back down if you overshoot and come across as too hierarchical, as contributing to the conflict, or as silencing members. In order of increasing intensity, your basic choices are to ignore and keep going, to attempt to redirect, to restate or reshape, to explore intent and reactions, to remind members of the group guidelines, or to directly ask or guide a violating member to act differently.

Prejudicial or Insensitive Comments

One situation in which we intervene more quickly and directly is when a member expresses prejudice, insensitivity, or hostility to or about another member based on some category, whether this is ethnicity, race, religion, gender, sexual orientation, or some other grouping. While we remain as nonconfrontational as possible, we quickly remind the group that each member is an individual, with personal choices and characteristics, and the purpose of the group is to help people make the changes they decide to make, and no more than that. We generally don't think of MI groups as places where we mutually explore larger values systems or work through prejudicial or limiting worldviews, except to the extent that doing so supports members making specific changes. In the same way that we don't divert MI groups to try to change members' personalities, we don't divert the group to try to change underlying cultural misperceptions, insensitivity, or prejudice. While these are worthy goals, they are distinct from the purposes of MI groups. At the same time, ignoring insensitive comments can also divert the group, so intervening and refocusing are sometimes necessary.

Working with a Co–Leader

As a group leader you have many responsibilities. You need to get the group started, keep it focused and positive, and lead members through exploring and resolving ambivalence. You also need to keep the whole group engaged, while keeping an eye on how time is used in the group. It is important to pay attention to the dynamics among group members as a whole and those between specific individuals in the group and any informal subgroups that develop. It is also important to track which members' issues or interests were not fully addressed in a given session, find a way to note and honor that, and see that they return, so their concerns can be addressed later. And you're just getting started!

Advantages of Co–Facilitation for the Leaders

Facilitating a group with a co-leader provides more options for managing group tasks. Co-leaders have greater ability to manage group dynamics and individual change simultaneously, more flexibility to handle negative interpersonal processes as they arise, and more opportunities to notice unspoken or unaddressed issues that would be useful to explore. Co-facilitating also allows more thorough between-session processing, conceptualizing, and planning. While it may seem less cost-efficient to have two leaders, co-facilitation often reduces the extent of outside supervision or consultation that is needed, increases the efficiency of the group, and lessens the likelihood that dysfunctional group patterns will potentially overwhelm the group. Anyone who has led groups in challenging settings long enough has probably had the experience of a group faltering or imploding. This experience can leave psychological scars on members and leaders alike. While the well-defined focus and emphasis on positive atmosphere may make this less likely to occur in MI groups than in some other approaches, having co-leaders can provide an important buffer if things start to turn bad, and serve as a helpful tool to get the group back on track.

Advantages of Co–Facilitation for the Group Members

Members of therapeutic groups perceive greater benefits from co-led groups (Kivlighan, London, & Miles, 2012). When co-leaders have similar ideas about the group but different skills and interpersonal styles, group members are more engaged and have less conflict (Miles & Kivlighan, 2010). Having two leaders allows for more attention to be given to members. Given their vulnerability at certain points during the change process, this can mean the difference between moving forward or remaining stuck. Another benefit of having co-leaders is that members get to experience interactions between the two leaders. When you interact with group members as a sole leader in a way that is consistent with MI spirit and practices, your style conveys important messages, but members may view this respectful approach solely as your role. When members observe two leaders interacting in an MI-consistent way, they seem to absorb the spirit of MI better by seeing how the leaders collaborate, negotiate, and understand each other, while working toward a common goal. When leaders display mutual respect, interest in each other's viewpoints, collaboration in making decisions, and support for one another's autonomy, group members witness valuable modeling of people interacting in an empathic yet goal-oriented manner. This is particularly the case when the leaders have different impulses or perceptions regarding group direction, yet respectfully work out a unified direction for moving forward.

Co-Leader Roles

Co-leaders can share leadership generally or take on different roles. For example, roles can be divided between structure and process elements. One leader may structure the session, introducing topical content, and managing focus and time, while the other may focus on building group cohesion and interactivity by linking members' interests and concerns, encouraging quiet members to participate and overactive members to step back, and redirecting members who become negative or tangential. Or one leader might focus on individuals and the other on group dynamics. Dividing tasks like this makes sessions more efficient and limits unproductive or confusing moments when leaders simultaneously lead in different directions on the same issue. It also cues members to tune into these different aspects of group work, advancing group development. As the group matures, co-leaders' roles may shift in planned or unexpected ways. This growth can also benefit members, who see these changes unfold in front of them.

Structuring Sessions

Engaging participants is a significant part of early group work. Participants may begin the group at varying degrees of readiness to change, interest in participating in services, and knowledge of what is involved in therapeutic groups. Some may have made significant changes in their lifestyles before beginning the group, and may be ready to jump in, to become involved with others and see what the group might offer. Others may describe problems in their lives but see the problems as external, not as issues that they play a role in maintaining through their own choices, or that they are able to change. Some members who have participated in groups previously may have a clear understanding of what is involved (or clear misunderstanding, depending on their previous experiences!), while others may never have talked with anyone at all about their struggles in life.

Given these variations, it can be challenging to start the group in such a way that all feel welcome, regardless of their readiness to make changes, interest in participating, or openness to sharing their experiences and ideas with others. Engagement obviously involves active participation of the members, but that doesn't necessarily mean jumping in immediately and wholeheartedly, becoming vulnerable by revealing struggles, or being willing to tell all. Involvement can be more subtle, especially early on. You might see a member nod as another member shares his or her story. A member may furrow her brow when you reflect another's concern. Or you notice a member making eye contact as another opens up regarding the struggles he is experiencing, or laughing when someone reveals a humorous truth about her life. The early goal is to engage members at whatever level they are ready for, so watch for opportunities to involve members bit by bit, allowing the group to unfold at a comfortable and unpressured pace.

There are several structuring strategies you can use to facilitate engagement.

Pregroup Social Time

Imagining group participation through the eyes of participants can give you useful insight into clients' perspectives. As professionals, we often focus on what happens during the formal session, but for members, sessions are set in the larger context of their entire experience with our setting, and that experience is set within the larger context of their lives. Although we may compartmentalize the group sessions from work that comes before or after, the boundaries around the opening and closing of sessions are less relevant to group members than to leaders.

One way to help members become more fully engaged in the group experience is through informal interactions before the session starts. We generally arrive at the group room 20 to 30 minutes before the session, get the room set up, then relax and talk with members as they arrive. During this time, we might talk about lighthearted matters, daily events and experiences, world events or local happenings, interests, and so on. Our focus is on aspects of members' lives other than the problem issues they wish to address. We are open about some things in our own lives as well, such as a sporting or cultural event we attended, or some hobby or interest. While this can help as an icebreaker, we think it serves a few even more important functions—relating to clients as people first, developing a connection before asking them to become vulnerable by discussing sensitive issues, flattening the hierarchy in the therapeutic relationship, and helping clients begin to broaden their focus beyond problematic aspects of their lives, onto their lives as a whole.

Opening Sessions/Warm-Up Exercises

Some group leaders like to open sessions with specific rituals or warm-up exercises. Such activities are not required, and you can just begin with conversation when groups are in working mode, or with a simple welcome and orientation to the session focus to start the meeting. However, if the group members seem to have difficulty getting started, you may want to move things along. You can use rounds to do brief "check-ins" around specific issues such as energy levels, agenda setting, and so on. You can invite reactions to the last session and any requests members may have about doing things differently. Alternatively, you might allow a few minutes for members to talk one-on-one with others about a goal for the coming week, or some other focused issue, to help them warm up to talking to the larger group. Jasiura, Hunt, and Urquhart (Chapter 15) describe more extensive activities based on "mind–body focusing," including guided relaxation. Overall, MI is not a particularly experiential approach in which change develops through experiences rather than discussions, so opening activities should probably remain fairly brief and of low intensity. However, simple warm-up exercises can be helpful as a bridge from the outside world to the group session.

Midmeeting Breaks

If your sessions are long, or if you are leading support groups divided into a didactic portion and a discussion/support portion, a midmeeting break can help facilitate transition to a new activity or allow a few minutes of downtime, so members can concentrate better for the remainder of the session. It can also serve as a variation of the pregroup social time, when members engage with one another individually and informally around personal interests and experiences, rather than only therapeutic issues. Snacks can help members be more comfortable interacting during this time, just as in other social gatherings.

Closing Sessions

It is important to reserve time to close sessions well, to allow members an opportunity to transition from the group interaction back to the "outside world." In addition, solidifying the lessons learned, perspectives gained (or abandoned), and experiences shared can help members gain more from group sessions. If you lead a structured group with specific session themes, this is an opportunity to highlight any messages you want members to take with them, and link the theme of the session back to the larger process of change members are undertaking. While summarizing each member's issues or progress is generally too time-consuming and leader-centered, it can be helpful to briefly affirm any clients who have made particularly noteworthy disclosures or progress. Your closing comments can also provide a preview of the next session.

While you should not "overdo" the closing aspect of sessions, it is usually best not to continue to explore client material up to the close of session. If you are aware of any unfinished business—an issue or theme a member wanted to explore but didn't; a bit of tension between members that did not escalate but also wasn't resolved; a member who explored an emotional issue that may still linger inside—this is your chance to acknowledge the matter briefly in order to reestablish normality or to let an unattended member know that you notice him or her and care. While issues cannot always be resolved, members usually appreciate the acknowledgment, and experience the group as safer because of it.

One option is to ask members to close by summarizing the highlights, thoughts, or changes they experienced in the session, and sharing something they can do between sessions to continue to move forward toward their change goals (which can include "thinking about it").

Preparing for the First Session

Pregroup Orientation

In Chapter 6, we discussed the purposes of holding a pregroup screening/orientation meeting with potential group members. This meeting can be used to refer individuals to other services, if they are unlikely to benefit from group participation, or if their involvement is likely to interfere with group processes to the point of risking harm to other participants. For those who go on to join the group, the meeting can increase their likelihood of success by decreasing dropout and increasing openness, hopefulness, and bonding with other members.

We recommend incorporating pregroup meetings, even if you do not have the luxury of screening clients and use the time only to help them prepare for group, and even if you are only able to schedule the meeting just prior to the first group session. The meeting can help you learn details that a person may be hesitant to share in a room of strangers and begin to build an alliance that helps to buffer the anxieties a person may experience in group. This connection and shared understanding can be especially helpful later if you need to redirect a dominating group member, or to encourage one who is hesitant to speak.

During the pregroup meeting, explaining the purposes and practices of the group helps the person prepare to participate in group sessions and to understand and commit to confidentiality about details other members share. Also discuss the limits of confidentiality, and any other ethical issues that need to be discussed up front (revisit some of these issues during the first group meeting, as well as anytime a new member joins). Share details around informed consent and communication with other providers. Although you may not have predetermined group guidelines (and we recommend developing these collaboratively as part of the early group process), discuss important normative issues such as attendance and timeliness, and any relevant agency rules around payment, participant rights, contact between members outside of group, apparent intoxication when presenting for group sessions, and so on.

Remember that this meeting is often clients' first exposure to you as a helper and to the concepts of MI and groups. Although there may be many details to cover and time may be limited, the meeting should be conducted in an MI-consistent manner, which includes exchanging information in an elicit–provide–elicit style that allows clients to get a feel for how you work. Though you may not want to go too far into clients' therapeutic issues or life challenges, it is helpful to communicate that the MI group is intended to help them make positive changes in their lives. It can be helpful to elicit a little information about clients' goals in order to prime them for later group exploration. Briefly exploring other relevant issues such as strengths or values, if there is time, can also be useful.

Framing the upcoming group in a positive light and conveying that people often find the group experience helpful and supportive can ease client concerns and raise interest, energy, and hopefulness. You can also briefly mention that although the group has a positive focus, there may be occasional moments of discomfort or tension. Let clients know that such moments, should they arise, are just part of the process of change, and that you will work through them together to get back to a positive focus.

Save time to elicit clients' experiences in previous groups, so that you can compare and contrast the upcoming group, if needed, and elicit their questions or thoughts about participating. Because clients may be slow to ask questions, your patience and genuine interest can go a long way to ensure that you don't seem to be eliciting their questions and ideas in a perfunctory manner (also use open questions, such as "What questions or thoughts do you have?" instead of closed questions, such as "Do you have any questions?"). You may even want to begin the meeting by telling clients to share questions or comments anytime throughout the meeting.

Before the meeting is over, give clients something to think about before the first group session. For example, you might ask them how they might like things to be better after participating in group, and what thoughts they have about steps to move toward those goals.

Finally, it can be useful to ask clients to commit to a specific number of sessions, perhaps four or more, before deciding whether the group is helpful and worth continuing. You can offer to schedule an individual meeting at that time to discuss the group experience if a client has considered leaving the group. Because clients may experience ambivalence and some discomfort related to group participation during the first few sessions, this communicates to them that such experiences are normal and are better considered after being given a reasonable time period to settle in. Discussing this now can reduce the premature dropout from the group that can undermine development of group cohesion and trust, and deprive members of a potentially helpful experience before it has a chance to work. You might offer an analogy such as how exercise can be uncomfortable and even painful at first, until our bodies become accustomed to it (or how medications can have side effects before the main effects emerge).

Preparing the Meeting Space

We arrange a circle of chairs before members arrive, ideally without conference tables or other barriers in the middle of the circle, particularly for psychotherapeutic groups. To the side, we place a table that can hold handouts and refreshments. Attendance sheets, supplies, and tissues can be placed there as needed. A clock should be visible, so that group members can track time left in the session and adjust accordingly. Moderate lighting is better than bright fluorescents, which can cause headaches and fatigue. If you are recording the interactions, have the equipment in place and ready but turned off until all members have agreed to such monitoring (which also should have been covered during the pregroup orientation). With support and psychoeducational groups, you may also want an easel and dark markers that are easily visible to all members. This may be very useful for the first group meeting, even with psychotherapeutic groups, in order to develop and record group guidelines for all to see and revise. If you use colored markers, keep in mind that some members may have color blindness, which most commonly is a difficulty differentiating between red and green. Of course, members may be managing any number of disabling conditions, and it is your responsibility to make sure that all aspects of group functioning are accessible to them.

Group sessions are more productive if they are private and protected from distractions. The group should meet in a separate room, with relatively good insulation from outside sounds, no reason for others to pass through the space, and no telephones, public address systems, or other outside intrusions. Leaders should not be on call or otherwise interrupted during the session. Members should turn off cell phones and music players for the duration of the session. It is easier to establish these protections up front than to address them as they arise.

Conducting the First Session

Challenges in Facilitating the First Session

Getting your group off to a good start is sometimes very easy and at other times more challenging. Some members may not talk. Others may talk too much. Some may complain or tell detailed stories, while others may minimize and remain superficial. There are many ways the new group may test your patience, optimism, confidence, and skill.

It is more important to do a few things well than to try to maximize the impact of a first meeting and risk having group members feel confused, unsafe, pressured, or exposed. The first task, rather than pursuing therapeutic change, is to develop a safe and supportive atmosphere that engages members in the group process. Progress toward change goals may safely take a backseat to establishing a positive, pleasant, and productive environment. It is an important achievement simply to get members to interact with each other rather than talking only to you as group leader. Having clients want to return (or at least feel okay about it), with a sense of trust in you and some hope that the group may be helpful, is more important than establishing therapeutic focus during the first meeting. Emphasizing social aspects over business aspects can help people feel respected and noticed. This lays a foundation for clients to use the group to help them change rather than to see it as a place where they are required to report on their lives (or misreport, if they feel unsafe).

The first task is not to pursue therapeutic change but to develop a safe and supportive atmosphere, in order to engage members in the group process.

Opening the Session

First impressions count. Even when you have met clients individually before the first group session, the opening of the first session is the start of developing a group identity and the many interrelationships that develop over the course of working together. Often, it's the little things that count. Relax. Breathe. Smile. Be friendly. Don't rush. Make people comfortable. You don't need to provide a long introduction or overview, just enough to provide a basic orientation and give clients a few moments to become acclimated to the group setting.

Similarly, don't jump right into forming group guidelines. Briefly introduce yourself as leader, and maybe share something personal that is not too private or detailed. Tell members you'll get back to discussing the group and work you'll be doing together after you get to know each other a little as people. Invite them to share something positive about their lives and something they do for fun, or a hobby or interest. Then, as people start sharing, do your best to shape the experience into an ongoing conversation between people rather than one person talking at a time, with no interaction. Make some links between people as you go along, and summarize similarities and your eagerness to get to know each other better before you transition to focusing on the "business" of the group. Although this may seem lighthearted and somewhat superficial, we believe it is valuable to first engage members outside of their problem area. It conveys the key message that people are more than their problems, which provides a foundation for the later work of broadening perspectives and building resources for change. It also develops positive connections between members that can help if tensions develop later. Although this conversation may be brief, it is important.

Group Overview

When members have gotten to know each other a little and conversation seems to have hit a natural transition point, it is time to discuss some of the business of MI groups. You can recap some of the highlights from the individual orientation meetings, such as the purpose of the group and the kinds of things focused on in MI groups. Although group members will have heard you discuss this already, a review is often helpful to underscore that everyone has been told the same things and to initiate the group with a shared understanding. It also can jump-start group cohesion, because members already have a common experience, even though this is their first interaction together.

Emphasize that the group is intended to be positive, that although people may have struggles or challenges and are free to discuss them, we focus more on looking forward than back, and more on making things better than on what's wrong or troubling. You may find it helpful to be explicit about this, along the following lines:

> "Some of you may have participated in other groups. This group may not be quite like any other group you've experienced—it will be somewhere in between groups where people only share their own stories and don't interact, and groups where people challenge one another and give each other advice. In our group, it is up to each person to decide what to change and rather than pressure any of you we will only support you in the way you find most helpful, and encourage you to do the same for each other."

Overall, members should experience the group as providing support, helping them gain clarity on what they want, and boosting their confidence and courage to make changes that will bring their lives closer to their hopes. They should find you helpful, keeping the group safe, while guiding the group to keep moving forward.

Several of our collaborators describe variations on opening strategies in later chapters, and we recommend taking a look at those for further ideas. As a guide, Valasquez, Stephens, and Drenner (Chapter 14) use the acronym OPEN to summarize the opening tasks of a group:

- Overview of group's purpose is presented: learning about members' goals, concerns, choices.
- Personal choice and autonomy are emphasized.
- Environment is described as one of respect and encouragement for all members.
- Nonconfrontational nature of the group is noted.

Decontaminating the Referral Process

Often, participants have been mandated or pressured to attend. These members have come to the group in such a way that they potentially contaminate the group with their aversive reactions to the referral process. They may perceive you as part of a hierarchy that is controlling them against their wishes (and you might actually be a part of such a hierarchy).

Depending on the degree of coerced participation among your group members, you can handle this in different ways. One way is just to proceed toward establishing a positive environment, and deal with this issue as it arises, in the same way you would address any other discord. If coercion is infrequent or mild, this may be your best option. Proactively addressing it early on is another option—one that might work better if pressure to attend is the norm and the consequences faced for not participating are severe (jail time, loss of job, children or family, etc.). It is always essential not only to be clear on any limits of confidentiality but also to identify your interests as group leaders, and differentiate yourselves from other professionals your group members may have encountered along the referral path (or continue to work with while they are in your group). Mention something along the lines of the following:

"Our main interest is helping people make their lives better. We know that some of you didn't come here entirely on your own and are in situations where you need us to report to others something about what you do here. We'll do what's best for each of you, with your permission, but our interest is not in forcing you to change against your will, or even deciding for you how your life could be better—only you can really say what would be better for you or how you might want to change. We're happy to share ideas, but our goal is to lead the group, so that you can best help yourselves and support each other, because each person and situation is different. We may not be able to do anything about consequences you might face if you don't participate, but our role is not to enforce consequences or keep you in line. We just want to help the best we can."

Of course, decontaminating the referral process is easier if you lead your groups as an independent entity, but clarifying your role and interests is useful even if you work within the system that is responsible for enacting consequences of violations of agreements or mandates. As much as possible, we recommend separating the role of group leader from any tasks that involve hierarchical reporting, reinforcement or punishment. For example, in addictions or criminal justice settings, toxicology screens can be done by others, who are not in the dual roles of helper and investigator or reporter. Group summaries can be limited to attendance and perhaps overall progress, without revealing details. Members can even be shown examples of reports or notes you might write (assuming that you have latitude to keep reporting minimal), or directly review notes you write about them. We believe that if you do not thoughtfully differentiate between the processes of helping and enforcing (or other hierarchical tasks), then you limit the ways your clients can be open and honest with you, and limit their possibilities for change. We believe it is best to acknowledge this with group members.

Group Guidelines

Once members have basic familiarity with the group, it is time to turn to group guidelines. We suggest using the word *guidelines* specifically, rather than the more hierarchical *rules*. We also suggest eliciting guidelines from members rather than providing them, although you can add important elements if they don't generate them on their own. Eliciting ideas for guidelines frames the group in a way that increases the sense of ownership among the members. Group cohesion increases as a result of working on a task together, before members focus on their individual issues. It also gives you a chance to guide them experientially on the style and spirit of MI, before getting into vulnerable personal matters.

First, ask for reactions to the overview of the group purpose and style. Then ask what practical guidelines might be helpful to focus group members in a positive, supportive, and forward-looking manner. As members introduce possible ideas, write them down for everyone to see, without asking group members to commit to any of them. Then, identify those guidelines that seem most important and least controversial, shaping the wording of initial group suggestions to come up with guidelines on which all can agree and commit to following. A few broad guidelines may be better than many specific guidelines, so combine similar suggestions into broader themes when possible. They are easier to remember and tend to emphasize the spirit of working together rather than compliance to rules and technicalities. Given that group participants may be referred due to rule violations in the first place, it is important not to risk setting up a dynamic that transfers their frustrations with other systems into the group environment. A core goal in MI groups is to give members a different experience to help them shake free from previous dysfunctional patterns, and setting up guidelines in a collaborative manner is one good way to start.

If members do not reach consensus on any of the proposed guidelines, propose trying out a variation "just for this session," and promise to review the guidelines again at the end of the session or at the beginning of the next. This process of setting guidelines incorporates empathic efforts to understand members' perspectives with guidance by the leaders, implicitly underscoring the group model. Feldstein Ewing, Walters, and Baer (Chapter 21, p. 392) suggest that this approach may also increase adherence to the guidelines "as members tend to be sensitive to violations of their own guidelines."

Typical guidelines are as follows:

• *Confidentiality*. Issues raised may be discussed outside of the room, but members' identities or specific experiences should not be shared. (Make sure to repeat the limits of confidentiality to which leaders must adhere, while reinforcing that you will not share personal information unless you have a signed release of information agreement with individual group members or are compelled by law.)

• *Respect*. Members may feel vulnerable about some things they share, and it is important to show respect for the challenges members face and their efforts to manage them. Examples of disrespect include interrupting, criticizing (even for "someone's own good"), pressing perspectives or opinions on others, tuning out or ignoring people when they are speaking, or ignoring a member in distress.

• *Turn-taking*. Group members are not forced to speak on a specific topic if they don't want to, but members should generally expect to take turns sharing their experiences and perspectives. Members should be aware of how much time they take, and remember to allow time for others.

Of course, many other guidelines are possible and important in different settings, including issues around attendance, participation, tardiness, relapse, and so forth. Several of our contributors discuss other issues related to group guidelines in their chapters.

Eliciting Members' Goals

With guidelines established, you might briefly turn to eliciting members' initial hopes for how things will be different following their participation. Some members may have goals identified for them by family, other practitioners, the courts, or other sources, whereas others participate simply on their own initiative. Even in mandated groups, however, each member has individual desires, intentions, and goals. Even if all members have a general goal of managing diabetes, for example, each person will have individual needs and specific goals—perhaps focusing on diet, exercise, medication, sleep, stress, or other health matters.

In addition, different members may have different group process goals: Some want the group to provide support; others want help to problem-solve, or want the group to challenge them in some way; still others wish mostly to listen to other members' stories and ideas, to draw from them for their own thinking. And of course, some just want to do what they have to do in order to meet the requirements of a mandate. Further complicating the matter, members who are not in the habit of identifying personal goals may not immediately be able to specify what they want from group participation.

All of this points to the importance of eliciting individual goals, often at repeated intervals over the life of the group. Practitioners often think in terms of agency goals or general therapeutic goals, such as recovery, medication adherence, or disease management. It is easy to forget to make sure clients have in mind their own clear goals that help to anchor group discussions and personalize any educational material you may introduce. Stopping to identify the personal importance of any newly introduced topic is well worth the time it takes, because it engages members and primes them to include information, examples, stories, or comments that they might otherwise not recognize as valuable and subsequently ignore.

Consistent with our overall approach, we think it is valuable to focus more on initiation goals—what the person is seeking to achieve, gain, or develop—than on cessation goals—what the person is attempting to stop, lose, or diminish. Focusing too much on cessation goals can leave the person adrift once the initial change is under way, and may increase the likelihood of relapse. Early in group process, before momentum is established, focusing on cessation goals can also have an energy draining effect that undermines members' sense of confidence about change. Even when the change primarily involves a cessation goal (e.g., to quit smoking), we think it is useful to focus on what members will do to replace the current habit. Rather than cutting back on sweets, members can focus on increasing the amount of fruits and vegetables they eat. Rather than quit arguing with their partners, members can emphasize their investment in a relationship and being respectfully assertive.

When clients have difficulty identifying initial goals, it is useful to help them move their focus from problems to goals:

LEADER (men's parenting group): Everyone's here in one way or another because of issues related to parenting, but it can be useful to get a little more specific about the goals for each of you.

BOB: For me, it's pretty simple. I'm in the middle of a divorce, and while we have agreed to share custody of our kids, we have pretty different styles. My soon-to-be-ex-wife is really organized, while I'm more laid back. She doesn't want to keep the kids away from me or anything, but she's worried that I won't handle getting them ready for school in the morning or doing homework and things like that, and right now she only wants me to have them on the weekends. I got her to agree to at least try 50–50 custody and told her I'd get involved in some parenting thing like this group for ideas during our trial period the next couple of months, before we have to finalize things with the divorce.

LEADER: So you think she might be overreacting a little, but you don't mind checking this out and seeing what tips you might pick up or developing plans that make her more comfortable with the idea of sharing custody.

BOB: Right. I don't really think there's anything wrong with the way I parent. We just have different styles. She's pretty uptight about it all and we've had our share of fights about it. But it seems better to do this now than fight over it and take the chance of having the judge limit me to every other weekend or something.

LEADER: So what things can you focus on that will be the most helpful?

BOB: Well, I do wake up pretty groggy and sometimes end up giving the kids rides to school when things don't go according to plan or the kids start fighting or messing around and miss the bus, so getting that sorted out would probably make her more comfortable.

LEADER: So you might want to focus on structuring mornings, and maybe even the evenings before, to keep things running like clockwork on school days.

BOB: Well, I don't know about running like clockwork, but even just making sure they have their school stuff with them and aren't eating breakfast bars on the school bus or have their hair sticking straight up because it didn't even get combed or something could help . . .

LEADER: That sounds great. So Bob is focusing on avoiding problems that in other situations might seem like pretty minor issues, but in his situation could feed into conflict with his ex-wife over his kids. Instead of just trying to avoid the conflict or tell his ex she's worrying over nothing, he's figuring out things he could do differently to get on top of the things and maybe even make his life a bit easier. What about other people? What could you change to make things better in your own situation?

Several of our collaborators discuss goal setting in later chapters, focusing on specific therapeutic issues. For example, Lane, Butterworth, and Speck (Chapter 17) discuss using the elicit–provide–elicit (E-P-E) strategy to home in on specific goals in a broader disease management group, and Feldstein Ewing et al. (Chapter 21) share how they use E-P-E in an almost game-like manner while setting goals with adolescents. For members who are unfamiliar with setting personal goals, ensuring that they have a good experience in the first session is more important than establishing direction. If they don't seem able to identify initial goals easily, you might work with them on simply expressing how they hope things might be better after participating in the group, and leave it at that. If even that is too much, ask them to think a little about it between sessions. Let them know there is no hurry to figure it out, because that is the purpose of the group sessions.

Closing the First Session

Whether you complete the various tasks we've described, or include additional tasks, at some point it is time to wrap up the first meeting, and it is important to close well. You can reserve time for this, or keep it brief, but it is helpful to find a way to leave some sense of orderliness and coherence rather than end randomly when the clock indicates time is up. If you have only a brief time, you can summarize the goals and processes established in the first group meeting, then open the floor to see whether members would like clarification on any issues raised or plans for the group. Always make sure to affirm the group for the first session whether things go well or (maybe especially) there are struggles in engaging or developing some sense of group identity. If you have more time, elicit members' perspectives on the first session, or ask for their reflections on things they appreciated about the session. However, if you open the floor for comments, make sure you have enough time to address any negative reactions that members may raise, at least to the point of understanding the concern and making a plan to address it in the next session, if there is too little time to explore as this session is wrapping up. Other possibilities for ending the group include addressing safety concerns members may have, discussing urges or other risks or threats that may cause concern before the next session, and possibly establishing a ritual for ending group. This might be as simple as a round of members saying what they'll do (or think about) before the next meeting.

References

Alden, L. E., Wiggins, J. S., & Pincus, A. L. (1990). Construction of circumplex scales for the inventory of interpersonal problems. *Journal of Personality Assessment, 55,* 521–536.

Chen, E. C., & Mallinckrodt, B. (2002). Attachment, group attractions, and self–other agreement in interpersonal circumplex problems and perceptions of group members. *Group Dynamics: Theory, Research, and Practice, 6,* 311–324.

Farrall, M. (2007, September). *Action for change: Motivational interviewing and drama in domestic violence and abuse.* Paper presented at Motivational Interviewing Network of Trainers Forum, Sofia, Bulgaria.

Hopwood, C. J., Ansell, E. B., Pincus, A. L., Wright, A. G., Lukowitsky, M. R., & Roche, M. J. (2011). The circumplex structure of interpersonal sensitivities. *Journal of Personality, 79,* 707–740.

Kiesler, D. J. (1996). *Contemporary interpersonal theory and research: Personality, psychopathology and psychotherapy.* New York: Wiley.

Kivlighan, D. M., & Angelone, E. O. (1992). Interpersonal problems: Variables influencing participants' perception of group climate. *Journal of Counseling Psychology, 39,* 468–472.

Kivlighan, D. M., Jr., London, K., & Miles, J. R. (2012). Are two heads better than one?: The relationship between number of group leaders and group members, and group climate and group member benefit from therapy. *Group Dynamics: Theory, Research, and Practice, 16,* 1–13.

Locke, K. D. (2000). Circumplex scales of interpersonal values: Reliability, validity, and applicability to interpersonal problems and personality disorders. *Journal of Personality Assessment, 75,* 249–267.

Locke, K. D., & Sadler, P. (2007). Self-efficacy, values, and complementarity in dyadic interactions: Integrating interpersonal and social-cognitive theory. *Personality and Social Psychology Bulletin, 33,* 94–109.

MacNair-Semands, R. R. (2002). Predicting attendance and expectations for group therapy. *Group Dynamics: Theory, Research, and Practice, 6,* 219–228.

MacNair-Semands, R. R., & Lese, K. P. (2000). Interpersonal problems and the perception of therapeutic factors in group therapy. *Small Group Research, 31,* 158–174.

Malat, J., Morrow, S., & Stewart, P. (2011). Applying motivational interviewing principles in a modified interpersonal group for comorbid addiction. *International Journal of Group Psychotherapy, 61,* 557–575.

Miles, J. R., & Kivlighan, D. M. (2010). Co-leader similarity and group climate in group interventions: Testing the co-leadership, team cognition–team diversity model. *Group Dynamics: Theory, Research, and Practice, 14,* 114–122.

Sadler, P., Ethier, N., & Woody, E. (2011). Interpersonal complementarity. In L. M. Horowitz & S. Strack (Eds.), *Handbook of interpersonal psychology: Theory, research, assessment, and therapeutic interventions* (pp. 123–142). Hoboken, NJ: Wiley.

CHAPTER 10

Phase II

Exploring Perspectives

Once members become engaged in the group process, whether this occurs in a single session or over a few sessions, it is time to move into the next phase of work, *exploring perspectives*. Often, people start groups under stress, narrowly focused on what is most irritating or the biggest obstacle. The goal of exploring perspectives is to help members place such stressors in the larger context of their lives through the process of exploring their situation, lifestyle, habits, ambivalence, and core values.

During this phase, you shift from strategies that engage members in the group process and build basic group cohesion, to strategies that focus more on members' perspectives about their situations. This transition may be unnoticed by members, because you are not changing your approach. In fact, you continue to convey acceptance, respond empathically, and seek to understand members' perspectives. With the subtle strategic shift from group building to exploration of their lives, members learn about each other's situations and perspectives, and may begin to question some of their long-held assumptions. This sets the stage for new learning and movement toward change.

> *During this phase, you shift from engagement to focusing on members' perspectives about their situations.*

Guiding Principles

Some principles help to guide your work in eliciting members' perspectives. Throughout this phase of work, taking a client-centered perspective is a particularly important first principle. As quickly as possible, try to develop a deep understanding of members' lives, perspectives, and values. The work in this phase provides the raw material from which to create new possibilities during the broadening perspectives phase, and primes members to bring forth their best selves by first connecting deeply with their current perspectives, feelings, values, and strengths. A superficial exploration of issues and perspectives during this phase can limit your ability to help members broaden perspectives and brainstorm change possibilities later.

Regardless of your experience or knowledge, it is especially important that this phase of work focus on eliciting members' perspectives, which may be slow to come at times, often hidden behind things they think they should say, ideas they've heard from other professionals or mutual help groups, or things they've read. While these are all potentially important sources to inform their perspective, it is important to help them dig a bit to find and share what they currently truly believe. MI works from the inside-out, so if members are only parroting others or sharing ideas they only halfheartedly believe, it will be tougher to help them expand their perspective later.

As you empathically explore members' perspectives, we recommend the second principle, keeping a *focus on the positives*. This means eliciting and exploring the positive reasons that people are in the group, the positive choices they are considering, and the skills and experiences they currently have and will develop that equip them to make changes. While individual MI sometimes focuses more on negative reasons for change, such as the problems that current habits create or choices that run counter to their values, these play less of a role in MI groups. On the one hand, the group environment tends to amplify internal and interpersonal dynamics, so focusing on negatives in the group, due to its semipublic nature, can quickly lead to shame, embarrassment, criticism, or debate, which are generally unproductive. On the other hand, the group environment can also amplify a positive focus. Strengths, hope, mutual support, and determination to improve things are important positive motivations to foster in groups.

An important time to focus positively is when members discuss negative events or reactions. It is natural for members who resent being "sent"

Guiding Principles for the Work of Exploring Perspectives

- Take a client-centered perspective.
- Focus on the positives.
- Bring the group into the moment.
- Focus on the present.
- Acknowledge suffering, but don't elicit grievances.

to group to feel coerced to participate. They may have grievances about the processes that led them to the group, often expressed early on as you initially engage the group. They may also have shame or guilt that is rechanneled into blame. As you explore perspectives, you may again hear these frustrations. It is important to acknowledge them, so that group members feel heard and understood, while you subtly refocus on the positive aspects of their participation. Often, you can do this in a casual manner. Sometimes a member continues to focus on resentments, and it may be more appropriate to give a more thorough summary:

> "John, you've been referred here by your doctors, who you see as pressuring you into coming to this group and making some pretty big lifestyle changes. Even though you seem a little annoyed by coming, you have been participating and sharing, and seem to have a lot of ideas about your future and how you'd like to live your life. I notice your high energy, and imagine that this will help you if you decide to make some changes. While I understand your aggravation, I wonder if you would be willing to put aside the way the doctors bother you for now, and focus on the possibility of changes that you see as potentially helpful?"

By acknowledging real concerns and frustrations without dwelling on them, and by affirming positive aspects of each member, you can diminish the relevance of other forces that initially pushed the member to participate. You can interact similarly with any negative focus that members may present.

A third principle that can guide your work is to *bring the group into the moment*. To some degree, this can be done simply by welcoming members and focusing their attention on the group session rather than the outside— for example, "How are you feeling tonight?" or "I notice that you seem relaxed this afternoon" or "What would you like to accomplish this morning?" instead of a welcome that focuses members' attention outside of the group, such as "How have things been since our last meeting?"

It is also useful to guide members to a fourth principle, to *focus on the present* when discussing their lives. While it is helpful to develop basic familiarity with significant situations and people in members' lives, lengthy storytelling can slow down group progress. Initially, members may be confused by your redirection back into the moment, and it can be helpful to give a brief explanation. For example:

> "Even though everyone has a long history before coming into the group, we generally try to focus on the present and on going forward rather than on details about things that happened in this past. And while it can be important to learn some things about one another's current lives, we will focus more on your own journey and possibilities to

make things better than on things that go on in your lives from week to week."

A fifth relevant principle of the exploring perspectives phase is to *acknowledge suffering, while not eliciting grievances*. Members bring their pain and troubles from life into the group. This suffering can color their perspectives on whether change is necessary, possible, or likely to result in a better life. It can compel members' attention and block progress. Fortunately, simply sharing it with concerned others is often all that is needed to put this in the background and allow the person to focus on making things better. You don't need to spend significant time analyzing suffering or its causes, or on the details of negative experiences. Usually, it is sufficient to reflect the feelings and the person's determination to move forward despite negative experiences.

Group Dynamics

During the engagement phase, members get to know aspects of one another's personal identities, such as hobbies, habits, and interests. As the group interaction deepens, more of members' *social identities* emerge, reflecting their typical patterns of relating within different social networks (family, coworkers, friends, etc.). Members have different habitual ways of relating to others, and these emerge and influence group process, recreating typical interactive patterns that exist in their everyday lives. These may be stronger and more influential in psychotherapy groups, but they affect psychoeducational and support groups as well.

These interactive patterns can contribute to remaining stuck (for example, less assertive members may have more difficulty reducing interpersonal stressors that then influence them to eat more, use substances, etc.; members with aggression problems may be easily triggered to conflict by reading hostile intent into neutral messages, etc.). Thus, a benefit of groups is that members learn new social and interpersonal skills in group interactions that can then be applied to those real-life relationships. Watch for dynamics that develop between members that may echo problematic dynamics in their social lives. Members' social roles and patterns can be examined, and interactions can be stopped and restarted on a more productive path. Initially, simply noting awkward or over-rehearsed interactions between members who are still new to each other is a useful strategy to explore their perspectives on social relationships. Later, as the group is broadening perspectives, you may swing back to these issues, if they provide momentum for change. While MI groups are not strongly process-oriented (the primary focus is not on in-session interactions and group dynamics), helping members perceive and change social patterns can be helpful, and sometimes failing to address such patterns means that a barrier to change remains stubbornly in place.

In successful MI groups, the group itself develops into a *positive social network* in which members participate, attach, and influence and are influenced. In order to promote this, continue to use strategies such as linking members, finding areas of overlapping interest, promoting their interest and involvement in other members' exploration and goal setting, and supporting one another. Group members develop a sense of group identity, and also their own social identity and role within the group, sometimes growing into new social habits, roles, and identities. This increases both their investment in the group and their openness to share their thoughts with other members. Often, members emerge with an expanded self-definition and new skills, and also greater confidence as a result of such transformative processes.

As members bond, develop a shared sense of commitment to improving things together, and experience mutual support, the group becomes more *cohesive*. To achieve strong cohesion, engage members as a group rather than as a collection of individuals, interweaving your focus back and forth from specific individuals to the group as a whole. Framing exercises or topics as things "we" do or explore together (rather than "you") is a subtle but useful way of contributing to cohesion. Consistently linking members via exploration of mutual content, themes, beliefs, attitudes, and hopes also builds cohesion. Keep in mind that cohesion is related to engagement, self-disclosure, investment, effort, and, ultimately, to group outcomes.

Therapeutic Factors

Four of the therapeutic group factors described in Chapter 2 are particularly important during this phase. These include *universality, acceptance, instillation of hope,* and *learning from interpersonal interactions.*

Early group engagement can change people from being isolated individuals into members of a collaborative group. As members move beyond initial engagement to more thorough exploration, they become more aware of one another's situations, issues, perspectives, and challenges. Through careful initial linking of members' issues and challenges, you can raise awareness of the *universality* of challenges, struggles and setbacks. As the exploration of issues and perspectives continues, linking members helps to develop connections between them and leaves them feeling less isolated and alone. It also helps them understand themselves better, because of the related examples they have to consider in other members' situations.

Often, group members' experience of sharing a common bond increases motivation, and problems become reframed more broadly as group members take on "our problems." Generalizing and tackling challenges as a group is a form of broadening focus that begins now and fully flowers as the group continues to develop. This can increase members' sense of *acceptance* by other group members. Optimism also increases as the focus subtly shifts from individual members' problems to the shared processes of change and as members experience the emotional support that is provided by the group. Because many members are initially demoralized, this *instillation of hope* is an important aspect of the help that groups can provide. While the attitudes and expectations of the therapist in individual MI can provide a sense of optimism that "this might work," witnessing the growth of other group members is a very powerful source of reclaimed hope. As the group continues to develop bonds and explore topics, members have an opportunity to learn from interpersonal interactions by developing and practicing social skills in a safe environment. Many who struggle with mental disorders, addictive disorders, chronic health problems, or criminal behaviors come to group with underdeveloped social skills or maladaptive social habits. Within the group, they have the opportunity to practice engaging in "small talk" while waiting for session to start or when departing. They also practice sharing perspectives, listening to others, giving feedback, and managing conversations with a group of former strangers. All of these opportunities for refining socializing skills can generalize to their lives.

Through mutual feedback about their ideas and effects on one another, members also benefit at the deeper level of relationships—learning how to build trust, share vulnerabilities, understand how others perceive them, and so on. This kind of learning usually occurs within the context of meaningful personal relationships with parents, family, romantic partners, and close friends. While members may have experiences with positive people in their lives, some struggle to overcome ingrained negative interpersonal habits that can be addressed in group, resulting in their learning to better manage the give and take of relatedness, recognize interpersonal sensitivities that trigger nearly automatic, nonoptimal reactions to others and recognize their own behaviors that negatively affect others.

Leader Functions

Managing Boundaries

You began establishing group norms as the group first engaged, and part of your attention should remain on managing key group boundaries over subsequent sessions. These include time management, membership in the group, member commitment to attending and participating in the group, and also shaping topical focus. Members may need guidance about attending every session or notifying the group if they must be absent for a particular session, arriving on time and remaining for the entire session, without outside distractions. Emphasizing how attendance and participation are important to others in the group draws attention to the importance of the larger group beyond the individual members involved. Such guidance can be given early in the group, before lateness or absences occurs, and can be repeated when a member is tardy or returns after an absence. For example:

> "Right now, we're focused on exploring each other's perspectives, and getting to know and understand one another. While we're doing this, it's important that we build the group together through shared experiences that increase understanding and trust for one another, and that's harder to do if people aren't always here and involved. We'll have a better experience if we all arrive on time, stay the whole time, participate as much as we can, and let the group know ahead of time if anyone needs to miss. How does that sound?"

Group Norms

During this phase, continue to develop group norms out of the agreed-upon guidelines and ongoing interactions, including norms about talk time and content. Notice the length of time spent focusing on individual members, and how members take their time or do not initiate their own turn. It is not important for every member to get equal time per session. Instead, they should develop a sense that everyone's issues will be addressed, at least briefly, and that although some members get more focus than others, all can benefit, and future sessions may focus more on different members. Help this along by linking content and themes across members, so that even if one member does not raise a particular issue, he or she remains involved when another member deals with a similar issue.

While managing turn-taking and talk time, also balance the amount of time you focus on individuals versus the group as a whole. Early on, relatively more time may be spent on individual members, with relatively less time spent on the group generally. However, as you reflect on the processes you observe in the group, members develop a better sense of the group as a whole and make more comments about group identity or processes over time. During the exploring perspectives phase, you might expect perhaps 70–80% of the focus to be on members, their interconnected issues, and common themes, with about 20–30% of the focus on the group as a whole, with its own characteristics, including boundaries, norms, types of content, and so forth.

Another area to balance is the amount of attention given to the past, present, and future. The eventual goal for nearly all of the focus to be on the present and future. However, there is usually some initial focus on the past as members explore what brought them to where they are now. Guide members to give just enough detail about their past, so that you and the other group members understand the current situation, but not in so much detail that attention to the past derails a focus on the present.

An additional group norm to be developed during this stage is for members to speak mostly on their own issues and how they connect to others rather than commenting on others' issues. While some may feel comfortable asking others about their interests and concerns, it is best not to allow any particular member to play a "junior therapist" role in the group. This does not mean that you should stop members from commenting on issues raised by others. Members should feel free to give feedback and share common experiences with each other but they should expect to balance their comments on others' situations with appropriate self-disclosure, and not go too far too fast. The following vignette illustrates how this might develop in a group during the exploring perspectives phase:

TOMÁS: So, all this makes me upset. The judge is breathing down my neck, my boss is threatening to fire me if I have more jail time, and my wife says she can't take much more of this. She's really piling on the pressure to do right and it's making it harder.

VANESSA: Wow, Tomás, you're really dealing with a lot of stress, but so is she.

TOMÁS: Yeah, it's been hard.

VANESSA: So what are you gonna do about your wife? Are you trying to make things better between you?

LEADER 1: Vanessa, it sounds like you're concerned about Tomás and curious about what he'll do to make his situation better. What does his story bring up that's related to your own situation?

VANESSA: Well, I'm feeling like the lady who has to deal with a situation that she didn't make but has to live with. I'm in the same boat as his wife. Even though I'm here to make my own changes, I'm also waiting to see what my boyfriend will do, and he's kind of a mess. He hasn't kept up with supporting me and the kids, and he's been to jail on and off, which means he's out of the picture a lot, and I have to deal with everything—raising the kids, paying for diapers and clothes, dealing with the bills, all of it. Sometimes I just think how unfair it is, and how he should make it up to me. So I can relate to Tomás's wife. I'm hoping Tomás does right by her.

LEADER 1: So when Tomás mentioned how his wife reacts, it reminded you of your own situation and made you want to give Tomás suggestions about how to treat his wife.

VANESSA: Yeah, it did. I just want him to do right by her, and I bet she'd support him more if he would at least tell her that he understands about the pressure on her, since she has to see that he really is trying to change.

LEADER 1: If your partner would really listen with an open mind, what would you ask him to do differently, and what would you do differently?

VANESSA: Well, I'd just like to know his plan to get out of the mess enough to be able to at least help out more, and I'd like him to acknowledge that I'm carrying most of the load right now even if I have to keep doing it while he straightens things out. If he'd just do that, I'd probably stop picking fights and probably be more supportive, too.

LEADER 1: So you're kind of waiting and watching to see what he does, then adjust based on that.

VANESSA: Yeah, but I guess that's something for me to think about, because if I keep waiting for him to change first, I might be waiting a long time.

LEADER 2: This reminds me of something we haven't talked about too much yet. It's good to be interested and concerned about each other. It's also important to pay attention to what issues get raised when someone shares a similar story. Reactions to other people's stories can be cues that we have an unresolved issue, sometimes one we're not fully aware of until the story triggers the reaction. So when one of us as leaders notices something that seems like that kind of reaction, like a suggestion for another member that seems to have some personal emotion behind it, we might ask about it, as it can reveal something that's important to work through.

SARAH: It sounds like the no cross talk rule in AA.

LEADER 2: OK, so in AA they say "no cross-talk." What does that mean?

JON: It means that you pay attention and learn what you can from each speaker when they share, but you don't comment on it. When it's your turn, you only talk about yourself.

LEADER 2: OK, so that's a bit different from what we do in here. I wonder if anyone else could help to define how this is different.

TOMÁS: It seems like here we each talk, and we listen to each other, and it's okay for us to share, if we're facing something similar, or have a discussion among us about ways that we have things in common, or even give feedback if the person is interested in it. But we should mostly focus on ourselves and what we're doing with our own lives.

VANESSA: Yeah, that's what I'm getting, too.

LEADER 2: Great. And, as we go forward in group, it's fine for us to talk about how things happen in here—how much time we spend on each person, whether there are connections that need to be discussed, and how you want the group to work. This is a place where we can talk about your concerns and plans, but also about how we as a group are functioning.

TOMÁS: That sounds great.

LEADER 1: Tomás, I don't want you to feel cut off if you want to talk a little more about the situation with your wife.

TOMÁS: Actually, listening to Vanessa reminds me how stressful this really is for my wife, and how she probably deserves to give me a little grief. (*Group laughs.*) But, seriously, I know she wants what's best and is worried, and she feels kind of helpless to do anything about it because it's my mess, like Vanessa says. I screwed up bad, no way around it. It's my mess to clean up, and my wife would probably handle it better if I was clearer with her about what I'm trying to do and how much I appreciate her support and patience.

In this example, one leader focuses on individual issues and the other on group processes. Leader 1 is concerned that Vanessa's comments may derail the process of positively exploring members' perspectives. She sees Vanessa's early comments as challenging and a little hostile, and she is concerned that these two members might not yet have a strong enough relationship to deal with this on their own, so she steps in to guide communications between members. She starts by positively reframing Vanessa's comments as concern for Tomás, then shifts the focus to address Vanessa's own situation. As Vanessa follows the lead, the leader broadens the focus to examine an interpersonal dynamic that seems to leave Vanessa stuck. Leader 2 chooses this moment to shift the focus from these two members to further developing group norms, eliciting input from members when possible, instead of defaulting to providing information, and tying the norms to the purpose of the group in supporting the autonomous change of each member. Once this process is finished, Leader 1 shifts the focus back to Tomás, who initiated the conversation, checking to make sure he didn't feel cut off by the temporary shift in focus, and Tomás responded by bringing his perspective on the group discussion back to his own situation.

Managing Emotions

During this phase, help the group members express some emotions, while keeping the overall level of emotional stimulation moderately low. You function as the safety manager of emotional expression in the group. With too much emotion, especially negative emotion, some members can become uncomfortable and retreat, perceiving that things could get out of control.

Others can become combative, trying to "convince" each other that they are wrong or shouldn't feel the way they do. Neither of these results in safety to express emotions within the group as a whole, or is particularly motivating. During this early phase, you can introduce the concept of sharing emotions gradually, encouraging openness but a little caution. Once bonds deepen and more trust develops, members will be able to express more emotions and manage the impact on the group more themselves, without requiring as much direction from you.

You function as the safety manager of emotional expression in the group.

One way you can begin to evoke emotions while keeping them at a safe level is to choose your reflective statements carefully. When members express intense feelings, you might reflect them at a somewhat lower intensity, or shift the focus from the target of the feeling to the feeling itself. You might also consider adding a nonemotional aspect to your reflection, putting it in context and eliciting group strategies for addressing intense emotions:

JON: I'm so damn mad I could kill that guy if he comes around me acting like that again. I'd beat him black and blue if I could get away with it, without getting arrested.

LEADER 1: So you're really angry, and at the same time want to avoid being consumed by rage and getting yourself into more trouble.

JON: I know. I know. That's my main goal. It's hard when people keep pushing you to your limits. How many times can you go there without crossing the line?

LEADER 2: What do the rest of you think? How do you deal with this kind of thing?

SARAH: I understand that. There are people in my life that could push me over the edge if I let them, but I can't go through that. I don't want to give them the power, you know?

JON: Yeah, you're right. I guess it might even burn him more if I just ignore him. He wouldn't be able to figure out what I'm up to.

TOMÁS: And the best part is, you'd have some satisfaction but you wouldn't mess up your own life that you're trying to fix.

LEADER 2: So it sounds like one possibility when we're in a conflict is to keep the focus on ourselves and what we're trying to accomplish. That can take a lot of strength sometimes, especially when it seems like people are doing us wrong. What are some other ways to deal with conflict or even to keep from getting drawn into conflicts in the first place?

Here, Leader 1 refocuses, from the member's anger to his presumed strategy to control it—a more productive, prosocial focus. Leader 2 broadens the focus to the entire group, drawing out others' strategies before summarizing the answers across members, then affirms them before narrowing the focus to elicit additional ways they can achieve the goal.

Fostering Client Self-Awareness

Another important leader function during this phase is fostering members' awareness of how they can reframe complaints, concerns, and problems into workable therapeutic tasks. People typically come into groups with an incomplete view of how or why things have happened in their lives, often perceiving that they're victims of others' bad choices, or have bad luck, or are destined to have chronic problems. They may be used to complaining about things to friends and have less experience in choosing to change something about their situation, especially when they think others are doing wrong. In exploring these perspectives, you hear them, understand them, and build an atmosphere in which members may begin to question and change long-held unproductive attitudes and beliefs. By helping members see their own choices and strengths more clearly, you help them view their complaints and situations as potentially addressable. You might also help them dismantle large problems into smaller components that can be addressed in steps.

MI Strategies

While many common MI strategies can be used to explore perspectives in a group, here we emphasize some of those that work well and reduce resistance. These strategies are appropriate early in group development, because they are unlikely to evoke conflict before members have established the bonds and trust in each other that enable a positive resolution to conflicts. We recommend waiting until later in a group's development to use techniques or strategies that may elicit negative emotions, and early on, to maintain a light, even humorous atmosphere that encourages further engagement as members begin to explore their perspectives in a new way.

Some of the more structured strategies we offer here may be particularly good for psychoeducational and support groups, and may be interwoven with unstructured discussion of the issues involved in psychotherapy groups. There are no specific formulas that we recommend. Try to think through the possibilities of each exercise, its purposes and ways of eliciting positive group processes and forward progress from members, and be creative in modifying how you use the ideas. Perhaps try a few different types and configurations of exercises described here to fit your particular group. The important thing is not to imitate these examples but to achieve the goal of increasing members' understanding of the value of exploring and addressing the situations that limit satisfaction with their lives.

Exploring Lifestyles

It is useful to explore members' lifestyles when a group is just getting started. Even if members share a similar problem or diagnosis, they don't yet know each other and may be hesitant to talk directly about vulnerable issues until they are more comfortable with each other. Exploring lifestyles is also a good focus in a single-session group, when you don't expect members to return as a cohesive group. The strategy is easily understood, is unlikely to generate defensiveness, and is a way to begin to understand members' life contexts.

Lifestyles and Habits

One way to explore lifestyles is to get a sense of how people are living, then expand the conversation to habits, possibly including the target behavior (if known), to see how these habits fit in the context of members' lives. This can be used in any type of group, because it is a simple conversational strategy.

How to Do It. You might start by defining the term *lifestyles* as the way we typically live, the things we typically do, how we spend our time, and the people with whom we spend time. Your questions that start the discussion might be: "Let's talk a little about lifestyles. How do you spend your time? What kinds of patterns are there in your daily life?" You can discuss this with the group as a whole, or break the group into pairs or small groups and ask members to talk with each other about it. Continue discussing this until good rapport is established and most members have volunteered some information about their habits. Then ask, "What about some of your habits, like your [insert shared problematic habit here, such as overeating, use of drugs, and so forth]? How does that fit in?" Explore how the behavior fits into their lifestyles, exploring both the positive and negative aspects of the behavior. Or, if focusing on health, ask, "How does your [habit] affect your health?" If you are leading a full-group discussion, reflect what you hear, both individual member statements and common themes, depending on group size and availability of time. You can also ask about the potential for adding healthy habits that are not fully established (e.g., regular exercise, medication adherence, adequate sleep) and how those could fit in. You might end this discussion by asking group members about their reactions to it and how it fits with what they want to get out of the group, reflecting and summarizing responses. Lane and colleagues (Chapter 17) share an example of exploring lifestyles in a group focused on chronic health conditions.

A Typical Day

Asking group members to share the details of a typical day is another way to get information on members' lifestyles and habits, but with even more detail. This activity is also good for all types of groups and works well either at the beginning of a group's development, or later, if group members are focusing too much on concepts rather than their actual behaviors, leading the group to be more of a discussion group than a therapeutic group.

How to Do It. Rollnick, Heather, and Bell (1992) offered an early version of this exercise in an individual consultation. They suggested starting with, "Can we spend the next 5–10 minutes going through a day from beginning to end? What happened, how did you feel, and where did your [habit] fit in? Let's start at the beginning." In groups, first explain the idea of this conversation to members: "It might help us to get a better sense of how each of you live your life in a typical day. Let's spend a few minutes with each person, and I'll guide you through telling us about your typical day." Help the first member who volunteers to tell a story of the day, focusing on feelings and behaviors. Summarize, then move to the next member, either in a round or simply by waiting for the next person to offer an example. As members' stories accrue, add reflections of emerging common themes to keep everyone engaged, such as "Stopping at a restaurant on the way home seems to be a trigger [overeating, drinking, smoking] for several of you so far. Let's see if that's true for others." It is important to check the reactions of other members or invite them to ask questions; otherwise, this activity may become overly focused on a single member at a time and leave others uninvolved. It is also important to guide the story of each person with your own questions, using closed questions as needed to narrow the focus, in order to keep things moving along. Another option, particularly with larger groups, is to use a worksheet that elicits typical morning, afternoon, evening, and nighttime activities, how problematic behaviors fit in, or places where new habits could be added. Once members have had time to write down notes, go through the worksheet as a group, and ask for examples of activities during each time slot and when problematic behaviors occur, or when healthy habits might be best introduced. End by asking group members for their reactions to what they've shared and heard from their peers. Another example of the typical day activity is described by Velasquez, Stephens, and Drenner (Chapter 14).

Exploring Ambivalence

Resolving ambivalence in favor of health or better functioning is a central purpose of MI. Often, people are stuck because they have contradictory thoughts and feelings about their situations and possibilities. They may mentally go back and forth, from one option to another, unable to decide, or having reached a tentative decision they seem unable to act. One of the strategies in MI is to help them organize their thoughts, so that they can perceive the "big picture" all at once rather than narrowly focusing on one aspect, then another, in a circu-

Help people to organize their thoughts so they can better perceive the "big picture."

lar fashion. This can also help move them out of the reflexively defensive posture in which many members begin the group, due to external pressures they have experienced. Exploring ambivalence helps them express all sides of their thoughts and feelings, rather than needing to defend the status quo side of their ambivalence when they think that everyone else is pushing the change side.

Introducing the Concept of Ambivalence

Members may experience a wide range of reactions about why they do and do not want to consider change. In individual MI you can easily monitor any emerging defensiveness and quickly change strategies to diminish it. In groups, this is more challenging to accomplish. Pro-change comments from a few members may elicit withdrawal, criticism, or anti-change comments from others. People who are eager to change may be perceived as naive or unrealistic, whereas those who are less eager may be perceived as threatening or "in denial" of their problems. Once a negative interaction begins, you may have to divert focus to address hurt feelings or resentments between members. This pattern is so common in groups that we recommend that you accommodate for it by introducing the concept of ambivalence early on, especially when you sense that although some members are eager to change, others are less eager.

How to Do It. We recommend openly acknowledging the challenges of making changes. You might start by stating that if change were simple and straightforward, members would have already done it, and that it is common for people to have mixed feelings about change. Even though they may want to make changes, members may be held back by other feelings or thoughts that keep them stuck, such as feeling unable to change right now. So the "open to change" and "don't want to change" parts of group members, and the balance between them, is important to understand and explore. State that you are not trying to force anyone to change anything, that you just want to help members get a better sense of their feelings and how those might be keeping them stuck. Members are often glad to be understood and relieved to have the matter out in the open.

If you wish to extend this preliminary discussion into a full exploration of members' ambivalence, make sure to accept the negative or status quo elements but eventually highlight the positive reasons to change, then elicit discussion of how members may overcome the temptations, concerns, or losses they may face in changing.

If you are unable to elicit a detailed discussion of ambivalence, or if you are leading a psychoeducational or support group, you might lead the group members in one of the following structured exercises. "Good things/not-so-good things" is a guided discussion that focuses on elements of the current behavior/situation that members like and elements they like less. "Ambivalence circle" involves a visual model of ambivalence and focuses on members' thoughts and feelings about change. "Group four-square game," a game version of a decisional balance exercise, considers the pros and cons of changing and of staying the same to help members reach an informed (and hopefully longer-lasting) decision about making changes.

Good and Not-So-Good Things

This conversational strategy works well when at least a few members have identified current target behaviors, whether similar or different.

How to Do It. Begin by summarizing the common themes. For example, "Several of you are struggling with smoking, and whether and how to cut back or quit. It might be helpful to explore the things you like about smoking. What are some of those?" Gather responses and briefly reflect on key comments, until the group seems unable to generate a new list of good things about the target behavior. After you summarize, say something like "There are some not-so-good things about smoking, too. What are those?" Gather responses, reflecting on them along the way, particularly those containing change talk. Summarize key points and themes, as well as change talk you've heard. Finally, offer a summary that highlights the ambivalence among the members:

"Most of you enjoy smoking. It's relaxing, gives you a break from stresses, and allows you to socialize with friends. On the other hand, you're concerned about your health. Susan is considering quitting because her father died of lung cancer, and that's not something she wants to go through. Rick doesn't have the same energy he used to, and can't play the sports he would enjoy with his sons if he didn't have breathing problems. Some of you don't like the example it sets for your kids, it's expensive, and you don't like the way you smell. How does that fit for you?"

Follow with open discussion, or use rounds to ensure that each member comments.

Circle of Ambivalence

This exercise shifts the focus from current behavior to the possibility of change, while still honoring both sides of members' ambivalence.

How to Do It. Draw a circle on a marker board or chart, or provide a handout. Divide the circle in half; label one half "open to change" and the other half "not open to change," as in the diagram below (or use "want to change" and "don't want to change," or even "change" and "status quo"—whatever works better for your group and conveys the basic idea). State that if our feelings about changing are completely balanced, the "open to change" and "not open to change" parts will be approximately equal:

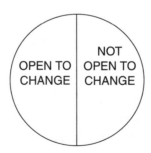

Tell the group that while some may have an exact balance between these parts of themselves, often one part is larger or more dominant in our feelings. Sometimes the circle of mixed feelings (ambivalence) might resemble one of these diagrams, with one side of the mixed feelings stronger or larger:

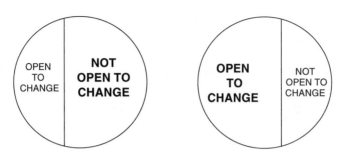

Ask members how these diagrams fit with their experiences. If your group members feel reluctant or demoralized, build their confidence by asking them to recall a previous change they made even in the face of challenges, and discuss how these diagrams and ideas fit that change. This reminds members that they have succeeded in making changes in the past, even though they had ambivalence about them. Spend ample time discussing these experiences and members' thoughts about what helped them make the change. After this discussion, you might offer the idea that change sometimes happens when the "open to change" side grows larger than the "not open to change" side. Mention that both parts exist at the same time, and that it may help them to make a decision about change to explore both sides.

Introducing the concept of ambivalence this way reduces defensiveness, helps members personalize these ideas, frames the possibility of change as something they may freely choose, and builds cohesion among members. Sometimes members take it deeper, into a discussion of underlying negativity about change and the oppositional stance they take toward change or the pressure to change. Several of our collaborators describe approaches to exploring ambivalence in their chapters, and Dunn, Hecht, and Krejci extend their discussion to exploring the functions served by behaviors in Chapter 18 on weight management.

Group Four-Square Game

This game, appropriate for psychoeducational or support groups, is a modified version of a decisional balance that allows members to voice all parts of their ambivalence in a lively and playful format. It is particularly well suited to groups in which all members have identified a similar problem, such as drug use or overeating.

Decisional balance, a cognitive therapy technique that helps people consider the pros and cons of changing and of staying the same, helps people carefully and consciously decide between two options. The way we approach this is not entirely neutral, but it honors the attraction to staying the same, while highlighting reasons to change.

How to Do It. Draw a box with four squares on a chart like the following:

	Pros	Cons
Stay the same		
Change		

Divide the group into two or four subgroups, depending on the size of the group, ensuring that there are at least two members in each group. *In the game, each subgroup competes to see which subgroup comes up with the best answers for each box.* For example, if you have four subgroups, then assign one box to each group and explain its meaning. If you only have two subgroups, assign one to the "stay the same" row and one to the "change" row.

Give each subgroup paper, tell members that you will time them, and that they should generate as many answers as possible for their box within 5 minutes. After time is up, call on each subgroup to report its answers, recording the answers and numbering them as you go. Count up the number of answers and congratulate the subgroup with the most ideas as the first-round winner. Have the members vote on the group with the "best" answers, and congratulate that subgroup as well.

Ask the whole group whether other items should go in one of the boxes. Summarize by reflecting the pros of staying the same and the cons of changing, and mention that these boxes represent temptations or "pulls" to keep doing things that may not be good for us in the long run. Summarize the cons of staying the same and the pros of changing, and note that these boxes represent motivation to change.

Debrief by asking members to mention one thing they notice on the chart that is meaningful to them. If they list something on the pro-change side, ask how they can use that to support making a change. If they list something on the status quo side, ask how they can overcome that or compensate for its loss by replacing it with something that fills the void.

If one of the status quo groups "wins" the game, you might elicit discussion on how people can overcome temptations when they are so appealing, or when there are so many. Make sure that if a status quo group "wins" by having either the most or the best answers in the game, it is not interpreted to mean that change is too hard or not preferred. Instead, reframe it as how our less healthy habits try to "win," as if they have minds of their own, and roll that into a discussion of overcoming temptations or accepting losses.

There are many other ways to explore ambivalence. Downey and Johnson (Chapter 13) describe a "pocket change" exercise, in which members write a change goal on a piece of paper to keep in their pocket. Martino and Santa Ana (Chapter 16) use an exercise called "on the fence," in which a member metaphorically sits "on the fence" while the group argues for or against change, facilitating exploration by the member. They also use an exercise called "warm seat," in which a member sits in a chair in the middle of the group to describe the positives of making a change, while other members take turns sitting in a facing chair to argue against change. This is intended to elicit additional change talk supporting the change by the member. Other chapters describe different ways of integrating a focus on ambivalence into MI groups.

Exploring Values

Members' values provide important guideposts for considering the importance of making changes. Most people think of *values* as convictions about what is important, meaningful, or good in life (e.g., family, honesty, or contributing to the world). Others think in religious or spiritual terms. Values can also refer to experiences we like, such as relaxation, excitement, joy or peacefulness (cf. Wagner & Sanchez, 2002). Members may talk spontaneously about their values (e.g., wanting to be trustworthy, to be a valued family member), providing you the opportunity to summon the better angels of their natures to guide them toward change. Exploring the deeper, often unspoken values of members can deepen the conversation, remind members of what they'd like to aim for and who they want to be, and encourage them to focus behavior changes toward living with greater consistency with their most important values.

Unguided, this type of discussion can raise a sense of negative discrepancy, as in "I'm not living according to my values, and I feel bad about that." We prefer to frame it positively: "Going forward, how could you live more closely to your values?" If any members make negative comments, you can reflect that no one lives perfectly in line with his or her values, and

> *"Going forward, how could you live more closely to your values?"*

that the intention of the discussion is not to make them feel bad but to help them focus on moving forward. This type of discussion is a particularly good fit for psychotherapy groups, but it can also be used in psychoeducational or support groups.

How to Do It. Introduce values similar to the description in the previous subsection. Emphasize that there are no right answers, and that most people have a mix of values, including ideals and preferences, between what they think they should do and what they really like to do. What is important for this discussion is to think about which things really motivate members in their day-to-day lives. Make sure to mention a few kinds of values that are not the typical "ideals" most people think of (e.g., having fun, being active, or having quiet time). Spend some time eliciting members' core values, and if members are struggling to identify them, ask, "What seems important right now at this moment?"

Give members time to think on their own, then begin to elicit a few values from a member. Ask the member to pick one value in particular and describe a time when that value served as an important guide. Often, emotion emerges during this discussion, and this is good and should be accepted (but don't draw too much attention to the emotion as it serves to deepen the experience and generally shouldn't become the primary focus of conversation). Encourage others to tell stories about times when their important values were key to experiences they had or decisions they made. In this context of activated emotion and deeper connection to important values, ask more about how values guide members' choices and actions. Ask how different values might work together, or how they might lead in different directions, and if any values are in conflict with one another, ask how it leaves them feeling or thinking. As you go along, make sure to link together similar themes regarding both the content of the values and how members go about using those values as guides.

Next, ask members to look forward and think about how they could live even closer to their most important values, using them to guide future choices. After discussing these positive, future-oriented hypothetical issues, ask members how their values could guide them regarding the issues they are facing now. Continue to link members' experiences in living consistent with their core values, as mutual empathy and group cohesiveness are amplified to the extent that you can help make these connections between members. Keep the focus on the positive, on moving toward greater congruence or harmony with values, rather than allowing the discussion to move toward the incongruence between values and behavior. Elicit members' reactions to one another's stories.

Some group members may immediately want to address a problematic behavior that may be the focus of their participation in group, but we recommend guiding them to defer that part of the discussion until you come to it. The intention is first to think broadly about values in a positive way, gradually narrow the focus to the more specific relationship between values and behavior, and only then to consider the specific problematic behavior in that context. Consider ending the discussion by offering a series of reflections of themes, perhaps with added reflective emphasis on statements of hopes or plans to bring members' choices and behaviors more in line with core values. Alternatively, ask members to share the stories or values of other members that most impressed them, and which ideas they might wish to incorporate. Finally, if appropriate, reflect on the deepening of experience and sharing that occurred during this exercise, which can be more "personal" than the previous exercises. If members opened up further, if trust seemed to deepen, or the group seems to have gained greater cohesiveness, mention those and how moving forward they can provide a springboard for the group to be even more supportive of each person.

Several contributors' chapters focus on exploring values, and Martino and Santa Ana (Chapter 16) describe a more structured approach to clarification of values and goals for individuals with dual mental health/substance abuse diagnoses.

Tips and Traps

Tips

First, listen more than you talk. It helps group members join the conversation, become comfortable speaking, and get involved. It also helps them begin to interact with each other rather than with you. It is also a way for you to model comfort with the group's pace of sharing, and it allows issues to emerge in a natural way.

Second, coach good listening skills among members. Shape and reframe their communications with each other to be increasingly respectful, supportive of autonomy, and affirming. As they communicate more, reflect common content and themes to link members.

Third, facilitate the development of group cohesion. Comment on (and support) the group's autonomy as it grows.

Fourth, use common language instead of group technical terms.

Fifth, when you are presenting bits of information, use MI strategies. Remember to first elicit what the group knows, and fill in the gaps with brief statements. Follow these up with more open questions.

Traps

A few traps can also occur during this phase of group. First, avoid presenting more than a small bit of information to get conversation flowing. Otherwise, you are likely to end up in a monologue rather than a conversation. Related to this, avoid the expert role of "information provider" or using jargon that sets you apart from the group. This stunts the group's development.

Don't jump into an activity without helping group members understand what you are asking them to do.

Similarly, don't get overly attached to a "curriculum" or session plan. While it can enhance your confidence to plan ahead, being with the group in the moment is more important.

Relatedly, don't fear what might come up in group. Your relaxed attitude and confidence about whatever emerges will encourage group members to share what's real.

The interpersonal tone of the group gets set early. Therefore, don't allow confrontation or attacks among members. If this happens, redirect and reframe the communication immediately.

Don't interact too long with any one member without involving the others, or allow a few members to dominate the conversation. Affirm their example of being willing to share, but involve others as soon as possible.

Progress Indicators

When members have shared some details and perspectives, and have a sense of "now what?" or of openness to exploring some new ideas and looking forward, the group has made progress toward change. This may happen over the course of a single session, or it might take several sessions to accomplish, depending on your setting, population, size of group, and other issues. Although it is important not to hurry the group forward, when at least half of the members seem ready to consider some new things, it may be time to transition into the next phase, *broadening perspectives*.

References

Rollnick, S., Heather, N., & Bell, A. (1992). Negotiating behaviour change in medical settings: The development of brief motivational interviewing. *Journal of Mental Health, 1*, 25–37.

Wagner, C. C., & Sanchez, F. (2002). The role of values in motivational interviewing. In W. R. Miller & S. Rollnick. *Motivational interviewing* (2nd ed., pp. 284–298). New York: Guilford Press.

CHAPTER 11

Phase III

Broadening Perspectives

By now, you should notice a shift in the group, from people still getting to know each other and directing their comments mostly to you, to group members having a conversation together. They may still interact with you regularly, but they have become familiar with one another's situations and perspectives and have begun deepening connections with each other. In exploring their situations, some may show a new openness, expressing thoughts such as "I never thought about it that way" and "I'd like it to be different, even if I'm not sure how." At this point, your group is likely moving on to the next phase, *broadening perspectives*.

MI groups approach issues from within clients' perspectives rather than trying to teach them to see and handle things differently. However, we don't work only with ideas or perspectives that members already hold, because this would limit the helpfulness of the group. Members are often stuck precisely because their perspectives have them boxed into self-limiting beliefs about their challenges and a lack of awareness about how they might approach their situations more productively. So the task is twofold: (1) Avoid the risks of trying to convince group members to see and do things differently, and (2) help them develop broader perspectives on the issues facing them, so that they discover or develop more productive ways of living.

By expanding their perspectives to include new ideas and interests, group members gain a greater range of possible choices. Helping them broaden their field of vision makes their problems seem smaller by comparison, increasing their sense of freedom. Through broadening members' perspectives, you keep the group moving forward by evoking direction and

199

momentum, enhancing investment and confidence in change possibilities. At the same time, attend to members who are slower to engage, perhaps still unsure of what to focus on, or who show signs of defensiveness. You might introduce the shift in your work together overtly. For example:

> "We've spent four sessions together and are getting to know each other and the challenges we face. Some of you have a pretty clear focus, and others are still unsure. We've spent most of our time talking about your concerns, the pressures you face, and a little bit about how you got here. Now let's spend some time looking toward the future, not to get ahead of ourselves, but to pick a star to steer by, like sailors used to out on the ocean, to avoid getting lost. In the group, we might explore each of your guiding stars, where you're heading. What are some examples of those?"

Whether you use sailing or some other example, using imagery that fits your group can help members shift to focusing on the future and imagining possibilities. Invite and link members' thoughts; accept their doubts or concerns about moving forward, but focus mostly on the possibilities.

Guiding Principles

While undertaking the tasks involved in the broadening perspectives, please keep some principles in mind to guide you. First, continue to maintain a *focus on the positives,* attending to the positive desires, needs, plans, and aspects of each member. For example, you might reflect to members who are still unsure about what changes they want to make, "While this scares you a bit, you're also open to the possibilities." For someone who seems stuck focusing on the history of the problem rather than on the possibilities for change, you might reflect and reframe, "It seems like you really want to understand this deeply and make sure you are well-prepared to make changes that work best for you." In addition to these general perspectives, a focus on the positive also includes intentionally creating an atmosphere

---

Guiding Principles for the Work of Broadening Perspectives

- Focus on positives.
- Focus on the future.
- Develop discrepancy.
- Accept defensiveness.

that naturally evokes positive emotions such as calmness, curiosity, joy, and acceptance. These positive emotions are not only themselves rewarding, but they also reduce the likelihood of strife within the group, evoke creativity among group members, and increase group cohesion.

The concept of broadening perspectives is adapted in part from Frederickson's "broaden-and-build" model of positive emotions (Fredrickson, 2004; Fredrickson & Branigan, 2005; Fredrickson & Losada, 2005). Traditional emotions theory suggests that negative emotions serve to focus attention on perceived threats and prime people to act (e.g., negative emotions such as anger or fear prompt people into fight-or-flight responses; cf. Nesse, 1990). Frederickson proposes the complementary notion that, rather than narrowing attention like negative emotions, positive emotions broaden attention so that people can perceive possibilities beyond the obvious ones and be more creative in solving problems. The "build" part of the model is that during times of stability between threats, positive emotions assist people to build resources that help them the next time they are under threat—building not only physical resources but also social bonds, cohesion, and interdependence among members of a group. Thus, while negative emotions serve to provide immediate protection in threatening situations, positive emotions serve to increase creativity and help people to build protective and supportive structures between threats.

Extending this to MI groups, not only does a positive group environment directly help members to escape downward spirals of negativity, it also helps them be more creative in fashioning better long-term solutions, and connects them to the wisdom and resources of the larger group. This expands the range of perceived possibilities and contributes to confidence about change (in that what "I" may not be able to do alone, perhaps "we" can accomplish together), prompting development of an upward spiral toward greater well-being (Frederickson & Joiner, 2002).

The strategies during this phase are those that help members open up to ideas beyond their previous, narrower vision of who they are and what options they have, while connecting them to the greater power of the group. Part of this process is to help members *focus on the future* rather than on the past or even on present circumstances. Guiding members to imagine together a number of future possibilities also helps them imagine a number of potential paths to get there. In essence, they are developing new goals for themselves that focus more on the vision they create for the future than on their histories.

It is helpful to *develop discrepancy* in a positive manner during this phase of group development. Developing discrepancy involves exploring the differences between clients' values and behavior, or between their preferred futures and present actions that may not lead toward their hopes and goals. While developing discrepancy, clients may sometimes experience

Helping members broaden their perspectives beyond a narrow vision of themselves and their options, while connecting them to the power of the group, facilitates significant change.

moderate tension that motivates them to change in order to "escape a dilemma" or avoid an undesired outcome. Yet developing discrepancy may also involve positively reenvisioning the future by piquing interest and curiosity, identifying the path most likely to lead to fulfillment and helping clients become motivated to seek that in place of their current lifestyles (Wagner & Ingersoll, 2008). We believe that this focus on positive discrepancy works better in groups. How can members' lives be better? How can they be more proud of themselves or more confident? How can they live more closely in line with their deepest beliefs and values? The discrepancy between their current behaviors and hoped-for future motivates people to close the gap, by either changing behaviors or letting go of their hopes for the future. The group's support can make it more likely that people resolve the discrepancy in favor of building a better future instead of downsizing their dreams.

In addition to the intrapersonal elements of discrepancy (relating only to the person at hand), you can also develop positive discrepancy interpersonally, across group members. For example, in sharing success stories, personal strengths, accomplishments, or personal goals, you can link one member's accomplishments with another's hopes, one person's areas for growth with another's strengths, and so on. Members not only provide support to one another but also inspire one another and provide detailed examples of possibilities to pursue, in a way that can have more impact than the hypothetical possibilities discussed in individual MI.

When group members first engage with you and with each other during the exploring perspectives phase, members may show some defensiveness about opening up to you and a room of strangers. During the broadening perspectives phase, you may see some return of tension when members consider making changes, which is common and can provide some of the fuel for change. However, many people can tolerate only limited amounts of uncertainty, and when they feel pressured or overwhelmed and the tension becomes too uncomfortable, they begin to debate, discount, or withdraw. Use MI strategies to reduce defensiveness if it reaches this level so that members feel safe and can refocus their attention on the possibilities of change rather than feeling they need to defend their autonomy in the face of pressure to change.

Accepting defensiveness may seem to be an unnecessary skill when the group is running well, but it may be needed at any time, because discord can arise seemingly from nowhere in groups. Members may sometimes silently stew while others are talking, then unleash their frustrations, fears, anger, or hopelessness when another member makes some seemingly innocuous comment. Managing negative feelings is a common part of group work. When negativity arises, staying relaxed enables you to approach its resolution thoughtfully. Remember that people commonly experience some reluctance when they stretch to consider solutions to their problems and implement significant changes in their lives. If you become tense, it limits your ability to conceptualize what is happening and the most productive ways to approach it. When you feel comfortable with some tension, members are more comfortable experiencing and working through the feelings and issues involved.

Group Dynamics

While using these principles to guide you, anticipate shifts in the group dynamics as you move through this phase. Typically, group identification grows, and cohesion and depersonalized trust deepen as the group builds a sense of homogeneity. We discuss each of these in turn.

As described previously, our social identity is focused on our relationships with others, such as family and friends, and our participation in formal or informal groups. Identifying with these groups lessens our sense of isolation, expands our "me" view to become part of a "we" that embeds us in social interactions that shape who we are, what we believe, and what we value. You can help members adopt the group as part of who they are by linking members' themes and experiences. Through this process of *group identification,* the group eventually becomes "us." Members view group sessions not just as places to go to accomplish tasks (or meet attendance requirements), but as "our group"—an entity with its own identity. Their bonds with one another deepen, and they feel a part of a community to which they can contribute. This further increases the group's cohesiveness.

As cohesion deepens and the group identity increases, greater trust develops, both individual trust ("Sandy seemed to understand what I was saying and helped me out") and broader *depersonalized trust* ("My group supports me when I'm struggling"). You can facilitate this by noticing and affirming helpful intentions among members. You can reflect group processes, such as times when members put their trust in the group to share experiences and perceptions about which they feel vulnerable. You might reflect that the person took a risk in sharing, or focus on how the group helps members to be more comfortable sharing vulnerabilities and resolving some of their problems. Your reflections help to protect budding group cohesiveness, until it grows beyond the need for a container.

Another element that builds cohesiveness and group identification is for members to perceive themselves as traveling together on a shared journey. It is not members' external similarity on age, ethnicity, or social background that is most important, but their sense of sharing core similarities and experiences with one another. You can help develop this sense of *group homogeneity* by evoking and reflecting similarities among members. While some of these similarities may be situation-specific (e.g., similar problem focus areas or goals), you can deepen this perception by linking members around their ambivalence about change, their mutual striving toward more satisfying lives, and their sense of commitment to take greater ownership of their lives and make changes to accomplish their goals. You can reflect more broadly on their shared experiences as companions along a pathway of change, and even more broadly on the path of life. Finally, it can help to emphasize ways that members' tasks are *interdependent,* in that they benefit from one another's perspectives and ideas and mutual support toward meeting their goals. Thus, when an individual member makes a gain in life, the whole group gains and members can celebrate the accomplishment together.

Therapeutic Factors

Most of the therapeutic factors remain relevant during this phase, and several become more prominent. Members and leaders provide mutual *guidance.* How guiding is handled is key to whether members take in and personalize new ideas, or discount, dismiss, or reject them. Next is *vicarious learning.* As some members discuss their methods for coping with or resolving issues, others may imitate their style of thinking and talking about issues, and try out their strategies. Affirming positive efforts or strategies in group does more than simply provide a boost for the member being affirmed; it highlights those strategies for other group members, inviting them to take note and consider the strategies for themselves.

Expressing emotions and experiencing others' healing responses allow some members to experience *catharsis,* the sense of relief following the release of emotional strain. This may reduce the risk of being stuck in regret, blame, fear, or sadness, and free people to take new actions toward change. While MI groups do not intentionally create cathartic experiences in order to break through emotional barriers or defensive conceptualizations, moments of catharsis do happen and can be productively incorporated into the group's progress.

MI groups also do not focus as intently on developing *self-understanding* as do other group approaches. However, people avoid change partly because they don't want to face frightening realities, and have to acknowledge that life has gotten out of hand and change may be needed to avoid the downward spiral ahead. It can also be difficult for members to enter unknown situations that require them to face what they have been avoiding, sometimes for years, such as being alone, being unsure who they really are once they stop playing out comfortable but dysfunctional roles, or coping without their usual crutches. While MI groups do not intentionally lead members to explore deeper existential issues, these may emerge spontaneously when members face the need to change their lives for the better. Exploring such issues requires comfort with being vulnerable in front of others, and it is advisable only once cohesion, trust, and hope are well-established. If existential issues arise too early, the person may not experience the group's support, and upon ending the discussion, may retreat from the group out of a sense of shame or heightened vulnerability. Also, such exploration may be too intense for other members, who may pull back and retreat to superficiality, because they are not ready to face similar issues themselves. However, when group cohesion, trust, and hope have developed, exploring existential issues can be powerful as members broaden their perspectives to consider not only new possibilities, but also expanded self-definitions and renewed senses of meaning and purpose. When this happens, group members can truly transcend previous self-limiting perspectives and beliefs.

Instilling hope remains an important therapeutic factor during this phase of group development. People become stuck partly because their perspective is limited by the presence of problems, conflicts, and hopelessness. Broadening their perspective involves developing an increased sense of possibilities and strengths, and a clearer vision of a better future. Members' perspectives broaden to include greater focus on these positive elements when they witness fellow members moving forward. As they try new options within the safe setting of the group, they gain hope about their own future.

Leader Functions

Several leader functions are highly relevant to the broadening perspectives phase. Again, with co-leaders, one might focus more on the MI strategies and eliciting content from individual members, while the other focuses more on group dynamics, therapeutic factors, and leader functions.

Managing Boundaries

Early in the group's development, managing boundaries involved logistical issues such as time management, attendance, and participation. Now, your attention shifts toward managing boundaries around members' group experiences and interactions. Differences in emotional expression and anxiety levels often emerge as the group experience deepens and moves beyond superficial interactions. Early optimism may be replaced by anxiety related to the challenges of making life changes. Some members may grow impatient and voice frustrations, while others internalize the anxiety and become quieter. Small differences between members may develop into larger differences. Some members may become more reactive to the occasional suggestion someone makes.

These developments are a regular part of the process of change in groups. Some represent members' reactions to their increasing awareness of discrepancy between how things are and how they could be, or between their desires and impulses and what they think they should be doing. Drawing attention to these reactions can lessen the likelihood that the group experience becomes overwhelming. Sometimes, this just involves reflecting reactions. Other times, it is helpful to affirm members' willingness to tolerate some discomfort, and their patience in working through issues that arise. Sometimes, light supportive humor can help break the seriousness of a moment, while at other times it is best to keep quiet and let the moment unfold, giving the ideas time to sink in.

Group Norms

As the group develops, you can promote a shift toward greater member–member interaction. One way is to defer answering a question and put it out for group comment, eliciting several reactions, and introducing the concept that "there are many good ideas" or "many ways to do it." Finish by asking the person who posed the question to react or summarize.

You can also promote members' interest in others' issues rather than focusing only on their own concerns. Until this shift happens, there is always a risk that the group will feel like a series of individual mini-sessions, in which members wait for a turn to talk about themselves and give only partial attention when others speak. A better functioning group is one in which members attend to their own issues but also show interest, compassion, and optimism regarding others' challenges. One thing you can do is ask members to give the speaker their attention, so that the person benefits from the interest and support of the group. Ask them to listen carefully for how the issues, concerns, or processes relate to their own. Guide them to talk to each other, while you reduce interactions with individual members.

In a well-functioning group, members attend to their own issues, but also show interest, compassion and optimism about others' challenges.

Additionally, by linking members' themes and experiences along the pathway of change, you increase their broader interest in each other. For example, you might link members' experiences of ambivalence:

> "Jon, you and Tomás have both talked about trying new things instead of drinking, and about your mixed feelings. And Denise, you said you have mixed feelings about taking your medications. It seems like several of you are focused on how to do what you think is best, even while you have mixed feelings."

You can also reflect on and promote unfolding aspects of group process:

- "I'm noticing that whenever someone brings up a really tough issue, everyone listens carefully and allows the person plenty of time to get through it."
- "This is a lively group today; I'm excited to see how you're working with each other! There's a good energy in the room as you talk about making some positive changes."
- "You're opening up an important issue—how to develop trust with each other and make the group what you want it to be. It's in your hands to create the kind of group atmosphere you think will help you get where you want to go."

During the broadening perspectives phase, norms solidify around providing support and advice to one another. Initially, when members interact, they may provide examples from their own lives or provide direction or even direct advice to other members. Later, as they become more attuned and listen more deeply, and with guidance and modeling from you, members learn to pause before assuming that their personal examples or advice are necessarily the most helpful thing for the person in the moment. Rather, they may learn to ask the person what would be helpful from the group, or ask permission to comment on something the peer has said. You can help this process along by modeling both listening and respectful responding, and making overt comments such as the following:

> "You might want to share an experience to help each other when you notice that someone is in pain, something that worked for you when dealing with something similar. And that's a great impulse to have. On the other hand, it can be hard for someone to hear others' success stories if they sound too much like advice. One way to check out whether the person is ready to hear you is to say something like, 'I have some

thoughts about your situation, but I want to make sure I understand it first. If you want support or ideas, let us know.'"

As the group develops, members focus more on their interactions with each other. Following your example, they may begin to comment on patterns of interactions. "Hey, I notice that when we all talk at once and get loud, Sarah looks like she wants to escape. Sarah, are you okay?" When the group is newer, members mostly tell stories about their interactions outside the group. When the conversation focuses on what is happening here and now in the room, however, greater learning and change may occur. You can facilitate this shift in group norms by modeling and making overt statements such as the following:

> "I notice that whenever a few of you seem a bit overwhelmed or frustrated with each other, someone else will change the subject to something lighter, I guess in order to reduce the tension. I wonder what we're missing by not continuing to explore the things that bother people. Have you ever noticed how people sometimes speak their minds more in tense moments than in lighter moments, as long as it doesn't become too intense?"

You can also focus on how to address thornier issues. For example:

> "I wonder if we could slow it down a bit. Tomás and Matt, you both seem a little frustrated. Why don't we take a few minutes to hear each of your perspectives, and then let's see if there's some common ground. Tomás, would you start by sharing how you're feeling, and what thoughts you have after hearing Matt share his concerns?"

A last group norm that is likely to change during this phase involves members taking more ownership of the direction of the group, developing a greater sense that "this is our group and we should make it what we want it to be." Some may comment that they are glad to get beyond the superficial and go deeper, that they feel safer sharing, and that they trust each other more. This provides another opportunity to link members around themes of what is useful about the group and what they'd like more of, setting the stage for them to discuss openly how they'd like the group to develop. It is common during this phase for some members to point out that others are not yet fully involved, or to request more sharing from members who have been quieter.

ROBIN: I feel pretty comfortable talking about personal things, but with you, Patricia, I never really know what you're thinking, and it makes me nervous.

DAVID: Yeah, Patricia, sometimes when you're quiet it comes across almost like you're sitting there in judgment. I wish you'd say more.

PATRICIA: What? I don't sit in judgment. It's just hard for me to say what I think. I usually think you're so brave to share how you really feel, because that's so hard for me. The last thing I'm doing is judging you!

ROBIN: Well, that's a relief. But, when you're quiet, sometimes your face looks . . . upset or angry maybe, and it's easy to feel like you are disapproving of what you are hearing.

PATRICIA: My face probably looks upset because I'm usually telling myself that I'm not doing the right thing in this group. . . . All of you seem so able to say what's on your minds, and I just don't know how to do that. I guess I need help, but I haven't known how to ask.

JON: Hey, Robin, I'm glad you brought this up. Patricia, I was thinking you were just kind of distant. Instead, it sounds like you've been stressed about holding yourself back, and you'd like to be able to open up. That's good, because I think we all want that. (*Heads nod around group. There is a momentary pause in the discussion.*)

LEADER: Patricia, what have you heard?

PATRICIA: Maybe they thought I didn't care or was even judgmental, because I'm stuck in my own head. Now, maybe people won't always think I'm angry at them or don't like what they're saying. I guess people want me to share more of my thoughts. I just don't know how to start.

LEADER: What does everyone think about that? (*Group members respond, affirming Patricia's reflections.*) It sounds like you've made a good start at opening this issue up. Now Patricia has shared that she doesn't know how to get started. . . . What do you want to do about that?

DAVID: Would it be helpful if we check in with you as we're having discussions?

PATRICIA: Maybe, but I might feel put on the spot and freeze up.

JON: How about if we just notice when you're being quiet and give you the option to share, but only if you feel ready? Remember when we first started—I didn't want to talk to anybody. It took a few sessions for me to realize that you're all good people, and I decided to take the risk to discuss some of my personal business.

PATRICIA: That sounds good, and I'll try to speak up a little more on my own, too. I really do think that's something I need to change, speaking up and standing up for myself overall. So if you promise not to laugh at me if it comes out wrong, I'll promise to try.

ROBIN: It's a deal! And thanks for telling us how hard it is for you to talk.

LEADER: So maybe you'll give it a try with something that doesn't feel too big the first time and see how it goes. And the rest of us will listen and be supportive, knowing that this is a little nerve-racking for you.

Attention to Emotions

During the broadening perspectives phase, increased expression of emotion will propel the group into deeper, more meaningful exploration. Just as reflection of emotion in individual MI is considered a complex process, developing a supportive atmosphere in which emotions are expressed, reflected, and shared in group is also complex. Although by this point the group members have built trust and cohesion, the group can still be threatened by a sudden, intense burst of negative emotion, especially if it is not satisfactorily resolved. Rather, the goal is gradually to increase the group's comfort with expression of emotions as part of exploring and broadening perspectives, while keeping anxiety at a manageable level across members. This process makes the group a safe place to express and resolve difficult emotions, which is an important part of making changes. Emotionality may even be a focus of change; some members may need to learn to express their feelings better, while others may need to tone things down a bit, taking others' reactions into account. The process of deepening, described in Chapter 8, is an essential part of facilitating the increased sharing of emotions and emotionally meaningful material.

At times, the group may reach its tolerance level for emotional expression, and you may want to lighten the focus (also discussed in Chapter 8). You can reflect emotions using words that slightly understate the intensity (e.g., "bothered" rather than "angry") to lighten the mood. You can also comment on the processes of sharing emotions that you note in the group. For example, you might reflect on one member's expression of emotion, while inviting other members to join in the discussion of managing emotions more generally:

> "Flora, your mother's comment really hurt you, and you thought it meant that she hadn't noticed the progress you've made. You're feeling tempted to get high again to numb the pain, but you also want to keep moving forward, no matter what others say. How have others managed this kind of feeling?"

When you comment on sharing emotions, you might provide a potential guideline to ease members' anxieties about the group becoming overly focused on emotion:

> "One thing that shows me the group has grown in trust is that several of you have revealed some intense emotions, and the group has heard

you. Sometimes when this happens, some of you might worry that the group is going to become like a big wave of emotion.

I'd like to suggest a possible guideline about that. When emotions are shared, we will continue to listen respectfully as we have been doing. But we will also make sure that before the group is over, each person who's shown some deep emotion will have a chance to wrap things up, so that you feel comfortable leaving here and aren't worried about being upset when the group ends. Also, we could do a brief 'check-out' with everyone before the end of group if there's been a particularly emotional conversation, because sometimes even if it wasn't your issue, it might push some buttons, and you might leave upset or worrying about the person who shared. How does that sound?"

In this way, you show comfort with emotion but pay adequate attention to safety. This type of comment sometimes leads to further discussion of what kind of group members want this to be.

Attention to Meaning

One aspect of broadening perspectives is helping members generalize concepts such as ambivalence, struggle, and readiness for change. When this is successful, members come to understand how placing their specific situation in a more general category can reduce their sense of isolation and frustration. To accomplish this, you can redirect members from ongoing discussion of the details of their difficulties toward more general themes related to ambivalence and struggle, importance, confidence, readiness. You can also reflect the meaning rather than the content of their conversations, and use this meaning level to link members thematically. Another option is to explore meaning and values explicitly, using a values exploration exercise or other activity.

Increased Transparency

As the group develops in autonomy and interpersonal maturity, you can increasingly reveal your thoughts about group dynamics and the choices you make as a leader, giving members the chance to observe the group on a meta-level. Beginning this during the broadening perspectives phase is important, because it may become a crucial tool to handle any continuing defensiveness or inertia. You as leader can then "speak the unspeakable," naming a process that is slowing the group's progress, especially an interpersonal process that is noticeable to all but off-limits for discussion under usual social norms.

"Devon, it seems like when discussion turns to child custody issues, it pushes a button for you. I'm not criticizing you about that, and I understand how angry you are that your ex's family's lies keep you from even seeing your kids unsupervised. You say that's it's just the way it is and talking won't do any good. I can respect that, and I think the group generally supports you talking about it when you want and keeping quiet when you don't. At the same time, I notice that you have some strong reactions when similar issues come up—shrinking down in your seat, shuffling your feet, and shaking your head. Then I notice other people stop talking about their situations, even if it seems important to them. And I wonder how people will be able to talk through the things they need to figure out. I don't think you mean to keep people from talking, so I wonder if you'd be willing to share a little about what going on for you when things like this come up, so we can see if there's a middle ground for all of us."

Group leaders using other approaches include some self-disclosure of their own feelings: "I notice I'm feeling uncomfortable as the group has circled back around to this issue of sharing versus distrusting again." However, in MI groups, leader self-disclosure about internal experiences should be used sparingly. There is always a risk that the group will revert to a pattern of members addressing you rather than each other. Because your job during this phase is to protect the group and propel its momentum in doing its work, your role is one of a participant-observer. However, choosing to comment on your own role, its evolution, and its limitations may help members break out of any overly fixed patterns of communicating.

MI Strategies

Most of the MI strategies during the broadening perspectives phase can be done with minimal structure, engaging members in conversations rather than exercises. The way we describe each strategy is just an example of how to develop the focus and achieve your purpose.

Heuristic Models

One useful strategy during this phase is to introduce a heuristic model through which members can view their ongoing habits and patterns. Heuristic models include the stages-of-change model, the ready–willing–able model, and models of adapting to chronic illness. Many useful models are available, and another model may fit your group better. Use positive models that you think will help members see things in a different light and allow their current perspectives to be illuminated.

When using this strategy, introduce one of these conceptual models after you finish your initial check-in with the members (we recommend using only one of these models in a given session, and maybe only one with any particular group). Think of it as providing some useful bits of information (mini-content) rather than education, followed by eliciting discussion and personalizing of the information. Experiment with how you present the mini-content sections and how you help members share their perspectives, whether in dyads, small groups, or as whole group in rounds or general discussion, until you find the right blend that gets the group talking and sharing. Finally, remember that discussion during all of these activities is intended to promote the positive group dynamics and therapeutic factors mentioned earlier in the chapter, and contribute to a positive focus on the future.

Stages of Change

A common heuristic that can be used across contexts is the stages-of-change model. Several published examples provide descriptions of using this model to help members frame their change process in a broader manner (Velasquez, Gaddy-Maurer, Crouch, & DiClemente, 2001; Velasquez, Stephens, & Ingersoll, 2005).

How to Do It. Ask members to think about a significant change they've made in their lives, and briefly elicit a few examples. Next, ask members how long it was from the time they first became aware of the issue to the time they began trying to change it. Usually members give a range of answers, including some who report years between awareness and a change attempt. Then ask how long it was from the time they first began trying to change to completing the change and feeling that it was all behind them. Reflect on commonalities, including any feelings of demoralization along the way. Mention that while their change attempts may have brought some frustration, what they went through is common. Mention that change is usually not immediate; rather, it occurs as a process over time, with occasional setbacks.

Ask whether members are interested in hearing about a different way to view their history and, if so, briefly introduce the stages of change, as illustrated in the accompanying box, perhaps using a wheel or spiral drawing of the model as you explain what each stage means. It can be useful to provide a bit of information, such as the finding that people often make several serious attempts before achieving change in ongoing habits (Prochaska, DiClemente, & Norcross, 1992). This can lower defensiveness as you assist members in recalling successful changes they have made, potentially boosting self-efficacy and optimism about the current issue. Members may report

Stages-of-Change Model

The stages-of-change model has five stages. In the **precontemplation stage,** people are not thinking about making a change. They may have never really considered it, or they may want to change, but don't feel confident, so they don't try. For example, someone who smokes knows that smoking causes health problems, but either he isn't too worried about it or doesn't feel like he can quit, or thinks he'll quit later.

When people start thinking about making a change, they begin the **contemplation stage.** During this stage, people may be unsure about whether to do anything different or just continue on as they are. There are both good and not-so-good things about their current habit or lifestyle as well as about changing. During this stage people usually have mixed feelings and go back and forth between different possibilities. It can be confusing to feel torn between options. So the smoker might go back and forth: Should he quit? Cut down? Not torture himself and just keep on smoking?

At some point, people decide to try to change and begin the **preparation stage.** During this stage, people think about how they can make the change, and begin making plans to do it. So the smoker might wonder: Should he try the patch? Medication? Go cold turkey or cut down gradually? Try hypnosis?

During the **action stage,** people implement their change plans and try out new habits or ways of being. They may look to other people for support or keep it to themselves for a while, if talking about it makes it more tempting, or if they want to play it safe. And they might not think of themselves differently. When smokers first quit, they might still consider themselves smokers, but smokers who are trying to quit.

During the **maintenance stage,** people try to sustain the changes they have made. Sometimes their identities change. So smokers might see themselves as ex-smokers and sometimes be tempted to light up when stress gets high or when they are around other smokers, but for the most part, they don't think about it all that often anymore. It kind of fades into the background.

Sometimes people have **relapses,** and cycle through the stages again. This is pretty normal. Other times, they may successfully change and just no longer think about it, like an ex-smoker who one day realizes he now thinks of himself as a nonsmoker.

---

that the model helps them, since viewing it from this lens makes change seem more achievable. Reflect key statements and emphasize that change is different for different people, but supporting one another's change attempts can make the difference between making small changes and achieving a life transformation.

Ask members how they see this model fitting for them, with the current target for change, if identified. Summarize common perspectives and highlight some differences, modeling nonjudgmental acceptance of how members see things. The summary provides a map of where the discussion has gone, but importantly, it should contain elements indicating where the group might go next with these ideas. It also helps to underscore dynamics such as group identification, homogeneity, and trust and interdependence (without using technical terms), while acknowledging personal choice and autonomy. For additional information on using stages of change in groups, see Chapter 14 by Velasquez and colleagues.

Ready–Willing–Able

Another heuristic, the ready–willing–able model proposed by Miller and Rollnick (2002), describes motivation in natural, nontechnical language.

How to Do It. Introduce the idea that people tend to change when they are "motivated." Ask members what this means to them. Elicit their descriptions of the three components of ready–willing–able, perhaps writing them on a board. Ask members to think about how ready, willing, or able they are to make the changes they are considering, perhaps on a scale from 0 to 10. Mention that getting stuck in any of these areas can be an obstacle to change. Reflect their perspectives on ways they are ready, willing, and able, and help them brainstorm ways to increase low ratings. If there is relatively little conversation, split members into pairs or small groups, and have them report back after they have some time to explore on their own.

Adaptation in Chronic Illness

Models for coping with chronic illness can be useful for groups in medical settings. Adjustment to chronic illness requires identity shifts and mastery of a series of nonlinear tasks (Cohen & Lazarus, 1979), and coping models fit the MI perspective because they avoid pathological labeling and focus on member-selected target behaviors and member-chosen processes that can lead to healthy change.

How to Do It. Present a brief description of the model. For example, in Samson and Siam's (2008) integrative model, adaptation to chronic illness is related to personal characteristics in five domains: (1) personal history and social context, (2) cognitive appraisal of the illness, (3) adaptive tasks, (4) coping skills, and (5) perceived outcome of the illness. This model uses technical language, which we recommend changing to simpler, descriptive language that suits the literacy level of your group. For example, personal history and social context can be referred to as "life experiences," and "family and cultural beliefs about illness." Similarly, cognitive appraisal can be referred to as "how your condition seems to threaten you, and the resources and alternatives you can think of to help." Adaptive tasks can be referred to as "things you do to compensate for your illness, such as changing diet or work or finding social support or spiritual meaning," and coping skills can be described as "the skills you use to accomplish those tasks, such as getting information, requesting help, setting goals and so on." Perceived outcome could be renamed "how much you're able to find your balance or regain a sense of things being normal." Ask members to give examples of how they see these playing a role in their adjustment to their condition. Elicit ways they could adapt to the new situation posed by their illness, and reflect themes across members. For example:

LEADER: I'm wondering if you might be interested in hearing about a model to understand your health that might help you move forward and return to having a more normal life. (*Group members nod heads "yes," "sure," "OK," etc.*) One way to think about your health is to look at how five life areas affect your health and how your health issues affect those life areas. The first is "life experiences." This refers to your personal history, things like your childhood, the people in your family and circle of friends who've dealt with illnesses, lessons you've learned over your life about health and illness, and what kind of situation you have now in terms of family, work, and social groups. How do you see your experiences affecting your health condition?

KATIE: I can really see that. My mom was a shut-in most of my childhood from her illness. I get scared that my diabetes will progress, and I'll end up in bed like she was.

LEADER: It's made you worry that your own illness might become disabling.

KATIE: Yeah, I really want to get it under control, so I don't end up like her.

MORGAN: I had almost the opposite experience. I'm the first one I know to have a serious illness. Sometimes it seems totally unfair that I'm struggling with heart disease at my age, when my friends are healthy.

TRACY: For me, my life experience has taught me to keep trying, not to give up. I try not to let myself get discouraged even when my sickle cell is causing pain and weakness. I know it will come and go, and I try to keep a positive attitude.

LEADER: So all three of you can see ways that your experience affects your ideas about your illness. What about others?

(*Conversation continues. . . .*)

LEADER: Another life area in this list is "adaptive tasks." What do you do to adapt to your illness? What helps you deal with it and work around it?

SUZANNE: For me, I pray to God to be relieved of the stress of having cancer, so that I can focus on getting the best treatment and not only on my fears.

SEAN: My doctor suggested that I learn meditation and yoga to reduce my stress. I didn't know much about them, but I took a couple of classes, and I was surprised how much more relaxed I feel when I do them each evening before dinner.

TRACY: Praying, meditating, yoga. . . . I need more practical coping skills. I have signed up for this service that helps with basics like getting a couple of meals delivered each week, and carpools for my kids' activities, so that if I'm having a bad spell, I can get away with doing less. So for me, getting outside help is important.

LEADER: These are some great examples. How about for others?

(*Conversation continues. . . .*)

End this discussion by asking questions in rounds that summarize what members learned, such as what they learned by thinking through these issues and hearing other people's ideas. The next round, ask which challenges this helped them identify. Then, ask what new things they might try. When all responses have been shared, end by summarizing key points and commonalities of content, and process themes across members.

Assessment Feedback

Assessment feedback is commonly used in adaptations of individual MI, in which a counselor provides assessment results and discusses their meaning with a client to enhance motivation to change. Early studies of MI groups involving assessment feedback and discussion with college students found that presenting feedback in groups was less effective than simply providing written feedback, perhaps due to embarrassment or defensiveness. Concerns were also raised that the group feedback could result in an unfortunate resetting of norms, working against motivation for change. However, a series of more recent studies using a semistructured small-group discussion format have incorporated assessment feedback without these unfortunate side effects by adapting the approach (Faris & Brown, 2003; LaBrie, Lamb, Pedersen, & Quinlan, 2006; LaBrie et al., 2008; see Chapter 5, this volume). In our own groups, we have included occasional selective assessment feedback, focusing on just a few elements of information. Martino and Santa Ana (Chapter 16) present another view on providing assessment feedback in their chapter on MI groups with dual diagnoses.

How to Do It. Routine clinical assessments, biomarkers of health or illness, or measures specifically gathered to produce feedback can all be used to generate the feedback. You might consider assessment that focuses on social functioning, such as the Inventory of Interpersonal Problems described in Chapter 7. You might also measure positive characteristics, using strengths measures that relate to job skills, resilience, "Big Five" personality factors, or interpersonal strengths.

Provide members with the same feedback elements, although their individual results will vary. The point is to provide members with new information and prompt new thinking. It may be helpful to distribute any written feedback in folders and instruct members to keep their own feedback private, while you discuss its meaning. Typically, you discuss each element with the group, define it, and explain its scale or categories. Elicit members' reactions to the assessed characteristics, risks, or strengths and how they think these may either help or provide challenges as members try to make things better.

When risk for future harm is part of the conversation, rather than focus on convincing people that they are at risk, the group conversation should remain factual—sharing the results, how those results relate to risks, and ways to reduce the risk. The group discussion can then focus on how members personalize the information. Often, some of the feedback is unexpected and can increase members' urgency about changing.

This strategy relies heavily on skillfulness in both reflective listening and the *elicit–provide–elicit* (E-P-E) conversational strategy. E-P-E helps to increase the extent to which clients take in and use the information, while also reducing the amount of information you need to provide. In this strategy, first *elicit* what members already know about a particular issue. In a group, this may be all that is necessary, because all relevant points may be raised by members. If that happens, it is a good time to affirm the shared knowledge base of the group and emphasize the value of looking to each other as sources of ideas. However, if important elements of the topic are not raised, *provide* that information for the group by "filling in the blanks." Also correct any misinformation shared by group members, while taking care to not embarrass any member. If a member shares an opinion masquerading as information, then affirm the member for sharing, while respectfully differentiating opinion from fact. Finally, after providing information, *elicit* members' reactions, particularly how the information applies to their own situation or how they want to use it. Personalizing information changes it from an inert fact into a motivator for action.

You may want to structure the
group so that it avoids negative group
processes, such as excessive observation rather than participation, or failing to focus on productive content
(Faris & Brown, 2003).

*Personalizing information
changes it from an inert fact
into a motivator for action.*

Looking Forward/Envisioning

Looking forward/envisioning involves guiding members to consider where
they will be or would like to be in the future. Different time frames may
be appropriate for different settings. For example, for members of a weight
loss group, envisioning their future at 1 month and 6 months may be more
appropriate than envisioning themselves 5 years out, whereas a longer time
frame might be better for a therapy group that focuses on overall lifestyle
change. One approach to looking forward is to have members imagine
themselves in the future, without having made changes, and compare that
to how the future would be if they made changes (see the example for
single-session, dual-diagnosis groups by Martino and Santa Ana in Chapter 16). You can also guide members simply to imagine themselves having
made a change, without a no-change comparison. This focus on the positive can build momentum and allow members to experience success in their
imaginations, instilling greater hope. This imagined success can have great
power and give members a sense that they are going somewhere positive.

How to Do It. Begin by introducing the future as a topic.

"Many of you have talked about the things you do to get along and
to deal with the challenges you face. Of course, it's important to be
able to cope with what life throws your way. It can also help to have
a clear vision of the future, one that pulls you forward and keeps you
focused on making your life more like you want it. We'd like to focus
on that future now. First, take a minute and daydream a little about
it. You might close your eyes and picture yourself at some point in the
future, the future as you would like it to be. Don't worry how realistic
it seems, just imagine how your life would be. Imagine how you would
feel about yourself, and about your success in developing the life you
want. [*Pause for an extended period of time.*] When you have a strong
image of what that positive future looks like, relax and open your
eyes."

As members look at each other again, invite them to share their vision. Provide guidance as the first few members share their changes, their thoughts

and feelings about it, and other things they noticed in imagining their future. Use rounds or open discussion to elicit each member's vision. Link members' content, themes, feelings or identities. If you have time to let the vision stand, don't get into practical ways of moving toward the future, just let the vision linger in members' minds and ask them to keep thinking about it, imagining it, and trying to flesh it out. If you are using this exercise in a single-session format, you might ask key questions, such as "What will it take to get there?"; "Which steps can you take now to get yourself there by then?"; "What help do you want from the group to get you started?" A third alternative is to split the difference, and ask members, "What's one thing you could do now to start moving toward that future?" Downey and Johnson (Chapter 13) share an exercise focused on eliciting mandated members' "hopes and dreams," and Dunn et al. (Chapter 18) discuss having members "choose their own adventure" in their discussion on weight management.

Reexamining Expectations

The purpose of this strategy is to help members define the assumptions and expectations they have about their lives, identity, relationships, and so on, and examine the extent to which these fit their lives now. The method is conversational.

How to Do It. This topic often emerges from a group discussion on negative emotions (e.g., anxiety, disappointment or shame) that are often related to unrealized expectations or expectations that no longer fit. You may evoke members' reflections on some of the basic expectations for their lives from childhood or adolescence by having them reflect and explore. Link similar themes, and ask members to consider whether those expectations or assumptions still fit, or whether they should be updated to fit their current realities. Elicit members' reactions as they consider modifying their expectations. Members often express a mix of relief and sadness at the idea of letting go of an old dream. Guide the group to discuss these updated expectations and reactions, and to imagine how these might help as they move forward.

Decisional Balance

Although we described a game version of the *decisional balance* strategy in Chapter 10, it is useful to revisit it to illuminate what may continue to keep some members stuck and unable to progress into action.

How to Do It. Using a conversational strategy, you can ask members to reflect on the current benefits/pros of staying the same, and similarly, the cons or difficulties of changing. Next, ask them to reflect on the cons of staying the same, and end with the pros/benefits of changing (this order builds momentum toward change by first addressing the concerns that may hold members back, then exploring the positive elements of making changes). If you used a decisional balance exercise before, ask members to reflect on differences. What movement have they made toward change, if any? How can they create additional forward momentum?

Exploring Importance and Confidence

In this strategy, group members explore why a particular change is important to them, and how confident they are that they can do it. Then they are guided to explore ways to increase their confidence and the importance of the change.

How to Do It. You can have members do this first on a worksheet, gather together in pairs, or explore together as a whole group. If you are working with the whole group, begin by asking members to identify one specific change or change strategy to discuss, (e.g., exercising at a gym or being more assertive with a partner). Help members outline a definable, achievable change over which they have some control. Then draw a line that extends from 0 to 10 on a board, give members a handout with such a line on it, or lay out an imaginary line in the room (or mark anchors on the floor with numbers on sheets of paper). Then explain that "0 means that the change you've selected is not at all important to you, while 10 means it is extremely important, whereas 5 is right in the middle. Think about the change. How important is it to you, on the scale of 0 to 10, to make this change now?" Ask members what number they gave (or have them line up by their number). After they share their numbers, ask each member (or sample a few from subsets of scores, such as low, middle, high), "What makes it that number and not a 0?" Asking them to indicate what makes it important to change elicits change talk. Summarize their answers, highlight change talk, and help to develop group identity and cohesion further by referring to the group as a whole for any summary statements that apply to all, and to "some of us" for themes that apply to subsets of members. This underscores the idea that different people have different values or reasons regarding the importance of making changes. Optionally, ask, "What might make your score a few points higher?" This allows members to think through things that would increase in importance, making it more likely they notice those developments should they occur.

Following importance scaling and using the same scale, ask, "How confident are you that you can make this change now?" Again, ask members "What makes it X and not 0?" As before, the only answer members can give will be some type of change talk, no matter how minimal. (*Note:*

Although rare, on occasion a person will give a 0. You reflect, "So right now, it's not important to you at all" or "Right now, you have no confidence that you could make that change"). Then ask, "What would help to increase your confidence by a few points that you can do this?" Reflect and link themes across members, and consider following up to determine how the group could help to increase members' confidence about making changes.

Consider using the findings as agenda items for moving forward, addressing thematic importance or confidence issues as they fit your group's needs. Several chapters in Part III include exploring importance and confidence, and Lane, Butterworth, and Speck (Chapter 17) give an example of a group leader helping members to clarify the difference between importance and confidence when members confuse the two.

Change Success Stories

Eliciting change success stories is another conversational strategy that can broaden members' perspectives by connecting them to their past successes, boosting their confidence about their current possibilities for change, and inspiring new change attempts.

How to Do It. Begin by mentioning that it can help to recall other changes members have made in the past. Ask them to take a few moments to think about two or three changes they have made. After a pause, ask them to consider sharing one of these changes; focus on how they started the change process and how they achieved the change. Elicit members' stories, make linkages between members' content and themes, and reflect change talk. After stories of successful change have been shared, invite group members to discuss what they can apply from these past successful changes to their current change.

If some members have difficulty identifying changes they have been successful at making, you can broaden the conversation to include any success or positive outcome they can identify (even if it wasn't necessarily a change), or even anything they did that made them feel proud. Members often discount past successes, so be patient and willing to find small successes (everyone has them). If a member still can't identify anything positive, honor this position and invite the person to listen and offer something later, if he or she wishes. In any case, avoid a situation where people feel bad for not being able to identify a success or positive achievement. This is actually fairly common when people are depressed or otherwise feel negative, and the message should be "It's okay if you can't think of anything right now."

Several contributors' chapters focus on eliciting change success stories. Lane et al. (Chapter 17) provide a case example of working with a member who does not initially recognize past successes. Martino and Santa Ana

(Chapter 16) creatively extend this exercise to include future hypothetical successes in groups for dually diagnosed mental health and addictive disorders.

Exploring Strengths

Exploring strengths fits well with broadening perspectives, because many group members are unfamiliar with considering and listing their strengths as part of moving toward change. Just naming their strengths and explaining them to each other, and hearing one another's feedback about these and other observed strengths, can increase confidence and willingness to attempt change. It can also increase group cohesion, trust, perceived homogeneity, and hope.

How to Do It. Begin by telling group members that when we are trying to change, it helps to remember all the tools we have at our disposal to help us succeed. One set of tools is our personal strengths. Ask members to consider their own personal strengths. You might give a few examples, such as "persistent," "courageous," "smart," "kind," or "compassionate." Ask them to take a few minutes to think of perhaps five personal strengths. Then, ask members to share some of their strengths, and how these strengths have helped them in past situations. Use a round, and as each person completes his or her own list, ask group members to add anything they think that person has overlooked and invite them to add these additional strengths to their mental list. To keep members involved, you can go strength to strength instead of person to person, and when someone mentions something such as "determination," explore how that strength has helped various members cope with situations or improve their lot. Next, invite members to discuss how they could use these strengths to improve their current situation. At the end of the round, comment on what you noticed in terms of group energy during the discussion, and ask group members to discuss how they feel after focusing on strengths (usually they feel more positive and motivated). Most of the chapters in Part III have examples that incorporate a focus on personal strengths.

Tips and Traps

Tips

First, relax and enjoy the group. When you focus on things you like about members, you convey an empathic presence without exuding pressure.

Second, use whatever tools you have to attend to both the process and the content. It is challenging to accomplish all the leader tasks and functions, and guide the group in its discussions, especially if you don't have a co-leader. Consider recording the session for review before the next session and making process notes immediately after the group, while your memory is fresh. If you have a co-leader, make time to discuss the group after each session and again, prior to the next session. These tools can cue you to attend to things you overlooked or couldn't get to in the last session and allow you to reexperience what is happening in the group, without having to manage it in the moment.

Third, begin to step back from the overt leadership you showed during the engagement and exploring perspectives phases, and "wean" the group slowly but steadily from its dependence on you always to provide the structure, topics, and interpersonal boundaries. By stepping back, you allow the space to open up for members to take on the leadership and direction of their own group, with you eventually becoming almost a consultant to their growth (enhancing their ownership of change and increasing activation).

Traps

The primary traps during this phase are flip sides of the same coin: moving too slowly or too quickly. If the group moves too slowly, it may rekindle ambivalence by remaining inactive too long. While waiting for some to "catch up" in readiness for change, others may get bored, drop out of group, or regress to less readiness. If the group moves too quickly, members' unresolved ambivalence may turn into resistance and demoralization. Additionally, group cohesion and trust may not build to the degree needed for the next phase. Use the accelerating and decelerating strategies discussed in Chapter 8 as needed, to find the right pace for the group.

Progress Indicators

For any particular group, the time spent in the phase of broadening perspectives will vary. Some groups remain focused on these tasks for several sessions; others make progress in a few sessions. When a critical mass of members seems ready to take action toward changes, then the group has begun the next phase of work, *moving into action*.

References

Cohen, F., & Lazarus, R. S. (1979). Coping with the stress of illness. In C. G. Stone, F. Cohen, & N. E. Adler (Eds.), *Health psychology: A handbook* (pp. 217–254). San Francisco: Jossey-Bass.

Faris, A. S., & Brown, J. M. (2003). Addressing group dynamics in a brief motivational intervention for college student drinkers. *Journal of Drug Education, 33,* 289–306.

Fredrickson, B. L. (2004). The broaden-and-build theory of positive emotions. *Philosophical Transactions of the Royal Society of London B: Biological Sciences, 359,* 1367–1378.

Fredrickson, B. L., & Branigan, C. (2005). Positive emotions broaden the scope of attention and thought–action repertoires. *Cognition and Emotion, 19,* 313–332.

Fredrickson, B. L., & Joiner, T. (2002). Positive emotions trigger upward spirals toward emotional well-being. *Psychological Science, 13,* 172–175.

Fredrickson, B. L., & Losada, M. F. (2005). Positive affect and the complex dynamics of human flourishing. *American Psychologist, 60,* 678–686.

LaBrie, J. W., Huchting, K., Tawalbeh, S., Pedersen, E. R., Thompson, A. D., Shelesky, K., et al. (2008). A randomized motivational enhancement prevention group reduces drinking and alcohol consequences in first-year college women. *Psychology of Addictive Behaviors, 22,* 149–155.

LaBrie, J. W., Lamb, T. F., Pedersen, E. R., & Quinlan, T. (2006). A group motivational interviewing intervention reduces drinking and alcohol-related consequences in adjudicated college students. *Journal of College Student Development, 47,* 267–280.

Miller, W. R., & Rollnick, S. (2002). *Motivational interviewing: Preparing people for change* (2nd ed.). New York: Guilford Press.

Nesse, R. (1990). Evolutionary explanations of emotions. *Human Nature, 1,* 261–289.

Prochaska, J. O., DiClemente, C. C., & Norcross, J. (1992). In search of how people change: Applications to addictive behaviors. *American Psychologist, 47,* 1102–1114.

Samson, A., & Siam, H. (2008). Adapting to major chronic illness: A proposal for a comprehensive task–model approach. *Patient Education and Counseling, 70,* 426–429.

Velasquez, M. M., Gaddy-Maurer, G. G., Crouch, C., & DiClemente, C. C. (2001). *Group treatment for substance abuse: A stages of change therapy manual.* New York: Guilford Press.

Velasquez, M. M., Stephens, N., & Ingersoll, K. (2005). Motivational interviewing in groups. *Journal of Groups in Addiction and Recovery, 1,* 27–50.

Wagner, C. C., & Ingersoll, K. S. (2008). Beyond cognition: Broadening the emotional base of motivational interviewing. *Journal of Psychotherapy Integration, 18,* 191–206.

CHAPTER 12

Phase IV

Moving into Action

The process of broadening perspectives helps members expand how they see their lives, opportunities, priorities, and strengths. Problems appear smaller and more manageable than when members had a narrower field of vision. Members perceive more opportunities for their future, and feel less constrained by past choices and their consequences.

With an increased sense of freedom, members may already be making spontaneous changes related to newly recognized opportunities. Some have a greater sense of hope and purpose. This elevation of emotion can increase willingness to try new things, and members often appreciate the group's support of their efforts. By this point, the group is usually cohesive; members share openly with one another, they are invested in one another's well-being, and any moments of disengagement or tension are fleeting.

All of these are indicators that the group has progressed to the last phase, *moving into action*. After developing broader perspectives on their situations and possibilities, members now narrow their focus and fine-tune plans for making changes. They increasingly act with purpose toward achieving their aims, adapt their goals and approaches in response to their experiences, and benefit from others' ideas and experiences in making changes themselves. By the end of this phase, group members should have implemented well-defined plans of action or made deep change in identity or perspective to the extent that ambivalence that previously held them back is transcended and has lost its inhibiting power. As group members make successful changes, they prepare for the group's termination and transition to life without the ongoing support of the group.

The work of the group as a whole occurs in a fairly predictable manner, as we have described. However, progress across group members is generally uneven. Some embrace making changes and take steps toward them, while others are still weighing possibilities. The shared nature of the group experience allows those who share successes to receive support from the group, and in turn serve as role models for others who remain stuck in uncertainty, often increasing their hope and momentum to move toward action themselves. In this way, group processes can help initiate and maintain momentum across members, beyond the momentum achieved with MI techniques alone.

Group members may express their movement into action in statements such as the following:

- "This week I stayed away from friends who use, and that helped me avoid temptations."
- "I thought about how Sam and Maria have been making big changes in their lives, and I felt more confident that I can make some changes, too. So this week, I started writing down what I'm eating, to see where I might be able to make some small changes."
- "I've been trying being more assertive, and so far, no one has had a bad reaction to it."
- "I still have to remind myself all the time to check my blood pressure and take my pills, but I used my calendar like the group suggested, and it was easier to remember."

Group members' variable progress means that you need to balance their individual needs with the progress of the group as a whole. Both aspects become prominent during this phase, yet neither should dominate the other in a smoothly functioning group.

Guiding Principles

Whereas earlier in the group, you focused on the positives of experiences, possibilities, and personal characteristics, it is now time to shift attention

---

Guiding Principles for the Work of Moving into Action

- Focus on actions
- Guide members to ask for what they need
- Encourage attention to group processes
- Focus on the immediate future
- Support self-efficacy

Balance tending to the individual needs of group members with the needs of the group as a whole.

to members' actions. By *focusing on actions,* even small steps, you keep the group focused on moving forward with change. At this point, members generally have strong relationships with you, the group as a whole, and each other. However, some may still find it difficult to identify or share what they may need with the group. When this happens, *guide members to ask for what they need,* bearing in mind that the group may soon be ending. It is time for members to discuss any unspoken concerns about making changes. Continue to encourage the group to *pay attention to group processes,* especially because these vary over time. As more members make positive changes, the momentum builds across the group, and spirits can be high; these times can make for a fun and excited group, or a peaceful and confident one.

By focusing on actions, even on small steps, you keep the group moving forward.

As members become more aware of the upcoming end of the group, some may express a desire to continue to have connections with each other afterward and also share their sadness at the upcoming loss. These thoughts and feelings merit attention as part of a healthy termination process for the group. Guide group members to *focus on the immediate future,* perhaps the next few weeks, to keep them keep moving forward on changes they are making. This can include discussions of how they would like to end the group, and how they will keep themselves on track in the weeks immediately following group termination. Finally, during this phase, take care to *support self-efficacy* as members take action to make the changes they have planned. Members may encounter obstacles or setbacks as they try new things, and it is important that they view these as temporary and resolvable.

Group Dynamics

As you act on these principles during the moving into action phase, continue to help members see that by working through issues together and using each other as resources, they can maximize their progress. Focus the group on *task interdependence.* For example, when some members have used the group well to move toward change, while others have proceeded independently, you might say:

> "Nearly all of you are at a point where you've made the basic decisions about the changes you want to make. Some of you have been trying new

things, taking action steps. When Johanna decided to stop drinking, she set that as her goal. Tom shared how he had to change more than just getting high, such as hanging out with different friends, avoiding certain events that would be really tempting, and even thinking about breaking up with his girlfriend who was still smoking. Around the same time, Keshia decided to stop eating snacks and to start walking to better control her blood sugar.

"So in all these cases, you made a decision to change something. What stands out to me, though, is what happened next. You three started sharing not only the decision about what to change and your plans for taking some initial steps, but also how you began to notice other things that needed to change to make these main changes work. After Tom shared, Johanna and Keshia, you both started to talk about additional changes you would consider to get to your goals, then in the next session reported to each other how things went. I noticed excitement among the rest of you about how all three of them added their experience together and came to support each other in making changes. What do you make of it?"

Ending with an open question that directs the group to pay attention to the collaboration of some members highlights the value of task interdependence and elicits alternative experiences from other members.

Therapeutic Factors

As the group prepares for action, two therapeutic factors that were prominent in broadening perspectives remain important. These are *guiding* and *vicarious learning*. As before, members share information they know or learn, but now the information tends to be based on experience. Once members begin making changes, they often encounter unexpected challenges and identify strengths they may have underestimated. When members share these, they are providing essential, tested information that the others can trust. This can result in concrete, constructive vicarious learning, such as when one group member adjusts her personal plans for change to take into account a challenge discussed by another. Thus, vicarious learning that was mere copying during earlier phases of the group can become iterative as members grow and improve through successive waves of sharing, adjusting, and taking actions.

Several other therapeutic factors become increasingly prominent during this phase, such as *altruism, self-understanding,* and the *expansion of hope*. Members often share altruistically, unselfishly giving their wisdom and support to peers, and experiencing the benefits of giving as well. They may experience increased positive emotions, including a buoyant mood and increased self-esteem. The act of giving without expecting reciprocity can be an uncommon experience for some members, and by highlighting it, you can further deepen and extend the acts of giving across members.

Similarly, members often explore more deeply their self-understanding related to taking action. Although they began to consider some of these issues during the work of broadening perspectives, they now may reflect more deeply on how their personal histories contributed to their problems. They may realize new things about how they create meaning in their lives. As a result of their experiences in the group, some give greater consideration to the ways they have been connected to or disconnected from others, and to the possibilities of making changes in relationships as well as in targeted behaviors. Some who experience anxiety that they may not succeed in changing may decide they have to take risks they never thought of taking—changing friends and leaving behind comforts and even part of their identity. Depending on the circumstances of the group, others may even have to face the possibility of dying if they do not succeed in changing.

These realizations and insights tend to emerge naturally as members move into action and take profound risks to make real change. Your task is twofold: to acknowledge and honor these important insights while you help members focus on maintaining their momentum toward change. While self-understanding is important, delving into self-exploration too deeply can derail the change focus of the MI group. Members' development of profound insights about themselves along the way is a bonus, but it is not the essential focus of the MI group.

Finally, as members make changes, *hope* in the group expands. Members share their optimism about taking what they have learned and applying it to other areas of their lives. Those who have not yet taken steps can experience the reflected glow of their peers' accomplishments, and believe to a greater degree that they, too, might succeed. This expanded hope can fuel a final push toward change for those who may be slower to initiate action.

Leader Functions

Your role shifts again in several ways during this phase.

Facilitating More Than Leading

In a mature group, members talk freely with each other, and the leader is less obviously involved in each discussion. Take on more of a guiding or consulting role with your group, perhaps initiating and ending sessions as usual but otherwise shaping group conversations subtly rather than participating in them. Step in primarily to open new topics, build linkages, and help members work together to gain greater optimism about their futures while they address the real challenges they face in getting there. You may continue to provide a summary of the group's process and content at the end of each session but, generally, focus more on supporting members in helping one another than on providing direct assistance yourself. The important aspect of the shift is that you focus more on what is needed to keep group members on track rather than supplying content prompts, all of the process comments, or all of the reflections that link members to each other. Now, members do more and more of those tasks for themselves.

Managing Challenges to Boundaries

Tending to boundaries, conflicts, and the upcoming termination of the group may not take much of your time, but still are important aspects of leadership during this phase. Group members who feel connected to each other may desire to continue these connections outside of the group. This can represent a breakdown of boundaries or may be acceptable, depending on the nature of the group. However, even if it seems acceptable for members to have a friendship outside of the group, it is important to consider the potential effects on other members and the group as a whole. Initiating contact outside of group can represent the formation of exclusionary subgroups that lead some members to feel left out. The group might become a less productive experience, because members are sharing information and experiences outside the group rather than within it. We prefer to discuss these kinds of developments openly with group members, guiding them to choose either not establishing friendships outside of group until the group ends or other choices that allow the group to remain the primary place where members interact and share with each other. These issues may be more relevant to psychotherapy groups than to support groups, but it is helpful to define the boundaries in any group, however open they might be.

Another potential challenge to boundaries may occur when some members make initial changes. Feeling like they got what they came for, they may be tempted to stop participating in the group. They may be excited by their initial experience with taking action and want to keep any awareness of the risks of backsliding to a minimum. Alerting the group to this potential challenge before it happens gives group members an opportunity to discuss the issue, and perhaps even to develop their own guidelines about it, such as the following example in a longer-term group:

TOMÁS: I'm feeling good, because between yoga, exercise, and sleeping better, my mood is miraculously better. It's been almost 3 weeks since I felt suicidal, or depressed even, for that matter. And I'm barely drinking. My wife seems happier or at least more hopeful. I never realized all these things went together like this.

JON: Wow, that's great. I still get angry, but I haven't been in any fights for a year now. But if it were me, I'd say, stick with the group still for a while yet.

SARAH: Yeah, Tomás, congratulations. We all know you can do it! That kind of gives me hope that I can leave cocaine behind for good this time. I haven't used for almost a month, but I gotta say that I'm still craving, especially when my friends call, and you know what they're doing. There's no way I want to end coming to group. And Tomás, I hope you don't either!

TOMÁS: I'm planning on staying for a while still.

NATASHA: How long *should* we come to group, if we've made the changes we wanted?

LEADER: What does everyone think? Remember, there are many right ways to use the group and make changes. So what do you want for the ending of the group?

JON: I've been in groups before with just a set number of sessions, like classes, and when it was done, you were done. Here, we don't have that.

NATASHA: But it makes sense to stop coming if you've achieved your goals.

SARAH: That's true, but I don't just come here so I can talk about my own ideas and experiences. I really like getting to hear everyone else's ideas and stories of how they are making changes. Even how their plans might not have worked. I always leave here with new ideas about how I can stay away from the crack, and build up other parts of my life to be better. So for me personally, I actually would like it if someone who's made great changes would stick around for a while. It helps me to hear it and see it. And besides, I'd miss each of you if any of you left!

TOMÁS: I kind of feel the same way. I'd like to stick it out with the group for a while longer. Maybe not the whole time, but definitely 3 or 4 more weeks.

NATASHA: Maybe we could have an agreement that if someone feels ready to leave, we all get a few weeks' notice. That way, nobody has to commit to staying forever, but we all know what to expect.

JON: That sounds pretty good. I can't see months down the road, but I can see weeks. Maybe if we want to stop coming, we can tell each other 2 or 3 weeks ahead. I'd want to get the chance to say goodbye and good luck, you know?

(*Heads nod around the group.*)

LEADER: It sounds like you respect each other, value each other's input, and really want to have a chance to prepare yourselves for any endings. It feels like everyone's connected, and that if anyone left, you'd really notice it. You want to honor that by giving a few weeks notice before you'd leave.

SARAH: Three, please. I'd prefer three.

TOMÁS: That sounds good. (*Other members say "okay" or nod their heads in agreement.*) It makes me feel good, too, to know that when I come each week, you're all rooting for me to succeed. That's never happened before for me. Saying that, I realize that the group is important to me. Very important. I've come to consider all of you my friends.

SARAH: Me, too, and I'm glad you're not leaving right away! I am wondering how I can deal with my craving, because I'm still pretty shaky on that. Tomás, how do you handle it when you feel like you might have a depressed mood coming on or are tempted to drink?

(*Group continues.*)

Normalizing Group Conflicts

Another potential challenge during this phase is the possible emergence of negative emotions or dissonance within the group. Some members may seem to withdraw, such as those who feel stuck and embarrassed because others seem to be thriving. Others may become more challenging, finding ways to minimize members' changes or question their ability to maintain change. One way to normalize and reduce tension is to reflect it as ongoing ambivalence that often resurfaces as people change. Your role involves attending both to the group as a whole, and to the ambivalent and struggling individuals. If the group is mature, it may be worth exploring the critical or withdrawn member's perceptions of how he or she is doing, and how the group might provide better support for the member.

Balancing the focus between individual members and the whole group is important in each phase of group work, but it may be crucial in this phase to avoid the disintegration of the group into subgroups, because members may become increasingly out of sync with one another as some members change and others struggle. It may be a challenge to maintain group momentum and energy when one or more members seem to be shrinking back from action. Moreover, at the individual level, it is important to help the person resolve ambivalence enough to move forward, to prevent hopelessness or a self-attacking perspective. The member who is slowest to move forward might resolve his or her ambivalence by dropping out of the group, rather than face it each week. Just as you might deal with the risk of termination by a successful group member who has made changes by bringing the issue up overtly, you can address the risk of dropout by the discouraged group member as well. For example, you might open up this conversation by saying:

> "We've talked before about how everyone makes changes at their own pace. I notice that a couple of you have expressed doubt that you could change, and maybe even think you're dragging others down. It might be tempting to quit coming to group when it seems like you're one of the few who are still unsure about change. If that's so, how can the group help?"

Some members may express negative emotions as the group nears its end. Withdrawing or acting dismissively toward others who have been a meaningful part of one's growth can be a defense against feelings of loss, fear, or self-recrimination for not having achieved what others have. When you notice that these conflicts exist but are not being discussed openly, you can turn positive attention toward the member who is frustrated by attempting to counter the development of negative emotions with the same kind of positive focus on change as earlier in the group. The person can then still envision a better future and move toward it. The end of group is only another transition, not the end of opportunity.

Alternatively, you can explore the negative emotions. With an experienced group, your comments about what you notice may be adequate enough to launch group members into a productive discussion of the meaning of their negative feelings and how to manage them. You could normalize these experiences as being common among people who know they will have to part. For example, it is common for soldiers to argue with their loved ones just before they are sent away for duty. Similarly, group members who have shared important experiences with each other now face their own lives apart from the group. In order to protect themselves from the loneliness they fear when the group ends, they may "reject" the group, or "fight with it" by creating conflict in the group, or withdraw emotionally.

Preparing the Group for Termination

Some members may have little experience with healthy, planned endings. People may have exited abruptly from their lives or died suddenly, leaving them no opportunity for reconciliation or closure. It is essential that groups, even those that have only a few sessions, give members the opportunity to reflect on the end of group, on what they have learned, and what they have meant to each other. The earlier vignette provided one example of how to open that conversation in relation to successful change by a member. You should also mention termination at several points, including the pregroup interview, the initial group meeting, during the broadening perspectives phase, and again in the moving into action phase. You might even remind the group about the previous discussions of termination, and ask them to revisit the issue now that they have been together for a while.

MI Strategies

As members work on the moving into action phase, it can be useful to blend conversational strategies with some structured tools, such as worksheets to help them plan *how* to change.

Below, we present several possible strategies for this phase of work. Depending on your situation, the size and readiness of your group, and the length of time you have available, you may select from among them in the most useful order that works for your group or work through all of them in sequence. As in previous phases, you can use these structured activities or a more unstructured conversational approach, whichever provides a better fit for your group. We describe merely one way to approach each task. Be creative in adapting, adjusting, or reworking tasks for your group. Remember that the most important thing is to keep group members engaged, making forward progress on their own changes, not completing assigned tasks.

Importance/Confidence Review

Reviewing group members' beliefs about the importance of change (the whys) briefly can lead to a thorough discussion of their confidence about changing. Even if they feel quite strongly that they should make changes, group members may lack confidence that they can change. Confidence is tied to several factors. Members must believe (1) that there is a plan that is likely to result in success, (2) that they can enact that plan, and (3) that they can stick with any longer-term elements of that plan. If these three elements are in place, members may feel quite confident about the changes they are making and have enhanced hope for their future, resulting in optimism that increases their energy to pursue goals. If any element is weak or missing, their confidence may be lower.

How to Do It. Assessing importance and confidence during this phase can be done simply, using the scaling approach (discussed in Chapter 11) to elicit change talk about each. Alternatively, you might introduce the review of importance and confidence conversationally, as in the following vignette, in which the leader also acknowledges a moment of altruism on the part of a peer, and the possibility for imitative behavior on the member's part, and finishes by focusing on specific actions the member could take in the immediate future to start making changes.

ANDERS: Even though I know it's bad for my diabetes, I just can't seem to stay away from sweets and bread and potatoes. Those are all my favorites, and they are exactly the things that increase my blood sugar!

ROSEANA: I felt the same way about cigarettes. I had already quit drinking, and that was my last pleasure. But that's the one that was hurting my heart. After that heart attack, it just wasn't worth it.

LEADER: You both enjoyed something that wasn't good for you. Roseana, it sounds like after your heart attack, it became more important to do something about smoking. How did that increase in importance translate into more confidence that you could quit?

ROSEANA: Actually, my confidence was still pretty shaky. I'd tried so many other times to quit.

ANDERS: Yeah, like I've tried to cut out carbs before, too. Many times.

ROSEANA: But this time, I think I changed inside. Somehow I took it more seriously. So while I was still in the hospital and craving like crazy, I asked for nicotine patches. And even before I went home, I asked about the stop smoking support line and got a bunch of brochures. The difference was this time, I actually read them. So instead of just saying "I'm quitting," I made plans. I even filled out a chart in one of the pamphlets about my craving situations, and what to do instead of smoking. So this time, I started out way more prepared. And of course, I still wanted a smoke. But I just kept telling myself, "You've already had a heart attack. The next one will kill you. Don't make that come faster than it should just to stick a cigarette in your mouth." I just had to keep myself focused on the goal, life. Staying alive, getting better. I'm not trying to preach or anything, but maybe something like that could be helpful for you.

ANDERS: I guess I haven't fully committed before. I've always said I'll *try* a new way of eating. But I haven't really prepared myself like you did. But the doctor says it could kill me, too. Diabetes seems less serious than a heart attack, but when she saw my test results this last visit, she freaked out. I could probably do better if I planned ahead more, like you did.

LEADER: (*to Anders*) So you really connect to what Roseana is saying. (*to Roseana*) And Roseana, thanks for sharing that story; it's really helpful. (*back to Anders*) So you're considering how some changes to your diet could help in managing your blood sugar. What would help to prepare you for that, and to feel more confident about it?

(*Discussion continues.*)

Hypothetical Change

Even after considerable discussion, some members may still hesitate to take action. Inviting those members to talk about change as a hypothetical possibility rather than an actual current change allows them to consider and reflect on actions without experiencing defensiveness, and can help broaden their perspectives even further, before honing in on specific changes they will implement.

How to Do It. First, summarize themes and content in the group discussion that lead you to believe at least some group members are nearly ready to change but might still be hesitant. Next, invite members to construct a "hypothetical" change plan. For example:

> "Many of you have taken some steps toward change and seem nearly ready to take on some of the bigger pieces of the changes you've been considering. Others are less sure. It might be helpful if we lay out hypothetical plans—*as if* you are ready to take action now, even though you might not be sure yet. We can let our imaginations run free, because you're not committing to anything right now. How does that sound?"

Next, guide the group discussion of the hypothetical plans, providing some of the typical components of change plans described in the next section. An alternative is to elicit these elements from the group as a whole (providing any components the group fails to generate), then ask members to form small groups or dyads to discuss hypothetical plans. When debriefing the exercise, you might ask who in the group might be ready to try out some pieces of the hypothetical plan. Next, after discussing those elements, ask who thinks the plan needs to be revised to be viable, and elicit changes that group members might want to consider.

Change Planning

When most members seem ready for action, it is time to narrow the focus of the group to the task of developing specific change plans that members will implement over the coming days, weeks, and months. While you can easily do this conversationally, many people benefit from having a record of their plan to review and update regularly, and to keep somewhere to prompt themselves even when they might otherwise not be thinking of it. Developing change plans can be done in a way that increases group cohesion and identity while emphasizing and autonomy and individualized planning.

How to Do It. Using the items shown in Figure 12.1 as a guide, ask members to develop a draft of a personal change plan. Give group members

---

Draft of My Change Plan

The changes I want to make (or continue making) are:

The reasons why I want to make these changes are:

The steps I plan to take in changing are:

The ways other people can help me are:

I will know that my plan is working if:

Some things that could interfere with my plan are:

What I will do if the plan isn't working:

FIGURE 12.1. Change plan.

about 15 minutes to work on these individually. Ask them to share their change plans, indicating how confident they are about their plans and about asking their peers for help. Ensure that each group member has a chance to share the plan. Guide the group discussion of how members might modify their draft change plan, use the change plan, or put it into action in the next week.

Another way to approach this task is to have a session in which you brainstorm these issues as a group, posing questions to the group, then allowing members to work on their plans between sessions and present them the next session, or work together in pairs on modifying and strengthening them first, then sharing them with the group. For example:

> "Tonight, let's talk about brainstorming change plans. Each of you has different things you're working on, but the idea is to just get the juices flowing in general, so we can all think up possibilities and hear each other's ideas. Here's a worksheet that covers the topics we can discuss, so you can get a sense of the things we'll cover. Feel free to jot down notes on it if you want, and I'll give you a fresh copy before we leave, if you want to continue to work on it between sessions. Change plans are works in progress—usually people keep revising them as they go along, so just relax and brainstorm possibilities. Why don't we start by going around the circle to address this first one, which should be pretty

easy. Just remind everyone as specifically as you can what changes you are working on."

Feldstein Ewing, Walters, and Baer (Chapter 21) further extend change planning by combining it with hypothetical change planning, information exchange using the elicit–provide–elicit strategy, and development of problem-solving skills with adolescents and young adults.

Strengthening Commitment to Change

Making a commitment to make specific changes to other MI group members can increase the likelihood that the speaker will make the changes (as long as the person doesn't feel pressured into making a verbal commitment just to meet a perceived demand). You might use this conversational strategy when a majority of the group members have clearly identified the changes they want to make, have taken steps toward change, and are just about to act on the more challenging parts of their change plan. Alternatively, you can turn this into a more structured exercise, as described below.

How to Do It. You might say:

"This group has come a long way. Most of you have clearly identified changes you want to make, and taken steps to get ready for changing. One of the final things you can do to give yourself the best launch into your new way of living is to make a clear statement of commitment to your plan.

"A clear statement would include what specifically you plan to do, when you will do it, and your commitment to it. For example, you might say, 'I am quitting smoking, starting next Monday, and I am fully committed to do anything it takes to stay away from cigarettes from then forward.' This statement indicates what will be changed, smoking; when it will happen; and what the commitment is. Try to be accurate. Don't feel like you have to say you are 'fully committed' if that's not how you feel right now. You can say, 'I am definitely going to try' or 'I think I'm about ready to try,' or whatever is most accurate for you right now.

"Let's divide the group into two. On this side of the room, let's have everyone who's sure they can make this commitment today. On the other side, let's have everyone who would like to make a commitment but needs a little more time, as well as people who aren't quite sure yet. For those who need more time, please work on a developing commitment statement that you can consider a draft of the one you might make when you are fully ready. If you aren't sure, write a statement about what you need to think through first, what steps you can take to move closer to a commitment, or what smaller steps you can take to get ready."

Allow members to choose a side. Ask members to work alone, then together, to write down a final version of the statement. When this process is done, reconvene the full group. Ask those who are ready to make a commitment to share their statements first. Reflect, or encourage members to reflect, each person's statement. Then ask those not yet ready to share their developing commitment statement. Reflect and debrief.

Getting Started

Taking steps toward large changes can result in continued change efforts. There is value in helping members "get started" with changes, even by taking a small step to create momentum. You can accelerate group movement toward change even if some members are still unsettled about it, because the small step is just a slight movement in that direction and does not require full commitment to the ultimate change goals. Every step tends to increase confidence and hope about succeeding at change.

How to Do It. Introduce the idea of the value of a small step toward change.

"Some of you are now ready to make changes or have already started, and others are getting closer to that while juggling everyday challenges. Even if you're not completely ready to make big changes, it can be helpful to take steps toward your eventual goals."

Ask the group members to form pairs or small groups. Tell them that each pair or group should spend 5 minutes discussing each person's potential changes, reviewing steps already taken, and coming up with two or three additional small, easily achievable steps in that direction, even if they are not ready to commit to any of them at this time. When the time is up, reconvene the whole group, ask members of each pair or group to present their ideas about small steps, then ask whether they would like the group members to suggest other possible ideas. Following this discussion, ask each group member to state one step he or she plans to try in the next week. If members are not ready to commit, ask them which step(s) they would be willing to consider further. Encourage the group to follow up with each other next session to see how the small steps went.

Learning by Proxy

Allowing members to share their struggles and successes so far can be a useful exercise to increase group cohesiveness and task interdependence, information exchange, and imitative behavior.

How to Do It. Comment on the progress you've noticed across members and how many are working to overcome challenges in making changes. Divide them into pairs that you select. Try to arrange pairs so that at least one partner in the pair has made good progress and taken noticeable steps toward change. Once they are in dyads, ask members to take turns listening to each other describe three challenges they are facing and a few steps they have taken along the path to change. After listening to the partner, the first listener writes down the challenges and the steps he or she heard. Additionally, members share a few things they learned from listening to the partner in the dyad that might apply in their own situation. Have partners switch roles and repeat the procedure, allowing them enough time to explore in some depth. Reconvene the larger group. Ask the listeners to give their partners the cards on which they recorded the partner's challenges and steps. Ask listeners to share what they learned from listening to their partners, focusing on how they might apply the ideas in their own situations.

Dealing with Setbacks and Challenges

As group members continue moving forward on their action, they often find that elements of their plans need to be adjusted. Success is accomplished not by developing the perfect plan but by persevering through challenges and creatively adapting to new developments.

If members were thoroughly engaged in change planning, they likely anticipated some of these challenges and made plans to overcome or work around them. However, actual frustrations are often more powerful than hypothetical challenges. At times, members may express these frustrations, lose confidence, and become pessimistic and critical. It is important to react in a positive way, remaining nondefensive in the face of criticism, even embracing the opportunity to address frustrations.

GABRIELLA: It seems like you are playing some kind of game where you won't give people direct answers.

LEADER: Like I could help more than I am.

GABRIELLA: Like you hardly help at all sometimes, even when you could.

LEADER: Well, that's definitely not my goal. How could I help you better with what you're trying to accomplish?

GABRIELLA: I didn't mean me, I just meant when people seem to really need some help.

LEADER: Okay, but I wonder if you could give me an example of how I might specifically help you better, and I'll keep your comments in mind the rest of today, while we're all talking, and check in at the end of group to get some feedback on how I'm doing with everyone.

GABRIELLA: Well, like last week, when I wanted some advice on how to handle my boyfriend when he criticizes me.

LEADER: Oh, I'm sorry. I thought you'd gotten what you were looking for.

GABRIELLA: Well, instead of telling me how to handle it, everyone kind of just left me with the idea that I'm supposed to just be honest and say what's on my mind when he acts that way. So I said this week, I'd let him know when he crossed a line. But then I did that twice this week and it blew up in my face, because he just got mad when I said he's always trying to control me and push me around, and he just needs to back off.

LEADER: So you feel let down now and upset, because it seemed like I gave you bad advice.

GABRIELLA: Well, you didn't really give me advice, but you didn't stop me from making a mistake either, and it seems like you probably knew my plan wasn't a very good one.

LEADER: Got it. Again, I'm sorry about that. From what you've said, it seems like this is something that will probably happen again, so what could we do now to make it better next time?

GABRIELLA: It's just that it seems so simple when we're here, and so clear, and then when he and I get into it, I just forget everything about what we talk about here. Then I just end up fighting with him instead of trying to make him see that I do want his input, but I just need to be the one who makes the final decisions about my own life.

LEADER: So you are speaking your mind more, which was a goal, and now you want to learn to do it more effectively. You've taken that first step, but now you want to do it better.

GABRIELLA: I hadn't really thought of it like that. . . . I guess that is right, I did say what was on my mind even if it didn't go over well.

ROBIN: And that's a big change!

PATRICIA: That's what I was thinking.

LEADER: So you did that. And it's frustrating that it didn't go like you hoped, but you also see that you were mostly able to do what you planned, though it was harder than you expected.

GABRIELLA: I guess . . . yeah, pretty much.

LEADER: And now you're thinking that if you could do it a little differently next time, and really feel confident in yourself and not get nervous or confused, you might be able to better explain that you're not trying to reject him, you just have to take more responsibility for your own choices, and you can't do that if you're just doing whatever he wants you to do.

GABRIELLA: It's almost like I could only deal with just saying something the first couple of times, and now that I know I actually can speak up, I can pay better attention to what I'm trying to say instead of just crumbling under pressure.

LEADER: And other group members see that as a change.

GABRIELLA: It's a really big change. It really is. I'm kind of surprised I could even do it.

LEADER: Well, I wonder, who else feels like it is a challenge to speak up and keep your head about you sometimes when facing negative reactions from people who are important to you? (*Other group members agree.*) Yeah? Well, I'm glad it came up, because these kinds of things can really derail plans when we're not clear on what we're trying to do, and confident that we can pull it off. Perhaps this is something we could focus on, maybe even practice a little bit.

In this example, the leader is accepting and warm toward a member who is criticizing the leader's work. Rather than pursue examples of what the leader supposedly did wrong or debate the accuracy of Gabriella's statements, the leader accepts the complaints and easily transitions to trying to give her what she needs now. The leader reframes a difficult experience from being a failure for which the member partially now blames the leader (and group), to being an important first step in a larger-scale change plan— and one that the member can be proud of while moving forward to taking the next step. The support of other group members is reflected by the leader both to reinforce this notion and to bring others into a conversation that has focused on one person for several interactions. The other members can recognize that they have contributed to this positive shift in momentum, and at the same time the leader generalizes the individual's challenge in order to make the time more productive for other members as well. Finally, the leader again reinforces that it is not only acceptable but also a positive thing for members to speak their minds in group, and that there is nothing to fear from openness and honesty. Lane, Butterworth, and Speck (Chapter

17) provide an additional extended case example on getting started, as well as additional information on dealing with setbacks and challenges.

Tips and Traps

In some ways, the moving into action phase can be the most rewarding as you witness members making significant changes and sharing important shifts in their perceptions of themselves. It can be challenging to foster the growth of group members and to maintain the group's cohesion and productivity, while also guiding the members through the process of termination. It is easy to overlook a return of significant ambivalence, even in someone who has begun to take steps toward change, or who has made significant changes. For many of the long-term habits, change may occur in fits and starts, and struggling to maintain gains is frequently an issue. Use complex reflections of feeling and meaning as some members stall while others succeed. It might be tempting to return to your leadership style from earlier sessions, when you might have filled the time with activities and structure rather than allowing the group to struggle a bit, while you facilitate progress more than you lead. Remember that this is the time to foster group members' autonomy in pursuing their changes and goals, and to help them approach the group's end in a proactive and planned way.

Continue to foster the growth of group members and maintain the group's cohesion while you also guide members through the process of termination.

Termination

Some groups are ongoing, with rotating members who exit as they reach their goals. Most MI groups, however, have a defined ending. Some members go on to participate in other services, while others end their participation in professional services. For all, however, the group ceases to be a part of their ongoing lives. They will no longer interact as a group, and many are likely to never encounter one another again, unless perhaps in passing.

In brief groups, members may not need much preparation for this termination. In longer-term groups, members often establish significant bonds with each other, with the leaders, and with the group as a whole, and the ending of a group is a life transition that deserves acknowledgment. Some members have histories in which endings with significant others have been abrupt and unplanned, often involving conflict or a sense of abandonment.

Thus, the termination of the group is an opportunity for them to experience an ending in a more planned and positive way. Acknowledging the group's time-limited nature over the course of group sessions can inspire members to participate more fully and be more prepared for the group's ending. Change planning, eliciting both the goals that they want to achieve before termination and those they want to continue to pursue after termination, also can help them approach the ending of the group more positively.

When the time comes for the group to end, members benefit from having some closing activity such as a celebration, graduation ceremony, or time to wrap up that allows people to share some summary perspectives. Given the importance of group cohesion and identity, these closing moments may focus more on opportunities for members to share their appreciation for one another and what they will "take away" from the time spent together than on reviewing individual progress achieved or lessons learned. Spending this time to reflect and share marks the endpoint of the group in their lives, and gives them the opportunity to carry it forward internally.

By this point in the life of the group, your participation is largely facilitative—opening and closing discussions, helping members keep on track, and making transitions. Extend this style into the group's closing moments. Inviting members to focus their final moments on themselves and each other, rather than on you as leaders or on the treatment program or agency in general, is autonomy-supporting. It is a subtle way to acknowledge that they are no longer your clients or group members, but fellow human beings on their own pathways that happened to intersect for a time, and now are diverging once again.

The following case example is a closing period of an MI support group for emergency "first responders" who struggle with traumatic stress. The leaders have just finished eliciting discussion of "how things will be 3 months from now if they are going 'according to plan.' " Inviting members to project into the future like this reminds them that while the group has played a role in their ongoing lives, the ending of group sessions does not represent the end of processes that have been initiated or strengthened. To close, the leaders shift the focus to having the members talk directly to one another about their experiences together and the impact upon them. The leaders stay out of the way of group members who are functioning on a deep level and offering one another their parting thoughts on how they bonded with one another, how their perspectives have shifted, and how they gained a greater sense of the universality of their experiences and greater pride in themselves and what they do:

LEADER 1: We wanted to see what you might want to share with each other about having gotten to know one another, or what will stick with you, before we go our separate ways.

DEVON: I think it's all been good, a positive experience for all of us. I was still on edge when we started, running around in circles in my mind about that little girl I lost in my arms. And this made a really good transition, not so much to let it all out, but to talk my way through it and step back and see the whole forest—remember what I'm trying to do, and all the people I *have* been able to help, you know? And I know I can't blame myself for times that it doesn't work out. I think I had to come to accept that. Not having that doubt about myself in the back of my mind, I can focus better, and in the work we do that can make all the difference, you know?

PATRICK: We're different in a lot of ways but we all have similar experiences and similar effects on us. Being here has been transcendental for me. To my fellow first-responders, I just want to say, keep your heads up—I don't mean that as a platitude, but for real. I am leaving here refueled. Reenergized. I have not felt like this for a very long time and I've really needed it. Thank you.

MICHELLE: I just feel so connected from listening to everyone's stories and experiences. It's an honor to have been "let in" a little into your lives, and that's a gift that each of you shared and I really feel good now.

IAN: Yes, you all are so incredible, so strong and even though a lot of us struggled, there's that sense of how important it is to make it through these things we're going through. We're kind of not existing on the same plane as everyone else; like Devon said, it's just so different when almost every day, you're facing death and seeing how such little decisions can make such a big difference—if you panic and turn left when you should've turned right, into the skid; if you decide to smoke that one last cigarette even though you're falling asleep; or if you thought your wife has all the kids with her and you just back the car out of the driveway without really stopping to check. Those little moments that change everything. You don't even think about it at the time, then you can never forget that little moment you weren't paying attention or made the wrong choice, or you are no longer around because of what happened. And we see the results of it, and try to make it turn out right but have to face that a lot of times we're just too little, too late. But what else can we do but try? That's what I've come to through listening to everyone. What else can we do?

(The group is quiet. The leaders let the silence linger, while Leader 1 scans the group with her eyes, silently inviting members who haven't spoken yet to join in.)

JAMIE: I just thought everyone was tougher than me. Everyone just wasn't bothered by it all. Or they just put it behind them at the end of the day and went out for the night, went to the bars or out with their friends. I had no idea that so many people in our work are so involved in our communities or really committed to making the most out of a relationship or dedicating themselves so much to their kids. I've really learned so much—after our sessions I would just go over things in my mind. How everyone was struggling in some way with similar things, but had such different perspectives and . . . I just really related to every one of your stories. There's something I got from everyone and it makes me feel more on track, stronger.

RAMON: Yeah, I'll definitely be thinking about each person in here for a long time. (*Other members nod and agree.*)

IAN: It's like we're finishing the group, but we'll still be together in our minds.

MARK: I've always talked to other emergency workers at parties or whatever. We just have seen so much, and we don't really have to say anything about it, you just know. But in here, we really did talk about it, not every detail, but the most important parts. Then we talked about what comes next—and refused to just get stuck in the mess it makes in our heads, like a lot of us were at first.

JAN: I've never talked to anyone about it. At work, you're too focused on what's happening at that moment, and there really isn't a lot of time to look back, let alone look into the future. And that has really helped in here. But I think maybe even more, it's just remembering who I am by getting to know who each of you are. All of us building something together, some kind of shared community. I think we're all people who try to make things better. Most of us were pretty drained before, but now it seems like we're ready to go again. Now I remember that our work is important, but isn't everything, and we have to still have our own lives and they're not something we squeeze in when we can, but really important to recharge and regroup so we keep having something to offer to the people who are unfortunate enough to have to meet us on our jobs.

LEADER 1: (*After a brief silence*) I really appreciate you all opening the window for us and letting us inside. It's been easy for us because you share so much. I appreciate how open and honest you've been. Some of you talked about being inspired by one another and that's definitely something I feel from our time together.

LEADER 2: I thank you so much for your time, for being yourselves. That you gave us your time and shared your stories is humbling. And it's uplifting how much work each of you put into getting out from under the weight of the events, refocusing your lives, and moving forward.

Thank you all for what you've given in your work. Good luck to those of you who are continuing on as responders and just as much to those of you whose lives are turning in a different direction. Either way, society owes you a debt of gratitude and we hope you continue to recognize the valuable role each of you plays, whatever path lies ahead. (*Group members agree and engage in small talk and share goodbyes as they begin to filter out of the room.*)

PART III

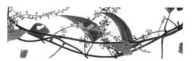

Applications of Motivational Interviewing Groups

In this part of the book, our collaborators offer examples of MI groups in different settings with different populations. Several describe the use of MI in combination with other approaches intended to address members' challenges better. Our collaborators discuss how they customize MI group techniques and strategies to fit the specific and varied needs of the people they serve in groups in addiction, mental health, physical health, and criminal justice settings. We recommend reading all of these chapters. Even if the clinical focus of a chapter is different from your work, each of the author teams approach MI groups in their own way, and you may find ideas or strategies that work for you in chapters focusing on populations or issues that are different from those of your group.

The first four chapters address different aspects of working with those for whom substance abuse is an issue. Downey and Johnson (Chapter 13) describe the use of MI groups with clients mandated to substance abuse treatment. Velasquez, Stephens, and Drenner (Chapter 14) present their experience using a combined MI and transtheoretical (stages of change) model group for addictions. Jasiura, Hunt, and Urquhart (Chapter 15) present a unique multimodal, MI-informed empowerment group for women with multiple challenges, including substance abuse, victimization, and oppression. Martino and Santa Ana (Chapter 16) apply MI groups to the challenges of dual diagnosis—helping group members with both addictive and psychotic disorders.

Two chapters address MI groups in health. Lane, Butterworth, and Speck (Chapter 17) present an overview of MI groups addressing a variety of chronic health conditions in medical settings. Dunn, Hecht, and Krejci

(Chapter 18) provide a description of MI/cognitive-behavioral therapy combination groups for weight management.

The following two chapters present MI groups for people with a history of criminal and violent behaviors. Carden and Farrall (Chapter 19) describe MI groups for men with a history of intimate partner violence. Prescott and Ross (Chapter 20) also address men in their description of MI groups for those with a history of sexual violence.

The final chapter addresses the use of MI groups with adolescents and emerging adults for a variety of lifestyle and developmental issues. Feldstein Ewing, Walters, and Baer (Chapter 21) describe the unique developmental challenges faced by this population, and how they use MI groups to address these issues.

All of the contributing authors are practitioners (some are researchers as well), and nearly all are MI trainers who are members of the international Motivational Interviewing Network of Trainers (MINT). While some chapters are by intact working groups, others are by coauthors who live and practice in separate locations. We chose them because they are MI group experts in their respective practice areas. Our thinking has benefited from their expertise, and we are pleased to be able to share their ideas with you.

CHAPTER 13

Motivational Interviewing Groups for Mandated Substance Abuse Clients

Sandra S. Downey *and* Wendy R. Johnson

"I'll do my 28 days, and then I'm out of here. But nobody's going to make me talk in this program." Dana's reaction is typical of women entering the therapeutic community in a minimum security prison. Inmates must attend at least the first phase of treatment prior to their release from prison. At the end of 28 days they may opt out, and this is what most new-comers intend to do. "It doesn't feel good to be forced into treatment. How could we make this time most useful to you?" The leader communicates acceptance that many of the women are angry about the mandated nature of the program. She also knows they worry about how, once released from prison, they will cope with life without returning to substance use. The leader hopes to convey this understanding and invite the women into an empowering and intrinsically motivating discussion. For several moments the leader elicits and reflects upon the shared perspectives of the group members. Becoming a bit more at ease, Dana hesitantly states, "Well, I do want visitation with my kids." Another member responds, "I know what you mean. I would do anything to see my kids and get them back some-day." Soon the women are discussing their hopes for the future and choices they might make. Contrary to her original plan to leave, Dana has begun a journey that will eventually result in graduation from substance abuse treatment and a decision to maintain sobriety for a more satisfying life.

251

The judicial system refers people to treatment in a variety of settings—inpatient and outpatient programs, group homes, halfway houses, prisons, and therapeutic communities. Coercive measures are often involved, making clients feel they have no say in their own change process. Random drug screens, threats of incarceration or longer sentences, and probation and treatment requirements can get in the way of establishing a trusting therapeutic relationship that fosters change. Clients often experience reactance to pressure to change, a natural tendency to defend their freedom when they perceive it is being threatened. They may argue why they do not need to be there, and why you do not understand and cannot help them. They may appear not to want to change, and seem to be in denial about their substance misuse. Instead, many clients who are keenly aware of the destruction substance misuse has caused them don't acknowledge it in a restrictive, mandated setting.

Working with clients mandated to group treatment presents specific challenges. Their anger and natural reactance may lead them to collude with other group members in resisting treatment and change. Sometimes, group members present a unified argument against change, making it easy for leaders to react authoritatively and compound the problem. Some clients seek to take control of the group or sabotage other members' efforts to participate. In prison settings, members who are open to change may present a cavalier attitude toward treatment in order to avoid being criticized by peers. Motivation to change upon release from jail is overridden by motivation to avoid conflict while incarcerated.

Another challenge arises when group members' comments run contrary to the spirit of MI. Members may pressure others and give unsolicited advice. Often, group members have preexisting relationships. Even in large urban areas, crime and drug networks are interconnected, and members may have complicated histories with one another. This can further undermine their willingness to share, and increase the potential for negative interactions or harmful repercussions.

Mandated clients frequently have multiple criminal offenses and relapse episodes. They experience poverty, underemployment, and homelessness. Many have endured trauma, domestic violence and co-occurring mental illness. Their families and friends also use substances and engage in illegal activities. All these factors undermine their confidence to change, even when the need to make changes is clear.

Finally, many of the settings in which these groups occur are themselves antithetical to the spirit of MI. Efforts to collaborate with clients and respect their choices can be undermined by a system that imposes negative consequences and limits choices. If not resolved, this values conflict can adversely affect the group treatment experience.

Fortunately, most group members hope for changes such as reductions in sanctions, regaining custody of their children, or living better lives.

Engaging group members in a collaborative process that reduces resistance and increases motivation can help them make changes because they *want* to, not because they *have* to. The following section illustrates how MI groups address the challenges that emerge over the course of mandated treatment.

Using MI in a Group
with Clients Mandated to Treatment

Group members often hold firm beliefs about injustices in the legal system and the relative harmlessness of certain drugs of choice. They may assert that substance use has not caused them problems and reject labels such as alcoholic or addict. The following vignette from an outpatient MI group with mandated clients illustrates how natural reactance and arguments against change can be prominent in group discussions. The leader uses MI skills to circumvent typical points of contention, engage members in a more helpful conversation, and inspire positive change. The MI skills are listed in brackets.

DAN: As soon as I get off probation I'm going back to smoking weed. It's ridiculous that it's illegal. It's never caused problems the way that alcohol has for people.

JUANITA: The government is a money-making racket. They want it to be illegal because that keeps money flowing. I've never seen anyone wreck a car or be violent after smoking pot.

LEADER: For you two, it's very frustrating that marijuana is illegal when it doesn't seem to cause many problems. What about others? What are your thoughts as you hear Dan and Juanita share their perspective on this? [expressing empathy with reflection]

MIKE: I've had to pay a lot of money in legal fees, and coming here is costing me more. I can't get a job because I'm a convicted felon, and coming to this group makes it that much harder. It's like they want us to fail.

TAMMY: Lately I've been so stressed. I have bipolar disorder and now I'm pregnant. I can't work and I have to raise this baby by myself. The only thing that helps is marijuana. I don't want to hurt the baby or go to jail, but I really don't know what I'm going to do.

SCOTT: I lost my license because of a DUI [driving under the influence]. So I'm supposed to work and get to all these meetings, and I have to ask other people to take me every place I have to go. My PO [parole officer] doesn't believe that I just made a stupid mistake one night.

LEADER: These are difficult challenges. On one hand, you'd like to smoke or drink sometimes and they can help you cope with stress. You're angry that the legal system is forcing you to stop. On the other hand, you are aware that because it is illegal, there are personal costs involved. You don't want to be on probation or go to prison or have problems getting a job. It's a tough dilemma to be in. [double-sided reflection]

MIKE: I haven't used drugs in 2 months and they're still making me come to this program. It's not that I mind coming here so much, but I could be out there making money and paying off my fines.

LEADER: Even with all of those obstacles, you found a way to get here to avoid further legal problems. You're trying to do what's best for you. And I'm curious about something. Is it okay to switch gears right now? [summarizing; affirming; asking permission; collaborating] (*Group members' heads nod.*) It's clear that some of you have made a decision and are avoiding drug use right now. That's not always easy to do. It might be helpful to others to hear what is working for you. [shifting focus to elicit change talk; affirming; exploring ability and steps to change]

DAN: I just keep to myself. I go to work and come home. I try to find things to do around the house, like working on the car that's been sitting in the yard.

The leader facilitates an emotionally safe atmosphere in a manner that increases the likelihood of change. Normal reactance is bypassed by allowing group members to voice their frustration. The leader reflects and clarifies their dilemmas, while drawing attention to their reasons and ability to change. The discussion also helps build confidence as the leader elicits and affirms their steps toward change. Finding an early opening in the conversation, the leader briefly summarizes, then shifts the focus to explore the change talk imbedded within the conversation. The group members are invited to consider the positive changes they have already made. What might otherwise be viewed in terms of compliance with authority is recognized as personal decisions and efforts to change. This shift helps to increase members' awareness of their accomplishments and build the self-efficacy needed for establishing and maintaining long-term change.

Guiding Principles for Implementing MI Groups in Mandated Treatment

We suggest a few guiding principles when applying MI to the unique challenges arising in mandated group treatment.

Embrace Resistance as a Pathway to Change

Despite the challenges of coerced care, it's possible to engage members in a process that can be life changing. Working collaboratively and respectfully provides clients with a new and empowering experience. Meeting resistance with empathy and acceptance allows group members to build enough trust to engage more openly in the group process. To do this effectively requires us to make an important attitudinal shift. We no longer view resistance as an obstacle to change. Rather, we embrace resistance as *a pathway* to change. Your task is to respond in a way that transforms the resistance into openness to change.

Expect Resistance

It's normal for mandated clients to feel angry about the demands placed upon them by the judicial system and to question their need for help. Some voice their frustrations or act them out. The challenge is to earn their trust while you elicit motivation for change.

Understand Resistance

Remember that resistance is a sign of discord within a relationship and does not mean a person is in denial or lacks motivation for change. Distrust, anger, sadness, and hurt are often at the root of resistance for mandated clients. This can arise from past experiences of abuse and betrayal, hostile interactions with treatment providers or authority figures, and being coerced to change. Group members may wonder, "Does this leader really care for us? Is she going to judge or punish us if we tell the truth? Will the group accept me and can I trust them?"

Resistance also arises from the fear of letting go of a source of emotional comfort. Many lack confidence that they will be able to cope with intense emotions and the stressors of life without substance use. Others fear the pain and hopelessness from failed efforts to change. With so much at stake, members may decide it is less risky to remain guarded and avoid change.

Respond Empathically to Resistance

Trust is established when group members *feel* understood. It's important to use reflective listening throughout each discussion. Make every effort to view the world through their eyes. At times, you may experience frustration in response to challenging group behavior. Use this feeling as a signal to check whether you are seeking to understand and reflect members' feelings and perspectives. It is essential to communicate understanding and acceptance not only in words but also in tone of voice and body language. Continue to express empathy when upholding program policies and setting limits with behaviors that interfere with the group process. MI skills help ensure that all members are approached with compassion and respect at all times.

Let's turn briefly to the distinction between *sustain talk*—speech that opposes change—and *resistance*—discord within the therapeutic relationship. With mandated clients, responding to sustain talk with disapproval or pressure can create resistance where there was none. Some leaders are concerned that responding empathically to resistance and sustain talk communicates approval of the behavior. However, true empathy avoids taking sides. It communicates acceptance of the person, not support for his or her behavior. Expressions of empathy are reflections of the clients' perspectives, not those of the leader.

> *When you experience frustration in response to challenging group behavior, check that you are seeking to understand and reflect members' feelings and perspectives.*

Offering double-sided reflections can capture the whole of the client's dilemma and increase awareness of all sides of the issue. For example, "Despite the potential legal risks, you would like to continue to get high." You can also assure members that the group is intended to provide a safe place where they will not be judged or pressured in any way. Explain that the group provides an opportunity to explore the role of substance use in their lives, so they can decide for themselves what they would like to change and how.

Following each group session, ask yourself, "How did I respond to resistance or opposing perspectives? What was I feeling, and what did my tone of voice and body language convey? Did members become more engaged and open to the possibility of change? How can I make things better next time?"

Seize Every Opportunity to Explore the Change Talk
(Note: It May be Hidden and It May Not Even Be "Talk"!)

Ambivalence makes it difficult for many people to change. There are often good reasons to keep things the way they are. Clients mandated to stop their substance use have an additional hurdle to overcome. While mandates provide a source of extrinsic motivation, they also create internal opposition that makes it even more difficult to choose to change. Avoidance of substance misuse after exiting the legal system requires that clients must come to their *own* decisions. The role of treatment is to facilitate the discovery of the personal benefits of avoiding substance misuse. This process enables clients to move from extrinsic to intrinsic motivation and to make a meaningful and lasting change.

Change talk represents a natural inclination toward positive change—the source of intrinsic motivation. You can tap into intrinsic motivation and thus elicit change talk by inviting members to explore the costs of substance use and possibilities of change. When trust is present, members share openly. Sometimes it is especially challenging to engage the group in a conversation about the personal benefits of change. When several group members express their anger or desires to use, listen for *any* tendency toward change. Offer a brief summary of the group's perspectives, then reflect the change talk heard. For example, "Even when challenges appear insurmountable, we sometimes experience a glimmer of hope. Victor has mentioned that despite his frustrations and multiple relapses, he hasn't given up. Tell us how you keep going despite these obstacles." Then invite the group to comment on what has been shared.

Motivation can be expressed in behavior as well as words. Noticing that group members continue in treatment despite not wanting to be there, you can reflect, "Although you love getting high, being here shows you value your freedom even more. How is your freedom important to you?" Commenting on their efforts allows members to discuss underlying values and desires.

Some group members stop using while on probation and intend to return to substance use once they have completed their legal requirements. Focus on the steps they are taking in order to complete their treatment, sentence, or probation/parole successfully. Elicit their growing confidence and the benefits they experience in avoiding substance use during this time. While engaging in effective treatment, some express hope that by the end of probation they will not want to return to substance use. Treatment can prepare group members to consider making a change in the future.

Affirm the Positives to Build Hope and Support Movement into Action

Clients in the criminal justice system often describe demoralizing experiences, as well as feelings of shame and guilt due to substance misuse. Help group members see themselves in a new light by reflecting and elaborating upon any reference or example pointing to positive characteristics and successes. Notice and affirm values, skills and talents, strengths and achievements, and efforts they make. Normalize their experiences and express empathy for their challenges, as well as their triumphs. Members discover a positive identity as they understand and accept themselves more deeply, and draw upon their skills and strengths. This provides a powerful source of hope and motivation for change.

Facilitating MI Groups in Mandated Treatment

Here we describe processes and activities that characterize the four phases of the MI group in mandated treatment.

Engaging the Group

The initial engagement phase for mandated clients involves the process of decreasing resistance and building trust, as we have discussed, as well as fostering supportive relationships between group members. The relationships among members provide the most significant source of support for change. Fostering group relationships helps members enjoy a sense of belonging and identify with each other's experiences. They also find comfort in realizing they are not alone in their struggles.

Building connections between group members can be accomplished in several ways. Invite members to discuss how they may relate to what others have shared. Ask how it feels when another group member compliments them in some way. Draw attention to their commonalities and invite them to explore further. This helps build group cohesion and highlights the mutual support members provide to one another. Taking time to build connections also provides an opportunity for members who share a history outside of group to get to know one another in a new way. Consider the following exchange:

LEADER: Lorraine, how does it feel to hear Shauna say that she admires your courage to go back to school? [enhancing self-efficacy; fostering supportive relationships]

LORRAINE: It feels good. I hadn't thought about it that way. I'm trying to overcome my fear of failing so I can be more productive. I'm thinking about being a veterinary assistant.

SHAUNA: I've wanted to do something like that for a long time. I know you have a job and kids to take care of, too, so it gives me hope that one day I'll be able to take classes as well.

LEADER: (to the group) Lorraine and Shauna have a lot in common. (to Lorraine and Shauna) You both have children and love animals. (Lorraine and Shauna smile at one another and nod their heads.) (to the group) Shauna, you mentioned Lorraine's courage. What else does it take to pursue our personal goals? [highlighting commonalities; elaborating on change talk]

The leader encourages self-reflection and draws attention to the affirmation and support that Shauna offers Lorraine. They share a meaningful exchange that can be personally gratifying. Then, the group members are invited to share their thoughts on the topic of personal strengths and hopes for the future. This could be followed by a discussion linking members' strengths to their current efforts to change.

You can also foster supportive relationships by helping members communicate with each other in a way that allows the safe expression of conflicting opinions. Remind the group that although we have many things in common, we are not all the same. Invite members to use "I statements" (e.g., "I think," "I feel," "I prefer") when expressing their views. This allows members to speak their minds without having to justify their beliefs. It also provides a mechanism that groups can fall back on when the topic gets heated or one member tries to tell another what to do. You can also intervene when one group member demeans another. Remind members that each person is valued and deserving of respect. You can empower the group by explaining that all members have an important role in maintaining a safe atmosphere.

Exploring Perspectives

Once trust and mutual sharing are established, members begin to explore perspectives on their current situations and the possibilities for change.

Clarifying and Addressing the Dilemma of Change

Group members typically have mixed feelings about the substance use that has created problems in their lives. Use of reflective listening while exploring members' experiences helps them clarify and begin to resolve the dilemma of change. It is also useful to explore the pros and cons of substance use early in the change process to help members acknowledge what they like about substance use and begin to explore the other side. At the end of the exercise, allow the weight of the discussion to fall upon the group. It can be painful to generate a vivid picture of the problems associated with substance misuse. Be sure to take time to process any feelings and observations that have emerged.

Exploring Personal Values

Reconnecting with one's values regarding right and wrong, remembering cherished relationships, and identifying what gives life meaning can have a dramatic impact on one's choices and behavior (Wagner & Sanchez, 2002). These realizations may have an even greater impact in mandated treatment, where the focus is often societal rather than participants' values. Exploring values helps members assess the extent to which their current behavior is in line with what they view as most important in life. Because people are often happiest when leading meaningful lives, in which they use their strengths and virtues for a higher purpose (Seligman, 2003), discussing values may lead to changes that allow group members to avoid substance misuse and experience greater fulfillment in life. The values card sort exercise (Miller, C'de Baca, Matthews, & Wilbourne, 2001) is one activity that adapts easily to a group setting.

Broadening Perspectives

As members begin to appreciate better the impact of substance use on their lives, explore what might lie ahead if substance use were no longer a problem. Helping members develop a specific vision of the future enables them to better achieve their goals and live by their values.

Building Importance and Confidence

Introduce activities that can help members explore the importance of making changes in their lives and build their confidence to change. Use of the importance and confidence scales is a good way to begin this discussion, and it allows members to explore *any* desired change in their behavior. This might be particularly helpful for those not ready to focus on substance use but willing to explore other areas, such as managing anger. The "pocket change" exercise in the accompanying box helps support any positive change group members are considering.

Looking Forward/Looking Back

Group members can develop a vision of change by exploring the past and looking toward the future. Members may explore who they were before problems with substances progressed and how things might look in the future, if they no longer used substances or had to report to an authority such as a probation officer. For example, if a member mentions athletics, ask questions such as "Tell us about your history in sports. How did you develop your talent? How did you feel when you won the championship that year?" [reflecting and exploring answers to avoid the question–answer trap]. When looking ahead, help members paint a picture by asking, "What do you most want to be doing a year from now? What will your priorities be? How will you be feeling about yourself and your life once you've reached your goals?" Identifying the worst that could happen if there is no change (e.g., ongoing legal involvement and incarceration, loss of family and self-respect), and the best possible outcome if change does occur (e.g., living a satisfying life with no justice system involvement) can help members further define the possibilities of the future.

"Pocket Change" Exercise

Invite group members to think of a small change they would like to make that may or may not be related to substance use. Ask them to write this change on a small piece of paper and place it in a pocket. Encourage group members to choose a change that is specific, measurable, and stated positively, for example, "I will walk for 20 minutes three times per week." At the end of the session, ask if the discussion pertains in any way to their "pocket change." Members are not required to share the change with the group, although they may do so if desired.

Members are asked to bring this "pocket change" to each group session and to share how the discussion relates. At the end of several sessions or upon completion of the group, members may share what change occurred with regard to this behavior.

Discovery of Hopes and Dreams

Exploring hopes and dreams may open members to the possibility of what they might accomplish in their lives. Interests that they have put aside can be rediscovered. Group discussions can explore questions such as "What brings you the most happiness in life? What are you passionate about? What have you dreamed of becoming? What gives you hope? What is your greatest hope?" This can help members set personal goals and identify exciting things to pursue as alternatives to substance use.

Example of Exploring and Broadening Perspectives

Revisiting our earlier example, in this segment the leader engages the group in an exploration of change.

DAN: I just keep to myself. I go to work and come home. I try to find things to do around the house, like working on the car that's been sitting in the yard.

MIKE: I don't go around anyone. I've been spending more time with my kids, though, so that's been great. Now that I'm not doing drugs my kids' mother is letting me see them more.

LEADER: Staying away from certain people and places helps. And you noticed there are some benefits to being clean, such as getting things done that you may have been putting off, and seeing more of your kids. What are others' experiences about what helps? [reflecting steps taken and benefits of change; eliciting further change talk]

JUANITA: I haven't used meth in a couple of months. I would have probably died if I didn't stop. I got down to about 96 pounds. I've been taking medication and that's been helping.

TAMMY: I don't want to have my baby in jail. They'd take it from me.

LEADER: There are other things in life that you care about besides using. These are things that help you to stay clean. What else might make avoiding substance use worth the effort? [summarizing reasons for change; elaborating on change talk]

The leader may continue using OARS to explore change themes. As you model OARS, you can also invite members to reflect what others are saying and to comment on (affirm) the values and strengths they see in each other, why and how they might change, and the difference this could make in their lives.

Moving into Action

Once group members build intrinsic motivation to change, many naturally find their own ways to initiate and maintain the changes they have chosen. As our example shows, often members have already made significant changes, sometimes due to the desire to avoid further legal problems. Group members can discuss options and develop a personalized plan to address their unique challenges, strengths, and desires.

Developing a Change Plan

Group members can develop a hypothetical or actual change plan, depending upon their readiness to begin making changes. Change goals typically include successful completion of court and treatment requirements; avoiding further legal, family, social, or health problems; reducing or stopping use of alcohol and/or drugs; avoiding risky and illegal behavior; preventing relapse; and finding happiness and purpose in life without misuse of substances. This is a good time to remind group members that the choice of whether or not to change is up to them. Encourage members to find what will most likely work for them.

Strengthening Commitment to Change

Once a plan is identified, group members can solidify their commitment to change and move into action. Eliciting commitment can include asking members, "What tells you that you are ready to make these changes? How do you know this is the right time? How will you be putting your change plan into action? What will you do this week? How will things be different or better in your life by the next time we meet? In one year from now?" [reflecting and exploring between questions]. This reminds them about their reasons to change and supports them in moving forward. Members can further solidify their commitment to change by identifying challenges that could interfere with their plans and exploring possible solutions. To deepen the group's learning, elicit at the end of each session what members are noticing about themselves as they reflect upon the conversation.

Keeping the Spirit:
Tips to Adopt and Traps to Avoid

Tips

There are many ways to incorporate the spirit of MI in groups with clients mandated to treatment. We offer the following tips to help group members move toward positive change as you lead them through the four phases of group.

Treat All Group Members as People, Not "Addicts"

Be as warm and welcoming as you would be toward friends and family who might visit your home. Have group members spend time getting to know each other, and make the group a fun place to be. Avoid referring to members as addict, alcoholic, or offender.

Recognize That the Group is Your Most Important Information Resource

Discussions that draw out group members' knowledge can be particularly rich and stimulating, and cover in an interactive manner the same content as a handout or workbook. Alternatively, resource materials and handouts consistent with MI may be used as springboards for discussion and sharing of ideas and experiences.

> *Be warm and welcoming as you would be toward friends and family who visit you in your home.*

Work Collaboratively and Offer a Menu of Options

Explicitly state that group members' ideas, wishes, and perspectives are not only encouraged but also vital to the group. Offer options for discussion, and let members know they are in the best position to decide what they most need from the group. This collaborative approach neutralizes some of the toxic effects of being mandated to treatment and is empowering for clients who have many restrictions placed upon them.

Remove Treatment Barriers

Remove common barriers that hinder the change process. When possible, be flexible about treatment requirements. For example, explore the benefits of a variety of self-help groups and other sources of support, and invite members to come to their own decisions regarding what might be most helpful to them. Similarly, removing any expectation that group members label themselves may be important for some. Clients can explore adverse consequences and come to a decision to stop using without taking on a label.

Share Information in an MI-Adherent Way

Acknowledge alternative viewpoints when presenting information. Avoid challenging members' beliefs, and allow time to discuss their reactions to what is presented. A comfortable exchange of ideas also allows members to learn from each other. Ask open-ended questions such as "How does this information resonate with your own experience of cravings and coping with them? What else have you learned about managing cravings that is not on this handout? Some researchers are finding that certain medications may be helpful in reducing cravings. What are your thoughts about this?" Inviting members to share their own ideas may at times also elicit frustration about being mandated to treatment and coerced to change. Strike a balance by allowing some time for a free exchange of ideas, then shift the focus to explore a less contentious and more motivating topic.

Show Your Optimism

Be sure to let members know they have the strengths and skills to make change happen, and that you and other members are on hand to work with them, and support and encourage their efforts. Maintain this hopeful and optimistic stance with all mandated clients regardless of their history or behavior.

Traps

Despite evidence that aversive methods fail to motivate meaningful behavior change (Ackerman & Hilsenroth, 2001; Miller, Benefield, & Tonigan,

1993), we sometimes unintentionally create discord or elicit passivity rather than forward movement. Common traps include the following.

> *Convey an unwavering belief that change is possible.*

Mistrusting the Group

Viewing members with suspicion or describing them as game players, manipulative, or even resistant reveals judgmental attitudes that can undermine your ability to build trust. Such attitudes block you from seeing and eliciting the inherent wisdom of the group and their capacity to know what's best for them.

Focusing on Deficits

We sometimes presume that members lack insight, knowledge, and skills, and we remedy this by structured informational programming. We can forget that people do not necessarily change because we want them to, tell them to, or show them how. When members do not progress according to our plan, we can become impatient and let negatives obscure the positives.

Safety Lapses

Letting members respond to others with criticism, put-downs, or offensive comments impacts the entire group negatively. Group members sense when they are being judged by their leaders or peers, and when it's not safe to be themselves. Allowing them to engage in distracting behavior, such as side conversations, limits the depth of sharing among members.

Role Confusion

Taking on a role more suitable for probation and corrections officers or, alternatively, siding against law enforcement, can be counterproductive. Policing for compliance and punishing slips and relapses also inhibit open dialogue.

Forgetting Your OARS to Elicit Motivation for Change

It takes diligence to convey empathy and explore change consistently through OARS. We sometimes lose focus on drawing out members' natural tendencies toward growth and change.

It may help to identify the traps that particularly challenge you, then consider what might help you to build trust and facilitate change more consistently and effectively.

Conclusion

Studies are beginning to demonstrate the efficacy of MI groups with mandated populations and incarcerated individuals (Easton, Swan, & Sinha, 2000; Stein & LeBeau-Craven, 2002). MI groups likely help us to engage those less ready to change, thus increasing the likelihood of positive outcomes.

Along with the growing evidence base, anecdotal support further demonstrates the value of MI groups with this population. It is common to hear clients spontaneously discuss the positive impact of the group experience in their lives. In one group, clients were invited to describe their experience of the group in one word, then elaborate on its meaning for them. Here are a few of their responses:

- Enlightening: "Instead of making a bad decision I choose a different course of action."
- Positive: "People feel more at ease to speak their mind and share their feelings."
- Relaxing: "The tension from the day is over. I leave here with a different attitude. Time flies."
- Mesmerizing: "Wow! I think about the resistance I felt the first day, and now I don't want to leave. Resistance comes from fear of being labeled drug addict or mentally unstable."
- Therapeutic: "We get to come in here and be around people—everyone with their eye on the prize: To do the right thing."

The following dialogue is with a client mandated to outpatient treatment as a condition of his probation. It is an excerpt from his first individual therapy session, after he had attended several MI group sessions.

CLIENT: I think it's really helpful. I've been to a lot of programs in my life, been to the mental hospital for getting in trouble growing up. I used to hate groups but I like this one a lot. It's just the people in there; it's a good support program.

THERAPIST: Part of what you like about it is meeting other folks and getting support. What else are you finding helpful about that group?

CLIENT: Just the fact that everyone can relate to my situation. We're pretty open in the group and I just find that really helpful. After the first group I was really excited about it. My probation officer noticed it. It's made our relationship better and all around it's made a lot of things better. There's definitely a difference.

THERAPIST: I'm wondering how things are different for you now.

CLIENT: I've been trying to be sober for a while. I've been doing pretty good, but coming to these groups is like a pat on the back. Makes me realize how good I'm doing. It makes me feel better about myself and it's just self-encouragement, and I love it. And it makes me want to stay on track. You know, coming and getting a fix, it's like its replacing drugs to come every Wednesday, talk about everything, go home, feel good, and when I have to work, I kind of want to go to work. Before I never wanted to. So I'm being productive. This feels good. If I work hard, you know, the sky's the limit. So it's motivating.

It is rewarding to know that this group experience makes a difference in many lives. We have watched in awe as our group members strive toward previously out-of-reach goals and renew their hope for a better life. Implementing MI groups has helped us avoid professional burnout. As a result of our experience using MI, our group work, like many of our clients' lives, has been in a word—*transformed*.

References

Ackerman, S. J., & Hilsenroth, M. J. (2001). A review of therapist characteristics and techniques negatively impacting the therapeutic alliance. *Psychotherapy, 38*, 171–185.

Easton, C., Swan, S., & Sinha, R. (2000). Motivation to change substance use among offenders of domestic violence. *Journal of Substance Abuse Treatment, 19*(1), 1–5.

Miller, W. R., Benefield, R. G., & Tonigan, J. S. (1993). Enhancing motivation for change in problem drinking: A controlled comparison of two therapist styles. *Journal of Consulting and Clinical Psychology, 61*(3), 455–461.

Miller, W. R., C'de Baca, J., Matthews, D. B., & Wilbourne, P. L. (2001). *Personal Values Card Sort.* Retrieved December 11, 2007, from *http://casaa.unm.edu/inst/personal%20values%20card%20sort.pdf.*

Seligman, M. E. P. (2003). Positive psychology: Fundamental assumptions. *The Psychologist, 16*(3), 126–127.

Stein, L. A. R., & LeBeau-Craven, R. (2002). Motivational interviewing and relapse prevention for DWI: A pilot program. *Journal of Drug Issues, 32*(4), 1051–1070.

Wagner, C. C., & Sanchez, F. P. (2002). The role of values in motivational interviewing. In W. R. Miller & S. Rollnick, *Motivational interviewing: Preparing people for change* (2nd ed., pp. 284–298). New York: Guilford Press.

CHAPTER 14

Motivational Interviewing– Transtheoretical Model Groups for Addictions

Mary Marden Velasquez, Nanette S. Stephens, *and* Kelli L. Drenner

This chapter describes a group treatment for cocaine abuse based on the transtheoretical model of change (TTM) and delivered in an MI style. The TTM has played an integral role in addiction treatment over the past 30 years, and MI complements the model and provides a way of facilitating change, even with clients who are resistant or not yet ready to change. We designed the TTM group as an alternative to existing models in which group members are encouraged to confront one another and group leaders rely on strategies that are authoritative and challenging rather than supportive and empathic. Our intent was to develop a treatment approach that is empirically sound, based on skills and strategies that can be mastered by clinicians who believe in clients' inherent ability to change, and tailored to meet clients "where they are" rather than where we would like them to be. The TTM group intervention, delivered in a client-centered, goal-directed MI style, utilizes activities and strategies to elicit specific change processes that promote successful behavior change.

Integrating the TTM and MI

Our 6-week, twelve-session approach draws from the *Group Treatment for Substance Abuse: A Stages-of-Change Therapy Manual* (Velasquez, Maurer, Crouch, & DiClemente, 2001). In this chapter, we present selected sessions that highlight how we utilize the MI OARS strategies of Open questions, Affirmations, Reflections, and Summaries in specific TTM-based group activities to help resolve ambivalence and create opportunities for member-generated change and commitment talk (i.e., statements of desires, abilities, reasons, and needs for change, and statements of being committed to change, as described by Amrhein, Miller, Yahne, Palmer, & Fulcher, 2003).

In order to understand the use of MI in the TTM groups, it is helpful to know a little about the TTM framework. Developed by Prochaska and DiClemente (1982), the TTM offers a way to understand, measure, and facilitate behavior change. The TTM's stages of change consist of: *precontemplation,* in which individuals are unconvinced that they have a problem, or are not considering change in the near future; *contemplation,* in which individuals actively consider change but lack short-term intentions to change; *preparation,* in which individuals have more proximal goals to change and begin to make commitments and develop initial plans to change; *action,* in which individuals change the behavior of interest and adopt strategies to prevent relapse; and *maintenance,* in which individuals solidify the change and integrate it into their lifestyle. Progression through the stages appears to be cyclical, with clients often making several change attempts before they achieve sustained modification of the problem behavior. Rather than viewing behavior change as an "all or nothing" event, seeing earlier, tentative steps as part of a dynamic change process is a more comprehensive and hopeful view of behavior change.

MI can be used in working with clients across all stages of change. For example, MI helps clients in the early stages to explore and resolve their ambivalence about change. MI can also enhance clients' intrinsic motivation to develop, initiate, and maintain behavior change efforts. For clients in later, more action-oriented change stages, MI helps to promote self-efficacy, reinforce accomplishments, and prevent relapse (DiClemente & Velasquez, 2001).

A second dimension of the TTM, the processes of change, can be conceptualized as the mechanisms or "engines" of change. These processes are activities, behaviors, and experiences that promote movement through the change stages, and fall into two clusters. The first cluster, the *experiential processes,* includes emotions and thoughts that are related to how a person views his or her situation and behavior. These processes are most relevant in the early stages of the change cycle. The second set, the *behavioral processes,* involves strategies and behaviors that are more important in the later change stages. Research indicates that certain processes are more salient in some stages than in others (DiClemente, 2003; Perz, DiClemente, & Carbonari, 1996). In addition, some processes span adjacent stages, whereas others are used in varying degrees in multiple stages. Therefore, by promoting movement through the stages of change, these processes can be utilized to help people "do the right thing at the right time."

Because positive change is enhanced by different types of processes in different stages of change, each TTM group activity focuses on specific experiential or behavioral change processes. For instance, in groups where most members are in earlier stages (e.g., precontemplation, contemplation, preparation), we emphasize exercises that help to elicit experiential processes such as consciousness raising or self-reevaluation. When groups have more members in later stages (e.g., action, maintenance) we emphasize activities that foster behavioral processes such as stimulus control or self-liberation. Although the processes of change provide direction and structure, clinicians can select sessions that facilitate use of processes that are most appropriate for a group's current needs (e.g., members' stage of change, length of time in treatment). The TTM manual provides some specific strategies and exercises that facilitate a particular process of change, and others that facilitate multiple processes. Two additional constructs, "decisional balance" (Janis & Mann, 1977) and "self-efficacy" (Bandura, 1986), are also integral to the TTM group intervention. We also incorporate additional strategies and exercises from other sources that fit the current needs of the group. Table 14.1 outlines and describes the experiential and behavioral processes upon which the groups are based, and provides examples of specific tasks or activities that facilitate use of specific processes.

Throughout the TTM group activities and discussions, the MI style and spirit create opportunities for group members to give voice to their personal values, goals, and reasons for change. Member change-talk—statements of desire, ability, reasons, and need for change—begin to occur more frequently, leading to member statements of commitment to making changes. The skilled practitioner will not only recognize member change and commitment statements but also respond to and reinforce them by using MI strategies such as reflections and open questions to further and deepen the exploration and elaboration of members' motivations for and intentions to make a change.

Running the TTM Group Using MI

In the following section, we offer tips and comments about our integrated MI–TTM intervention, with session examples and bracketed notes about OARS utilization.

TABLE 14.1. MI Group Exercises for TTM Processes of Change

TTM process of change	Description	Promotes movement from which stage(s) of change?	Group exercises
Experiential processes			
Consciousness raising	Gaining knowledge and insight about behavior patterns	Precontemplation Contemplation	• Identify personal stage of change • Describe a "typical day"
Dramatic relief	Experiencing and expressing feelings about unhealthy behavior	Precontemplation	
Self-reevaluation	Exploring how behavior may conflict with goals/values	Precontemplation Contemplation	• Discuss assessment results • Explore values • Discuss pros and cons of using
Environmental reevaluation	Exploring how behavior may negatively impact others and environment	Precontemplation Contemplation	• Discuss relationships • Discuss others' concerns
Social liberation	Exploring alternatives and social supports for change	Contemplation Maintenance	• Locate potentially supporting resources
Behavioral processes			
Self-liberation	Considering new ways of being that increase confidence	Preparation Action Maintenance	• Develop an action plan • Recommit after a slip
Helping relationships	Receiving support from helpers and significant others	Preparation Action Maintenance	• Identify social support networks • Consider new relationships
Stimulus control	Avoiding or altering drug use cues	Preparation Action Maintenance	• Identify ways to reduce temptation and risk *(continued)*

TABLE 14.1. (*continued*)

TTM process of change	Description	Promotes movement from which stage(s) of change?	Group exercises
Behavioral processes			
Counterconditioning	Substituting healthy behaviors for unhealthy ones	Preparation Action Maintenance	• Identify healthy ways to change
Reinforcement management	Rewarding positive behavior changes or recognizing positive consequences	Action Maintenance	• Identify healthy ways to reward self-change

Starting the Group

In the first group session, we introduce members to the MI spirit and point out that this group experience might be different from others in which they have participated.

> "In this group we use a motivational approach. This means that we will avoid confronting one another or being the expert on another's life— instead, we'll help facilitate change by listening to and supporting each other. We are here to learn more about you and any changes in your drug use you may be considering, and although we have knowledge about and experience with successful drug change processes, ultimately, if there is any changing to be done, you will be the one to do it."

Thus, from the beginning, we emphasize that we will not coerce or try to force change. We note that although we are the group leaders, each member plays an important role in supporting other members. Importantly, the essential MI principle of expressing *empathy*—understanding the choices, feelings, and concerns of another—is emphasized in this first session and serves as the foundation of all subsequent sessions.

> "We know that an atmosphere of empathy, acceptance, and respect makes the group more helpful for its members, because research indicates that this kind of approach is much more effective than a confrontational one."

During this initial session, we find that presentation of elements in the acronym "OPEN" helps develop a shared group culture.

- Overview of the group's purpose is presented: learning about members' goals, concerns, choices.
- Personal choice and autonomy are emphasized.
- Environment is described as one of respect and encouragement for all members.
- Nonconfrontational nature of the group is noted.

Including these elements in the introduction promotes a positive group alliance and helps to counter potential tendencies to confront, criticize, or challenge other members that may have been learned in other groups. Over the course of the group sessions, members incorporate the nonjudgmental and affirming manner modeled by the group leaders as they reflect feelings and concerns of other members and support their growing sense of self-efficacy.

Reflections and Open Questions

Throughout the group sessions, we often use two MI strategies sequentially: *reflections* and *open questions*. A combination of these strategies in a group setting can be utilized to provide structure and direction to the group dialogue. We begin with a brief reflection of a point made by a group member, followed by an open question that incorporates part of the reflection *and* provides a clear avenue for constructive discussion among other group members. Sometimes this strategy can help a group maintain focus and direction, and contain members whose long histories are recalled in "war stories" that disrupt the positive flow of the discussion. At other times, this approach provides structure for members who are sidetracked by anxiety or tangential thoughts, helping them to get back on track. In this example from the "Relationships and Concern" session, which promotes the use of the *environmental reevaluation* process of change, the leader briefly summarizes points made by some members, then moves the session forward with an open question that elicits constructive comments from other group members.

LEADER A: What are some other ways that people have expressed concern? [Open question] Like some of you have said, people walking out of your life, nagging you, or like [Group Member A] said, talking about his mother's hopes for him. What other people in your lives have concerns? [summarizing; open question]

GROUP MEMBER B: I have my wife . . . her unconditional love for me . . . but you know, if you abuse this drug, you're gonna hurt somebody. If there's anybody out there, anybody that cares a whole bunch about you, they don't want to see you go down, and that's exactly what you're gonna do if you abuse this drug . . . no question about it.

LEADER A: That's what [Group Member B] was describing, "going down" [reflection that connects one member's comment to another member's concern]

GROUP MEMBER B: If I could turn back time, you know, a lot of things would've been different.

GROUP MEMBER C: But I really don't like to turn back time, because that's made me who I am. I really don't think I'll ever do coke again. I really don't think I ever, ever, ever, will do coke again.

LEADER A: If you had to choose the most important reason for what you've said, "I don't think I'll ever use coke again," what would it be? [open question to elicit change talk]

GROUP MEMBER C: My most important reason will probably be me. I mean I want to do it for everybody else, but mostly for me. I want to quit. I missed a lot. I can't explain how much I missed. Everything was on *my* time. I'm gonna do what I want to do. I just had that attitude. I missed so much. So it would be for me and my future.

LEADER B: So this time you really want to do it for you. . . . You feel like this is for you. You were missing out on life when you were using cocaine. [reflection of change talk]

Constructive Affirmations

In a group context, affirmations are useful to highlight and acknowledge collective behaviors or accomplishments of the group, as well as those of individual members. Although affirmations are a powerful means of conveying appreciation, respect, admiration, and support, they are cheapened when delivered in an undiscriminating or disingenuous fashion, and they lose their impact when delivered too frequently. We believe that the most useful affirming statements are judicious, genuine, and specific. We convey affirmations in a warm and sincere manner because those that are rushed, tossed out casually, or delivered without eye contact come across as superficial. This "style" aspect of an affirmation is especially important when working with members whose life experiences may have made them especially sensitive to perceived hypocrisy and empty praise. Some of the most effective affirmations describe a specific behavior (e.g., "The way you stuck with your job last week despite your boss's unpleasant attitude must have been really hard—that took determination and courage" or "Putting money aside for your child, even though you had to cut back on other purchases, is really admirable") rather than an intention, decision, or attitude (e.g., "Your deciding not to use next week is really great" or "That's good that your attitude is positive"). This latter type of affirmation does little to build intrinsic motivation, and it can come across as an admonition or an encouragement to please (e.g., "Tell us what we want to hear").

> *The most useful affirmations are judicious, genuine, and specific.*

Reflections on Reflective Listening

When reflecting client statements, we have found that less is often more. Instead of maintaining an empathic focus on a member's concerns, longer reflections tend to make instructional points or dominate the discourse. In contrast, shorter reflections convey a real understanding of the member's remarks and have greater impact. Thus, at times, the power of a reflection is increased by using only a word or two that intensify the meaning and impact of a member's statement. In groups, reflections crystallize key points raised by members and strategically serve as punctuation marks that help to clarify and draw attention to selective member responses, such as change and commitment talk.

> *Shorter reflections have greater impact.*

LEADER B: You said some important things, you're saying that on the one hand you were using cocaine so you could feel part of life . . . but then you realized that over time, you were actually . . . [affirmation; beginning a reflection of ambivalence]

GROUP MEMBER C: I was already important to the right people. With these other people, it was just a false sense of importance that I had. But the people that mean the most, those that are going to be in my life forever, I was not giving the attention to. . . . You don't even have to say a word. You look at them and say, "Man, she's really disappointed in me" or "My son knows what I'm doing," or like little stuff like that, I mean, nobody has to say a word, then it just clicks one day and you have to let it [the cocaine] go.

LEADER A: It clicked. [simple reflection]

GROUP MEMBER C: You have to make a decision.

LEADER A: It is almost like you were saying, there's going to be a turn, it's a turning point. [complex reflection—intensifies meaning and captures change talk]

GROUP MEMBER B: Oh yeah!

Summaries

Summaries have special utility in our groups. While we intersperse summaries throughout the session, each meeting also ends with a process summary that takes into account themes and issues expressed by each member. In this ending summary, we acknowledge struggles, but the primary focus is on the change talk and commitment language that have occurred throughout the session. In this example from the "Relationships and Concern" session, the leader uses a "collecting" summary to highlight a common theme among group members and ends with a powerful reflection of feelings:

LEADER A: You know, there's a real commonality here about losses and pain—about hurting your self-image, losing self-esteem, and certainly losing money. A real sense that there has been more than enough pain and it's time to turn things around. [summary]

GROUP MEMBER B: It kind of feels bad when the folks, the people you love, see you.

GROUP MEMBER C: Yeah, when they see you, you feel guilty.

LEADER A: You feel ashamed and don't want to feel that way anymore. [reflection]

Elicit–Provide–Elicit

The "elicit–provide–elicit" strategy can be used in groups when provision of information—or even judicious advice—is indicated. The first step is to elicit what members may already know about an issue (e.g., "What have you heard about health concerns related to cocaine use?") or their permission to share knowledge or a concern (e.g., "Would it be okay if we looked at some information that has been helpful to many?"; "Could we take a few minutes to talk about _____?"). This type of respectful approach generally lowers resistance and almost always results in a positive response, which in turn creates a more open attitude toward the subsequent information. This query is followed by the provision of information or concern (e.g., medical conditions associated with cocaine use), then an open question is asked to elicit thoughts about the information and turn the dialogue back to the members (e.g., "What stands out most for you about this?"; "Which, if any, might concern you most?"; "What are your thoughts about that?"). This technique invites group members to reexamine facts they have previously learned or to consider new information and incorporate elements of it as appropriate for their needs and circumstances.

Identifying and Exploring Members' Stage of Change

One exercise that is particularly useful in promoting consciousness raising in the group setting is to describe the stages-of-change concept, ask members to assess their own stage, then explore what that means to them in regard to change. This can help to create a sense of momentum in which change is understood as a dynamic process rather than a static "Either I have changed or I have not" conceptualization. It is also a good exercise for "breaking the ice" in early group sessions, because it allows members to share their own personal view of their substance use.

Consistent with the MI spirit of collaboration and autonomy, after first asking members about their interest in this topic, then describing the stages of change with everyday examples, we turn the dialogue back to members by asking open questions such as "What are your thoughts about this?" or "How does this fit for you?" This staging concept is readily understood, because members typically are very interested in both sharing where they currently are in the cycle of change and reviewing their previous "positions" in the stage cycle. Overall, this topic elicits much discussion and creates an early opportunity for members to actively engage in the group process. Members' responses allow us to reflect our understanding and acceptance of their situations, concerns, and goals, which in turn strengthens group cohesion. This focus also provides a chance for us to invite quieter group members into the discussion. We have noticed that in subsequent sessions members often continue to refer to the stages, remarking how useful they are in helping them conceptualize their current situation and make choices.

In introducing stages of change, we read vignettes from the TTM manual to the members and ask, "In what stage of change is the individual in that vignette?" This particular vignette is about a client in the action stage:

LEADER A: *(reading vignette)* "Marcus is proud of himself. He has gone for 2 weeks without taking a drink. He has started 'hanging out' with some new friends at work who don't drink either and his work has improved, and his boss even noticed a difference. When he threw out all the alcohol from his house a few weeks ago, he wasn't sure if it would last. Even though he's been tempted to stop by the bar after work, instead he has jogged in the park every evening." What stage of change is Marcus in?

GROUP MEMBER A: Action!

GROUP MEMBER B: Action.

GROUP MEMBER C: Maintenance.

GROUP MEMBER D: Both of them. He's quitting the use, but he's also avoiding the triggers.

GROUP MEMBER E: He's reinforcing himself.

GROUP MEMBER F: He's putting himself in a position where he is not allowing himself to be . . . you know, to hang out with the friend who drinks.

LEADER A: He removed some of the temptations. [reflection]

GROUP MEMBER F: Right, right. Well, it's basically maintenance *and* action. . . .

LEADER A: You do the same things that you were doing with the action strategy, but (when) you . . . do them so long they become a regular part of your life. Action becoming maintenance. [reflection; demonstration of the stage of change identification exercise evoking multimember participation and engagement]

GROUP MEMBER H: I'm thinking about it [about changing].

LEADER B: You're in the contemplation stage —you're thinking about it. [reflection]

GROUP MEMBER H: Thinking about it, a change. The only way I can change is to start to prepare myself to start to talk about it in the group session.

LEADER A: It almost sounds like there's a little bit of preparation there— "one of the things I can do." One part of your plan will be to talk about it in these sessions. Who else . . .? [reflection; open question turning issue back to group]

GROUP MEMBER C: I will say I'm in action. I mean, I quit using. I have . . . different sets of friends, my negative and my positive friends. And when I was doing my negative things, my positive friends called me. I told them, I'm busy, I can't talk to you at this time, because I was using, but I can talk to them now because I'm doing something about it. I just want to leave my negative friends and try to fix it with my positive friends.

LEADER A: You've done some changing, you've taken some action. Who else? [reflection; open question as an artful intermission that returns topic to group]

GROUP MEMBER F: Can you be at two [stages] at one time?

LEADER A: Tell me about it. [open question that explores member's perspective]

GROUP MEMBER F: Contemplation and um, preparation. Okay, I am thinking of quitting, wondering how it might affect others, maybe . . . maybe trying small changes. Kind of in that stage a little bit . . . where "let's not drink a 12-pack a day, let's just see if you can drink socially." I want to drink, but I don't want to smoke [cocaine], but I know if you're drinking you're gonna need the smoke.

LEADER A: You're starting to cut down, you're thinking about cutting down on your alcohol use, and kind of in preparation for not using cocaine.

LEADER B: Thank you for that example—that part is so normal—to be in different stages of change with two different behaviors. We can be in preparation and switch back to contemplation, or you could be in contemplation and "jump over" preparation, back in action. [affirmation; summary]

GROUP MEMBER F: Well, it would also be precontemplation, 'cause I'm thinking it is okay to drink, but I really deep down know I shouldn't because if I do I know it is going to lead to something, so in my mind I'm telling myself I really don't have an alcoholic problem, I only have a cocaine problem.

LEADER A: You know the word that describes what you're talking about is *ambivalence*. Ambivalence is so common in the contemplation stage. "I know I want to change this, I'm not sure I want to change this." It sometime feels a little bit like confusion. [providing information; reflection]

GROUP MEMBER F: Oh, yeah! Confusion! (*General laughter*)

LEADER B: It's kind of like a dance, kind of moving from side to side, and back and forth. [complex reflection using metaphor]

GROUP MEMBER C: You're waltzing!

LEADER B: You're waltzing. [simple reflection]

Note how members' responses build on one another and how the group leaders guide members through the self-assessment process, mostly using simple reflections. We recommend making the stages-of-change model a central part of early sessions, because it provides both a shared vocabulary and helpful insight that promotes group cohesiveness.

And Last, but Not Least, Lessons Learned from Our Members

Members have told us that they benefit from occasional reminders—either from a group leader or a group member—about relating to other members with the MI spirit and style of respect, nonconfrontation, and support. They generally appreciate these refresher remarks and receive them almost with a sense of relief, because they are absolved of the need to confront, persuade, or judge each other. Many members report that not feeling judged by their peers or the leaders is a new and helpful experience.

In some sessions, discussions are generated by handouts and written exercises, which are kept in a folder for each member. Because some members are living on the edge—marginally homeless, estranged from family, and struggling with multiple life stressors—we keep the folders onsite and give members copies to take with them if they wish.

Finally, a common challenge for substance abuse treatment groups is how to reduce relapse-related attrition. Although research indicates that several quit attempts generally precede the final quit, individuals who have recently relapsed are often demoralized, embarrassed, and reluctant to return to their treatment programs. The MI approach, based on expressions of empathy, acceptance, optimism, and encouragement, conceptualizes relapse not as a failure but as an opportunity for learning. Members who miss several sessions because of a relapse and then return to the group have told us that the "spirit" of the group was what made it possible for them to rejoin and resume the change process.

Assessing Group MI Treatment Fidelity

We have used the Motivational Interviewing Treatment Integrity (MITI) behavioral coding scale (Moyers, Martin, Manuel, Hendrickson, & Miller, 2005) to assess leader fidelity to MI in our TTM groups. The MITI assesses treatment quality by coding two global MI concepts, "empathy" and "spirit" (collaboration, evocation, and support of autonomy). Several types of leader verbalizations, which can also be coded and used to assess MI fidelity, include closed and open questions, simple and complex reflections, MI-adherent remarks (e.g., affirming, asking permission to give information or advice, expressing support) and MI-nonadherent remarks (e.g., advising without permission, confronting, arguing). Although the MITI has previously been used to code individual MI sessions, independent coders were able to use it reliably to assess our group treatment. Results from this coding review indicated that the group intervention was highly adherent to MI principles and strategies (Velasquez, Stephens & Ingersoll, 2006).

Conclusion

This combined TTM group intervention respects the autonomy of group members who may be at different stages of change, and it offers a variety of activities and exercises designed to promote and solidify commitment to behavior change. It also fosters an atmosphere of mutual support and caring. We find that the client-centered, goal-oriented style of MI is a natural fit with a group context, because the principles and strategies of this approach allow consideration of individual member concerns and circumstances, as well as address the explicit group goal of cocaine use behavior change. Group members respond well to the use of MI in the TTM groups, and leaders enjoy the challenge of using their MI skills in more complex situations. At the same time, because using MI in the group setting can be challenging, we recommend that you become skilled in practicing MI in individual sessions before moving into MI group work. While the MI approach with individuals has been described as "waltzing," we think that using MI in groups is more like "conducting a symphony." Each member plays an individual instrument and contributes to the collective melody of the group, and at the same time responds to the conductor. The conductor, in turn, gently guides the instrumental interactions, as well as the overall orchestral composition.

> *Leading groups in an MI style is like conducting a symphony.*

References

Amrhein, P. C., Miller, W. R., Yahne, C. E., Palmer, M., & Fulcher, L. (2003). Client commitment language during motivational interviewing predicts drug use outcomes. *Journal of Consulting and Clinical Psychology, 71,* 862–878.

Bandura, A. (1986). *Social foundations of thought and action: A social cognitive theory.* Englewood Cliffs, NJ: Prentice-Hall.

DiClemente, C. C. (2003). *Addiction and change: How addictions develop and addicted people recover.* New York: Guilford Press.

DiClemente, C. C., & Velasquez, M. (2002). Motivational interviewing and the stages of change. In W. R. Miller & S. Rollnick, *Motivational interviewing: Preparing people for change* (2nd ed.). New York: Guilford Press.

Janis, I. J., & Mann, L. (1977). *Decision-making: A psychological analysis of conflict, choice and commitment.* New York: Free Press.

Moyers, T. B., Martin, T., Manual, J. K., Hendrickson, S. M. L., & Miller, W. R. (2005). Assessing competence in motivational interviewing. *Journal of Substance Abuse Treatment, 28,* 19–26.

Perz, C. A., DiClemente, C. C., & Carbonari, J. (1996). Doing the right thing at the right time: The intersection of stages and processes of change in successful smoking cessation. *Health Psychology, 15,* 462–468.

Prochaska J. O., DiClemente, C. C., & Norcross, J. C. (1982). In search of how people change: Applications to addictive behaviors. *American Psychologist, 47,* 1102–1114.

Velasquez, M., Maurer, G. G., Crouch, C., & DiClemente, C. C. (2001). *Group treatment for substance abuse: A stages-of-change therapy manual.* New York: Guilford Press.

Velasquez, M., Stephens, N., & Ingersoll, K. (2006). Motivational Interviewing in groups. *Journal of Groups in Addiction and Recovery, 1*(1), 27–50.

CHAPTER 15

Motivational Interviewing Empowerment Groups for Women with Addictions

Frances Jasiura, Winnie Hunt,
and Cristine Urquhart

Dear Nameless One . . . I dare not speak your name,

I used to think you saved my life. You came to me like a rescue mission when I was down. I could go to you and find a friend. At first it was like a honeymoon, all lighthearted and no more depression. But that was just the start. So slick, so smooth you are. I hardly noticed the way you worked into my dreams, my waking life, my very soul.

You became like a jealous lover demanding more and more of my time, my money, my health.

The weirdest part was that you were inside me pulling the strings and I was working hard just to keep up and keep you in my life. I was stealing and lying, and then lying to cover up the lies. All out of control.

Over the past months, with lots of help, none of it from you I might add, I've struggled and found ways to distance from you, to take back my days and nights, my feelings, even the rough ones, my thoughts, my self-respect. You will always be in

*my memory brain, but I now know you are truly dangerous and
recognize your footsteps if you try to approach.*

*I give thanks every day for my sanity and contentment, my
spiritual core, and my desire to go positive. You are never again
my friend and you are never again welcome in my life.*

Letters like this one, from a client to her drug of choice, are sometimes read
aloud in our intensive day-treatment group program for women with multiple psychological, health, and social challenges. The group incorporates
MI, cognitive-behavioral, and embodied approaches. We pair MI spirit,
principles, and strategies with a feminist empowerment philosophy to help
women address their challenges. They can emerge from this experience
with a positive peer group and new skills, confidence, and commitment to
change.

Women with complex health and social concerns may benefit from
multiple, integrated interventions for trauma and substance abuse (Harris
& Fallot, 2001; Najavits, 2002). Women's healing often happens through
their relationships, especially healthy connections based on empowerment
and reciprocity (Covington & Surrey, 2000). The centrality of the collaborative relationship in MI is consistent with a relational model of understanding women's experience of substance use. There are other parallels between
the spirit and principles of MI and women-centered, trauma-informed care,
including respect for autonomy and an emphasis on empowerment and
choice (MI and Intimate Partner Violence Workgroup, 2009). Studies have
shown that MI reduces women's substance use problems and related health
concerns (Yahne, Miller, Irvin-Vitela, & Tonigan, 2002; Floyd et al., 2007;
Ingersoll et al., 2005).

Recent studies have suggested that MI-informed group interventions
for women are helpful. LaBrie and colleagues (2008, 2009) found that
small groups using MI and personalized feedback helped college women
with alcohol problems to reduce their drinking. Another study integrated
MI into a group program for young homeless women who had multiple risk
factors, including substance use, violence, and trauma (Wenzel, D-Amico,
Barnes, & Gilbert, 2009).

Our women's day-treatment program mirrors the intensity of a residential setting, while reducing barriers to women's participation in addiction
treatment, including child care and cost (Healthy Choices in Pregnancy,
2002). Women in our groups often have long histories of polysubstance use,
gambling, violence committed against them, and involvement in sex trade
and other harmful situations. Barriers to engagement include distrust of
professionals, previous failures in educational/treatment settings, undevel-
oped skills for managing challenging interpersonal situations, discourage-
ment, and powerlessness. Many of the women also struggle with poverty,

trauma, inadequate housing, and child care problems; are under-educated and unemployed; and have compromised physical and mental health. Some have been court-mandated because of child protection issues. They are often hesitant to join a women's group, and later reveal their mistrust of other women. Regular attendance is a significant challenge when members return to chaotic lives and unsupportive relationships.

Women's addictions often have significant historical/cultural roots. *Empowerment* is "relational action where mutual attention, empathy, engagement and responsiveness . . . reconceptualize power" (Goodrich, 1991, p. 20). Women lack empowerment when they become externally defined and marginalized through the oppression of addictions, poverty, trauma, and abusive use of power. They can internalize negative identities based on society's rejection of, or indifference to, their life experiences, which frequently include mental illness, prostitution, drug abuse, and unhealthy parenting of children. They often have low self-esteem, amplified by the discrepancies between their values and choices they have made, and turn to unhealthy coping strategies as survival mechanisms.

This chapter highlights the role of MI within the group for women, offering examples of MI relational and technical elements woven throughout the group process, from engagement to closure. We base our interventions on MI spirit and principles, seeking to balance individual needs and group involvement, while evoking movement in the direction of change by eliciting and reinforcing change talk and commitment. Guided by the spirit of MI, leaders and group members are challenged to put aside their reflex to fix others, and instead to take every opportunity to strengthen members' autonomy and choice, while building collaboration within a subculture of women who tend to distrust each other and anyone in authority. As participants live their lives while attending the group, their clarity around priorities, concerns, and capacities can shift over the 4-week period; their motivation often is supported and strengthened by the group. For example, one member decided to engage proactively with child protection authorities and offer random urine screens. When she reported back to the group how she did that, and the positive outcomes, other members took notice and appeared to "borrow her self-efficacy." We foster a positive group climate with compassion, power sharing, and recognition of every effort toward teamwork.

Our opening scenario illustrates how every group interaction offers several alternative directions to consider. In our example, this member is taking action steps by writing and reading her letter, declaring the costs–benefits of drug use and of change, and announcing her movement from ambivalence to commitment. She offers a transformational shift in self-perception by claiming the strength and determination that live in the statement "You are never again welcome in my life." In this moment, we might respond by eliciting, strengthening, and supporting her change talk and commitment. Alternatively, we might notice that the letter has sparked internal processing among other women in the group. Because this group has strong cohesion after an

> *Foster a positive group climate with compassion, power sharing, and recognition of every effort toward teamwork.*

intensive 3 weeks together, we return our focus to the group to strengthen mutuality and active participation, thanking the woman for sharing, and inviting members to journal for a few minutes to allow time for autonomous processing. As we return the group's attention to the letter writer, we might ask members to summarize what they heard in the letter, thereby reinforcing change talk, then ask the letter writer, "What did we miss?" and "Where does this leave you now?" Following this, we might encourage mutual exploration of similar experiences in the whole group.

MI in Pregroup Screening and Orientation

We meet individually with each potential group member for the dual purposes of engagement and screening. During this 45-minute interview, we hope to activate the woman's optimism about the group and set the stage for collaboration by connecting with her as the group leaders. We also screen for her readiness to participate in an intensive day-treatment program. We assess several admission criteria, including prior group experience, safety concerns at home, support, ongoing individual/trauma counseling, intention to attend every day, resolution of barriers to participation, and severity of withdrawal symptoms, if any.

An abbreviated sample interview follows, demonstrating relevant MI components (in brackets).

LEADER: Welcome, Donna. It's great to meet you. . . . (*more introducing, welcoming*) Your counselor sent over this referral form that you completed together. It looks like you're interested in attending our women's empowerment group. We're wondering what you've heard about it? [eliciting]

DONNA: Well, not a lot, really. My counselor says it would be good to have more support instead of just seeing her once a week. I have a friend who has been telling me about it for a long time. . . .

LEADER: Have you seen the group poster, Donna?

DONNA: No.

LEADER: This is a list of topics that other groups have chosen to focus on.

We're wondering what areas, if any, might interest you if you were to attend group? [agenda setting]

DONNA: Well, everything on this list is what I need. Relapse prevention, grief, abuse, assertiveness, healthy relationships, just about everything.

LEADER: Other women have said the same thing, Donna . . . and it's not a surprise, because this program was created by women for women. It's about finding healthier ways to manage real life situations. [providing information]

DONNA: Yeah, it got so bad . . . they took my kids and I want to get them back, but now welfare just pays for my one room in someone's house. (*Starts crying.*)

LEADER: So it feels like things are spinning out of control; your kids aren't with you . . . you really want to get back on the track. And you made it here today. [complex reflection; affirmation]

DONNA: Yeah, and it was my own damn fault. Nobody made me drink and drive. Nobody made me get into coke. It was just living the life and fun, fun, fun!

LEADER: So it was fun for a while . . . and now you're picking up the pieces. [complex reflection; affirmation]

DONNA: Yeah, it gets a real hold on you, that damn coke, and even when I don't want it, I still want it.

LEADER: Tell us about your decision to stop this time. [direction and eliciting change talk]

DONNA: Three weeks ago, the anniversary of the day my brother died, I realized that I was wasting my life, and I didn't want to do that anymore.

LEADER: Sounds like that was a turning point. . . . [complex reflection] How have you stayed stopped? [direction and evoking strengths, strategies]

DONNA: Well, I've been smoking pot but not much, and I've been staying by myself and not going downtown and basically, just trying to deal with the cravings and the nightmares.

LEADER: So you want this time to be different, and you want to complete the program if you start it. (*Donna nods.*) So help us here, Donna. You've tried other programs, and have a sense of what works and doesn't work for you. Tell us more about that. [supporting autonomy and eliciting collaboration]

DONNA: I don't know. I really miss my kids and worry about them a lot. And I didn't say much when I was in the other treatment centers. I used to be exhausted and worried about everything, and very depressed. Now I'm at least talking about it and maybe that will help.

LEADER: So already this feels different. You're talking more, not going away to a treatment center, wanting to find ways to stay connected with your kids, taking better care of yourself, staying connected to your counselor. You know a lot about what helps you stay away from coke. [affirmation; autonomy; collaboration] You mentioned smoking pot. Tell us more about that and what about other drugs, prescriptions, gambling, and so forth. [evocation]

DONNA: Well, I always take antidepressants, but my doctor prescribes those. Then I do smoke a little pot to help me chill out, and I do have a beer now and again, but those are not really why I'm here. It's all about the coke, the number 1 worst nightmare.

LEADER: We really appreciate your honesty, Donna. That will go a long way in making this time different. [affirmation] During the month of this group we ask everyone, including ourselves, to intend to stay clear of alcohol and illegal drugs and use prescriptions only as prescribed. If someone does use while in the program, leaders look at each situation individually. Sometimes we have had to ask a member to start again. [Providing information] What's your take on that? [eliciting]

DONNA: Oh yeah, I'm okay. I really need to get my kids back. I really need to do it this time. And it will give me something to do every day instead of watching TV.

LEADER: Throughout the 4-week program, we encourage women to keep working with their counselor on ways to make your life work, handle urges. . . . It sounds like this is important to you, Donna. [reinforcing change talk] You're thinking you would use the group to anchor your days so you can manage the cravings and stay away from coke. It might help to start with a small project now, so you're not just waiting for the program to begin—what do you think? [asking permission]

DONNA: Sure, what is it?

LEADER: We recommend a small journaling project that you can start today and bring with you the first day, where you write about three questions: (1) Why do you want to quit?; (2) Have there been times you tried before?; and (3) What makes this time different? [evocation; direction]

DONNA: That sounds great. It might make me feel better to have something productive to do. . . . I'd like to make this really work for me, so I'm never again in this terrible situation.

LEADER: Okay, it's a go. We are excited you will join us in the group,

Donna. We'll call you next week to touch base. . . . Is it all right to leave a message at this number? . . . We'll see you a week from Monday, and don't worry about bringing anything [notebook, pens] with you. . . . We'll have all that and some snacks too. [providing information] Anything else you're wondering about . . . anything we've missed? [collaboration]

Facilitating MI Empowerment Groups for Women

Engaging the Group

Structuring and Facilitating Women's Empowerment Groups

We offer these closed-enrollment groups, 4 hours per session, 5 days a week for 4 weeks. The time investment and closed structure help to build the delicate group cohesion, safety, and mutuality needed to support members as they face difficult situations, entrenched beliefs, and strong emotions. To maintain clear group boundaries, we do not counsel members individually, but we do encourage them to continue with individual counseling. Groups are held within a setting of other community services in order to safeguard anonymity, confidentiality, and safety. We ask members to keep the location confidential.

Members partake in both individual and group exercises to strengthen autonomy within a supportive group context. We use group rounds, where a pass is always an option, to give every woman an opportunity to speak and be validated. We stimulate varied learning styles through both individual and group activities and across reading, writing, speaking, art, and movement domains. Each session includes skills building in body–mind focusing, such as conscious breathing, guided relaxation, short meditations, and movements that promote ease in the body. To foster group cohesion and build collaboration, we avoid agenda-driven, expert-based, didactic instruction. We find these

> *To foster group cohesion and build collaboration, avoid agenda-driven, expert-based, didactic instructions.*

embodied approaches help to deepen focus, reduce individual trauma reactions, quiet drug urges and thoughts, and lay the foundation for change. Throughout the day, we monitor the attention span of group members and offer short, frequent movement breaks, along with two longer outdoor respites. Group members have consistently expressed appreciation for this structure, which provides the safety and containment that are vital for trauma-informed work, guided by the MI spirit of partnership, acceptance, compassion, and evocation.

Facilitating Group Cohesion and MI-Consistent Group Process

While engaging the group, we coach members not to respond to each other during check-in or check-out rounds. This temporary prohibition of "cross-talk" short-circuits unsolicited advice, questions, digression into stories/experiences, and other MI-inconsistent responses. When exploring perspectives, we encourage interaction, while helping members notice when peer persuasion and unsolicited advice elicit resistance to change. As the group develops, we strengthen affirmation and reflective responses, and encourage more interaction, skills practice, awareness, and responsibility. In daily breaks, conversations can fall back into familiar, aggressive communication patterns. In group, we coach members to revisit these conversations with new skills. An MI style of guiding and emergent skills development help the group as a whole to become more MI-consistent. The synergy that seems to develop leads to greater willingness among group members to trust one another and the group process, which leads to rekindled hope and focus on change. The culture itself begins to shift.

Both the relational and technical elements of MI are pivotal throughout these women's empowerment groups. We elicit and reinforce change talk within a collaborative approach that reconstructs "power over" into "power with," "power to," and "power from within" (Starhawk, 1987). We affirm helpful group behaviors, include the group in all possible decisions and responsibilities, and seize every opportunity to elicit and make visible each woman's innate desire to be well, responsible, and compassionate. An MI style of warmth, acceptance, empathy, and gentle direction is crucial as we roll with multiple resistances, ever-shifting readiness, volatile responses, and dynamic relationships, while evoking change talk and encouraging cognitive-behavioral skills practice. MI spirit, principles, and skills aim to build *the group* as the hard-won container of trust: in the leaders, the structure, and themselves. That trust is quickly betrayed if members suspect that we view ourselves as "the experts" or any member as "needing to be rescued or fixed." We offer members genuine recognition as they readily assume responsibilities in the group and experience themselves as reliable and generous. At the same time, we are tender with their battle wounds and deeply respectful of their will to survive.

Managing Conflict

Members consistently describe how, in their lived experiences, anger and frustration often disintegrate into conflict, unresolved endings, verbal abuse, and violence. Disagreements within the group can quickly escalate into withdrawal, sarcasm, or verbal aggression, and trigger trauma reactions and subsequent drug urges to ease the distress. Our own "righting reflex" is often triggered. When conflicts first arise, we slow the discussion down and ask members to direct all communication to the leaders, not to each other, and engage in active listening and conflict containment. We coach members to practice previously learned conflict strategies, such as "I" language only, sticking to the issue, and direct expression of needs. If a woman chooses to leave the circle in the heat of conflict, we respect her boundaries and self-care, ask her to return shortly, and call for a short break. We invite each member to debrief in the check-out round, to rank urges to use drugs, and to commit to return the following day. Group members experience healthy, nonviolent resolution of conflict, supported by relaxation tools to contain intense reactions.

Starting the Group

Ideally, groups begin with eight to 10 members in order to maintain a feasible cohort size, with an anticipated 25% dropout rate. We create a warm atmosphere with light food, background music, and a circle of chairs around gifts from previous groups that offer a sense of continuity and belonging. Bridging from the individual screening interviews, we warmly welcome each woman as she enters the room on the first day, and begin group by acknowledging the many decisions and courage needed to attend. Addressing unspoken safety concerns, we begin with individual journaling and invite members to privately list and rank their concerns about participating in the group. We offer assurance that journals are private and can be locked away between sessions. We facilitate several quick and fun icebreakers. We prefer a name familiarity game, in which everyone, including ourselves, attaches a positive adjective to her first name, such as "Hopeful Hazel." This simple exercise initiates a subtle shift in self-perception toward the preferred self and can build momentum toward change by tapping into positive emotions. Members often return to these names.

Next, members brainstorm what they would like to share with each other, and frequently choose to disclose ages of children, "drug of choice," previous treatment programs, support groups, hobbies, birthplace, and relationship status. We use open questions, affirmations, reflections, and summaries (OARS) to link common themes among group members. Isolation further softens when members identify and address common barriers to attendance, such as transportation and child care. The simple procedure of asking members to inform the group in advance if they cannot attend appears to decrease nonattendance. We acknowledge anonymously when some members are mandated to attend, and help members openly explore boundaries around confidentiality, anonymity, information safety, reporting requirements and procedures. Members brainstorm their expectations and "burning issues" for the program. Posted on the wall, this list of topics fosters group cohesion, serves as a compass for the group, aids in time management, and invites members to address their highest priorities.

Members brainstorm group guidelines intended to foster healthy boundaries, safety, and collaboration. These are also mounted on the wall and reviewed weekly to offer safe footing in times of conflict. One typical group developed the following guidelines: respect for others (including punctuality), confidentiality, talking in turn, no interrupting, no finishing sentences, no side talk, no fixing one another, staying on topic, no eating, cell phones off, no talk glorifying the drug lifestyle, no socializing outside of group (reviewed after 2 weeks), attending every day, and remaining substance free. The final two items on this list are often flash points that provide a fertile opportunity for members to experience facilitated dialogue. While a member voices her heartfelt intention to attend every day and remain drug- and alcohol-free, she may lapse. We explain that, taking into consideration the overall well-being of both the individual and the group, we have sometimes needed to ask members to begin the program again.

Exploring Perspectives

The group sessions include daily check-in and check-out rounds, limited to 5 minutes per person, in which we reinforce change talk and practice skills. We use the elicit–provide–elicit strategy to cultivate a collaborative learning environment. We elicit a group summary from members' at check-in, in which the day's topic/theme emerges; this theme can be supported but not driven by the Healthy Choices in Pregnancy program manual. We elicit members' prior understanding of the identified topic, then provide/facilitate knowledge and skill development through written material, discussion, practice exercises, and personal goal setting. By welcoming all perspectives throughout the work, we offer an opportunity to develop personal agency, tolerance, curiosity, and openness, and increased capacity to develop new lifestyles and practical solutions.

A final check-out round focuses on individual concerns, confidence level, and action plans, which are revisited in the check-in the next session. We leave enough time in the check-out round for problem solving after each member ranks urges to use drugs and concerns about personal safety. We invite members to review privately their initial "list and rank" journal entries, to notice any shifts in the scaling numbers, and to share them if they wish. Each day ends with a meaningful ritual created by members.

At the beginning of each week, check-in may reveal new issues that require immediate attention, or positive changes that reflect increased coping and communication skills. At the end of each week we invite members to prepare for weekend difficulties that may arise in the void of not attending supportive group sessions. Weekends provide reality checks and rehearsal for when group ends.

Group members often express little hope as they enter the group and share shattered experiences of incomplete and often abusive endings they have experienced. Once they begin to benefit from the group's predictability and safety, they begin to wonder aloud how they will manage/maintain changes and momentum when group ends. As the group progresses, we offer encouragement, collective problem solving, and resource sharing to support skills transfer beyond the group. Members revisit their original list of topics, bringing heightened urgency, skills, presence, and trust to sensitive areas of grief, loss, abuse, trauma, and sexuality.

As we continue to explore these women's perspectives on their lives, we focus on their individual situations and lifestyles, their personal values, the fit between their values and lifestyles, and the ambivalence they feel about the various challenges they face in restructuring their lives. As the women become more open and trust continues to deepen, they begin to bond together as a group, beyond being a collection of individuals. When we sense that cohesion and trust are high enough, we turn to broadening perspectives.

Broadening Perspectives

We integrate MI, cognitive-behavioral, trauma-informed, group process, and embodied awareness approaches to build safety and skills, empowerment, and readiness as we move into this phase of work in which women feel understood and ready to consider alternative perspectives. We bring new ideas to group members, to broaden their understanding of addictions. For example, women find it helpful to explore various models of development and change, and importantly, the larger context of society's role in women's issues. A variety of techniques are useful when delivered using an MI counseling style. For example, we help women do functional analyses and decisional balances for specific behaviors such as drug use, harm reduction, or abstinence. We use visual aids and exercises to elicit cognitive-behavioral skills practice in problem solving, assertiveness, communication, conflict resolution, and healthy relationships. We incorporate MI strategies such as envisioning a better future, exploring members' sense of importance and confidence about making changes, and exploring their strengths and supports. With permission, we offer increasing feedback and coaching in the OARS communication skills. The group gains momentum for change as members experience success in applying strategies for wellness, relapse prevention, and drug urges. Members are invited to post the written or drawn products of exercises to remind them of the selves they are striving to be.

In one group, a woman shared that she had had cocaine urges all night long. She paused, then added "except when I didn't!" Through the rest of the group, whenever she noticed her overgeneralizations, she would remember "except when I don't." This is an example of a group member practicing her developing skills in the group with immediacy, openness, transparency, and trust. In instances like this, we affirm movement toward change goals and invite other members to notice how this effort during group activities is a part of their active work toward the better lives they are seeking. As we ourselves and group members recognize and reinforce behavioral, emotional, and physical shifts within the supportive group environment, these changes become the "new normal" and are more easily maintained.

Moving into Action

While daily attendance *is* action for these women, some move into action on larger issues right away, while still exploring other concerns when the group ends. Members share a range of difficulties, from those that are small and easily resolved to daunting, intergenerational challenges without clear solutions. For example, our letter writer, who opened this chapter, identified her need for skills and support to accept and manage difficult emotions; to let go of abusive relationships including drugs; to access her natural creative abilities; to find a healthy community; to deal constructively with conflict; and to prevent relapse and manage drug urges, thoughts, and feelings. To build self-efficacy, we encourage members to identify their spheres of influence and attempt smaller, simpler changes during the first half of the group. Sometimes, hypothetical planning is the most appropriate way to help members imagine how to change a longer-term behavioral pattern. We introduce the idea of "trial changing." In a group round, we invite the women to imagine the smallest changes they might implement for just a week. We ask them whether they are ready to commit to this "trial," and we offer more support and planning to those who remain uncertain. We work with all levels and fluctuating readiness for change, and reflect the kernels of change talk in hesitant and fledgling statements that show tiny movements toward healthy change. As the group continues, we address more sensitive topics and guide dialogue toward hypothetical changes for more comprehensive challenges. We encourage a group member to invite her peers to help her brainstorm ideas for next steps. After writing all possible ideas on the board, she is then invited to select the "top three" that seem most likely to fit for her. These rounds and participatory exercises provide support and new perspectives, while building momentum for change and teaching a process that can be carried forward beyond group. We acknowledge women's strength to talk about challenging behaviors, knowing that people talk themselves into change. When one group member takes on concrete change efforts, she offers her peers a vicarious experience of hope and tangible success.

Closure and Exit Strategies

Anger and frustration often erupt in the intensity and hard work of the last 2 weeks. We empathize and look for opportunities to practice communication and coping skills. We use OARS, reframing and emphasizing personal choice and control to defuse heightened feelings, and we encourage members to set themselves up for successful completion.

In the final week, each member writes a program summary to clarify what she experienced and learned, and her next steps. She identifies and scales her progress and knowledge in at least five areas: relapse prevention, self-care, communication, healthy relationships, and helpful self-talk. This written evaluation helps her solidify her action plans, provides important program feedback, and is a bridge back to her referral counselor. We meet with each member individually for 15 minutes to review her program summary, acknowledge gains made, and offer feedback on written pre-postassessment measures. Ideally, resources are in place to facilitate her next steps, which may include further treatment, peer support options, education and training, or job readiness programs. Members offer each other appreciation and concrete, constructive feedback. Each group plans its ending and marks this passage in its own unique way, including the design of distinctive completion certificates. Some groups have chosen to have potluck dinners; to release balloons; and to invite referral counselors, community support people, and family members to their ceremony on the final day.

Outcomes of the Group

Participants write about the impact of the group; the following is a summary of typical comments:

- "Every day I give thanks. It was a life or death struggle for me, and now I have a handle on some healthier choices for dealing with problems."
- "I'm more realistic and can even see things from different points of view."
- "With others in the group, I learned to feel more trusting and could see our similarities. It's easier to talk out loud now instead of holding it all in, as if I were the only one who felt this way."
- "I can use my new learning and life skills every day and feel more in charge of myself."

- "I'm more aware of the ways I work myself up into anger or negative judgements, or down into despair, and therefore can be more conscious of avoiding old, harmful routines."
- "My core values give me strength, courage, and reassurance, even in times of trouble, so I can honestly say I like myself."

Conclusion

We have witnessed the transformative possibilities of these MI-informed empowerment groups within this population of marginalized women. Women invite us into their most tender, hidden, and raw places, exposing shame, guilt, self-loathing, destructive internal voices, and a deep resignation to life, side by side with good humor, buried hope, compassion, and resilient core values. The women often experience a resurgence of hope as they interact in a life-affirming culture where they feel heard and honored, often for the first time.

The MI framework fosters empowerment by helping them envision a better future and initiate concrete action steps toward it. It provides the women a language for framing new possibilities and a process for letting go of old attachments and burdens that inhibit change,

Women often experience a resurgence of hope as they interact in a life-affirming culture where they feel heard and honored.

while honoring the paths that have led them to this point. Integrating MI into a group format creates a spirit of generosity, positive emotions, and energy for change that can lead to these transformational shifts in identity. The groups allow the women to gain "new normal" experiences in healthy relationships and female friendships that, with adequate support, they may transfer to their families and social networks. Within this context, despite long histories of poverty, trauma, addictions, unemployment, isolation and abuse, these women muster the resilience, courage, and determination to create better lives for themselves and their children.

Such groups are challenging to facilitate. Proficiency with using MI skills and spirit with individuals is an essential prerequisite. With so much going on every moment, co-facilitation is a necessary and separate skill set. Humility, humor, immediacy, and fluid co-facilitation are required to compensate for the inevitable misses and bumps along the way. It is well worth the effort, however, to see women accomplish what they often previously believed was impossible. While future research and clinical innovations will improve services by revealing even better ways of helping, we hope that this current example of integrating MI into an empowerment group provides useful ideas to consider as you work with those who may need something more than traditional outpatient services in your area.

References

Covington, S. S., & Surrey, J. L. (2000). *The relational model of women's psychological development: Implications for substance abuse* (Work in Progress, No. 91). Wellesley, MA: Stone Center, Working Paper Series.

Floyd, R. L., Sobell, M., Velasquez, M. M., Ingersoll, K., Nettleman, M., Sobell, L., et al. (2007). Preventing alcohol exposed pregnancies: A randomized control trial. *American Journal of Preventive Medicine, 32*(1), 1–10.

Goodrich, T. J. (Ed.). (1991). *Women and power: Perspective for family therapy.* New York: Norton.

Harris, M., & Fallot, R. D. (2001). *Using trauma theory to design service systems.* San Francisco: Jossey-Bass.

Healthy Choices in Pregnancy. (2002). *D.E.W. program facilitators manual.* Victoria, British Columbia, Canada: B.C. Government Press. Available at *www. hcip-bc.org.*

Ingersoll, K. S., Ceperich, S. D., Nettleman, M. D., Karanda, K., Brocksen, S., & Johnson, B. A. (2005). Reducing alcohol exposed pregnancy risk in college women: Initial outcomes of a clinical trial of a motivational intervention. *Journal of Substance Abuse Treatment, 29*(3), 173–180.

LaBrie, J. W., Huchting, K. K., Lac, A., Tawalbeh, S., Thompson, A. D., & Larimer, M. E. (2009). Preventing risky drinking in first-year college women: Further validation of a female-specific motivational enhancement group intervention. *Journal of Studies on Alcohol and Drugs, Supplement, 16,* 77–85.

LaBrie, J. W., Huchting, K., Tawalbeh, S., Pedersen, E. R., Thompson, A. D., Shelesky, K., et al. (2008). A randomized motivational enhancement prevention group reduces drinking and alcohol consequences in first-year college women. *Psychology of Addictive Behaviors, 22*(1), 149.

MI and Intimate Partner Violence Workgroup. (2009). Guiding as practice: Motivational interviewing and trauma-informed work with survivors of intimate partner violence. *Partner Abuse, 1*(1), 92–104.

Najavits, L. M. (2002). *Seeking Safety: A treatment manual for PTSD and substance abuse.* New York: Guilford Press.

Starhawk (1987). *Truth or dare: Encounters with power, authority, and mystery.* San Fransisco: Harper.

Wenzel, S. L., D'Amico, E. J., Barnes, D., & Gilbert, M. L. (2009). A pilot of a tripartite prevention program for homeless young women in the transition to adulthood. *Women's Health Issues, 19,* 193–201.

Yahne, C. E., Miller, W. R., Irvin-Vitela, L., & Tonigan, J. S. (2002). Magdalena Pilot Project: Motivational outreach to substance abusing women street sex workers. *Journal of Substance Abuse Treatment, 23,* 49–53.

CHAPTER 16

Motivational Interviewing Groups for Dually Diagnosed Patients

Steve Martino *and* Elizabeth J. Santa Ana

Many programs for treating patients with co-occurring severe psychiatric and substance use disorders rely on group interventions to develop patients' motivation to address their dual disorders (Drake & Mueser, 2000; Goldsmith & Garlapati, 2004). MI has been recommended as a best practice for motivating individuals (Drake et al., 2001; Minkoff, 2001; Ziedonis et al., 2005), but the literature offers few comprehensive descriptions about how to implement MI in groups in dual-diagnosis specialty programs. This chapter presents a model for MI groups for dually diagnosed patients, focusing on MI groups in the acute care phase of dual-diagnosis treatment.

Conceptualizing MI Groups

Our main assumption in conceptualizing MI groups for dually diagnosed patients is that while we provide the components of MI, group members also are involved in a group dynamic that serves to mutually enhance their motivation for change. In MI, motivation is seen as an interpersonal phenomenon that emerges from the transaction between the leader and patient. Miller and Rollnick (2013) refer to this motivationally enhancing interpersonal style as *MI spirit,* which involves the key components of partnership, acceptance, compassion, and evocation.

For group therapy, Yalom and Leszcz (2005) suggest that universality, imparting information, and instillation of hope are the most salient and active ingredients that lead to behavior change in the early phase of treatment. These three factors foster a group climate in which members experience commonality, support, and encouragement that promotes their efforts to change behavioral problems (Kivlighan & Holmes, 2004).

In MI groups, we recommend cultivating these group therapeutic factors and core elements of MI spirit simultaneously to maximize a motivationally enhancing therapeutic environment. Specifically, we suggest normalizing members' universal experience of ambivalence about change and encouraging them to explore their mixed reactions and other common experiences in group (partnership), as in the following vignette:

LEADER: (*to group*) Many of you may have mixed thoughts and feelings about being here and the problems you are facing. For example, some of you may not only be angry, believing you don't need to be here, but also wonder if your hospitalization could be an opportunity to address your psychiatric or substance use issues. Others may feel relieved to be here, yet be quite uncertain about how you can change overwhelming problems. Let's talk about your reactions to being hospitalized and the issues you are facing.

GROUP MEMBER A: I was pretty angry that my wife gave me an ultimatum. But now that I am here, I think it's for the best, for me, and for my marriage.

LEADER: (*to Group Member A*) At first you were feeling angry about coming to treatment. Now you feel a bit more at ease about being here, because there are some things you hope you will get out of treatment, especially for helping your marriage.

GROUP MEMBER B: I was really angry, too, when they committed me to the hospital. But my manic–depression and drinking were getting out of hand and if I kept going like I was, I probably really would have killed myself.

In addition, you can emphasize the multiple, interacting problems that dually diagnosed group members often face in recovery, and the freedom each of them has in deciding which behavioral changes they pursue (acceptance), as in the following exchange:

LEADER: (*to group*) This group is a place where you can talk about any issues that concern you, whether those are related to psychiatric, addiction, relationship, or other areas. While you might take into account what other people have told you, this group is designed to help you decide what problems you believe you have and what, if anything, you might want to do about them. The group operates by a general principle: Changes you make that come from within yourself will feel better and last longer than those you that you believe have been forced upon you.

GROUP MEMBERS: *(Multiple members nod in agreement.)*

To further tap into universal experience, use structured activities to generate a common theme or focus on change-eliciting topics (e.g., identifying personal strengths and how members might apply them to their dilemmas) to build members' motivation for change (evocation):

> "To help you consider what, if anything, you want to change in your life, this group includes several activities. Each time we meet, I will explain the activity and then ask you to take part in it to the extent you feel comfortable. Today, we are going to talk about. . . . "

Regarding information sharing, we recommend establishing the ground rule that group members may provide only solicited advice or ask permission as a prelude to advice giving, which the recipient is free to accept or reject (acceptance). This also applies to the use of objective feedback from assessment measures, sometimes used in MI groups to help members consider how their current behavior may be problematic for them (evocation). As one example, members may be given information about how their symptoms are consistent with a particular psychiatric condition; they are then asked to consider this information and their reactions to it.

Ask all members to consider how information shared by others might apply to them or affect their motivation to change rather than concentrate feedback solely on one patient (partnership). Model how to listen to members' reactions, and encourage members to reflect their understanding of each other's perspective (partnership). For example, a patient named John received feedback about having a major depressive disorder. His psychiatrist recommended he take antidepressant medication. John was ambivalent about taking the medication.

LEADER: John, you feel two ways about taking the medication. Part of you hopes that your depression is due to your drinking and drug use. Another part of you thinks that you drink and use drugs because you have been depressed, and that's why you have found it so difficult to stop.

JOHN: I just don't want to have to rely on another drug to feel better. I hate the idea that I can't beat this on my own.

LEADER: *(to group)* What do other people hear John saying?

GROUP MEMBER A: John, you sound like you are worried that you'll replace one addiction with another.

GROUP MEMBER B: And that if you take the medication, somehow that means you are weak or even crazy.

JOHN: Yeah, you both are right. Sometimes I do feel like I'm going crazy and taking medication will only prove that. But my way isn't working and that's how I ended up here [dual diagnosis program].

To promote hope about the possibility of change, we recommend facilitating structured activities that elicit members' ability to change. These include examining past successes; looking forward, assuming that behavior change has occurred; or brainstorming feasible change planning strategies (evocation). At the conclusion of activities, help members consider what steps toward any aspect of behavior change they might feel ready, willing, and able to make, even if this means agreeing to explore psychiatric or substance use issues without a commitment to change them (acceptance). At the end of the group, have members reflect on the helpfulness of the activity and the impact it has had on their motivation for change (partnership).

MI Groups in Acute Care Settings

Implementing MI groups in acute care dual-diagnosis programs requires considering the context in which the group occurs. Inpatient and intensive outpatient programs typically offer patients multiple group treatments (e.g., goal setting, coping and relapse prevention skills building, symptom management, psychoeducation about psychiatric medications and symptoms, discharge planning), as well as several case management services (e.g., linkage to self-help programs, assistance with entitlement applications and transportation needs, referrals for housing and vocational rehabilitation, coordination with health care providers). An MI group is only one of several groups that patients may attend. In addition, patients in these programs typically vary widely in the type and severity of their psychiatric and substance use disorders, resulting in heterogeneous group membership. Moreover, members vary considerably in the behaviors they wish to address (e.g., psychiatric issues, substance use, treatment/medication adherence, relationship problems). Further compounding these challenges are the open admissions policies of programs wherein patients may stay for several days to weeks, which result in changing group membership from session to session, differences in the number of members who attend group, and often only one or two opportunities in which to work with patients. Finally, a substantial proportion of dually diagnosed patients may feel coerced into treatment, either through involuntary admission to an inpatient setting or due to external pressures that make program participation a "requirement" of their treatment plans. They may feel reluctant to change and be disproportionately referred to MI groups given their low levels of motivation. MI groups should be structured to accommodate these realities.

MI groups in acute care settings combine processes designed to engage group members by using structured activities. All of the structured activities in MI groups are designed either to evoke why change might be important to the members, drawing out reasons that support change or that create the desire or need for change, or to develop members' confidence in their ability to change, optimism that their lives can improve, and commitment to the change process. The leader usually implements one activity per group session. Below, we describe these activities in relation to the phases of MI groups.

> *Structured activities explore why change might be important and develop members' confidence in their ability to change, optimism that their lives can improve, and commitment to the change process.*

Engaging the Group

We recommend several strategies to address the issues described earlier and to promote an MI style of interaction between you and members and among all members. First, given the multiple groups available to patients in comprehensive dual-diagnosis programs, we recommend that participation in an MI group be voluntary, consistent with MI spirit. Patients may attend the group to explore their resistance or ambivalence about changing, without having to make a commitment to change their substance use or psychiatric-related behaviors. We have found that when patients may choose to attend MI groups, they can consider motivational issues in a less oppositional manner. This also reduces the risk that patients with low levels of motivation might discourage other members from approaching change, which is a possibility when groups are "stacked" with participants invested in their status quo behaviors (Walters, Ogle, & Martin, 2002).

Second, introduce in each group in an MI culture-building preamble that (1) details the goal of the group, namely, to explore issues that may affect motivation to change some aspect of their behavior; (2) notes how ambivalence or reluctance to change behavior is normal; (3) presents as a ground rule reaching one's own conclusions about the need to change behaviors, without confrontation or unsolicited advice by the leader or group members; and (4) describes how a structured activity assists members in considering topics that may affect their motivation for change (Foote et al., 1999). This preamble provides clear guidelines for how group members are to work together, a particularly important feature for patients hampered by psychiatric and substance abuse symptoms and cognitive impairments, who may be working together for the first time.

Third, we recommend that you use highly engaging activities that actively involve members in the exploration of motivational issues, thereby accommodating problems of attention, concentration, and fatigue that potentially result from symptoms, medications, or participation in various other program groups and individual meetings. These single-session activities do not require prior MI group attendance, and they may be implemented in any order that makes the most sense for the majority of members (e.g., exploring the importance of change, building confidence). Activity selection can be guided by input from other program therapists who work directly with the members. Ask them to provide you with one- or two-sentence written referrals about the nature of the member's primary motivational issues (e.g., wants to drop out of the program, feels marijuana use is not a problem, is ambivalent about taking medications for mania) and any other critical matters that might be important for the leader to know (e.g., suicide risk, impending court appearance, housing crisis, major health problem).

Fourth, we recommend that you actively facilitate group discussion. You should introduce the group and the activity, guide members' participation in it, redirect members to the common topic as needed, and promote an MI style of interaction among members. Thus, you function much like a conductor, selecting activities, culling mutual understanding and support among members, and strategically orchestrating the evocation of change talk, while handling resistance as needed. Finally, given these multiple leader tasks, diversity of patient problem areas, and limited opportunities to work with members in group and over time, we believe that the group should be kept to 10 or fewer participants and that each group should last at least 50 minutes.

Exploring Perspectives

Acute care MI groups consist of structured activities that help patients focus on relevant behaviors they might consider changing, and explore why behavior change might be important to them. These activities serve to help ambivalent members carefully weigh their opposing thoughts and feelings, or to prompt members who are reluctant to change to consider what might make change worthwhile.

Mixed Bag

Ask members to think about a behavioral issue related to their dual-diagnosis recovery that they are uncertain they want to change, such as attending treatment regularly or taking medications. Ask members to report voluntarily the mixed bag of thoughts and feelings that support either changing or remaining the same. As members speak, record their statements into two categories on a board: reasons to change or reasons to stay the same. Once collected, members write down the reasons that apply to them under columns representing the two positions and discuss what they conclude from the relative balance.

On the Fence

Ask members to think about a problem behavior (e.g. wanting to use drugs or alcohol vs. not wanting to use) that pulls them in opposite directions (change or maintain behavior). Divide members into two groups that physically face each other. Whereas one side's task is to argue for change, the other side is to argue for status quo behavior. Next, have a volunteer sit between the groups, as if "on the fence" about the issue. The volunteer describes the dilemma, then in a back and forth process, the other members make their arguments, with the volunteer sequentially responding to what members on each side have said.

Warm Seat

Once again, members have an opportunity to talk about a behavior related to the dual disorders they are ambivalent about changing. Place two chairs facing each other in the center of a circle of the group members. A volunteer sits in one of the chairs (the warm seat) and describes his or her dilemma to the group. Other group members enter the circle one at a time and sit in the opposing chair to argue why the member should not change (sustain talk). The member's task is to counter these arguments directly or to ask for assistance from other group members when he or she feels uncertain about how to respond to the sustain talk.

Sorting It Out

Adapted from an activity that uses packages of cards (Moyers & Martino, 2006), this activity involves preparing in advance a worksheet that lists important life goals and values (e.g., be physically fit, be loved by those close to you) or relevant goals for patients who struggle with major psychiatric disorders (e.g., stop hearing voices, have a clear mind). Ask members to write at the top of the worksheet behaviors that might contribute to their current dual-diagnosis problems (e.g., drug or alcohol use, remaining in an unhealthy relationship, medication nonadherence). Next, define personal goals and values as highly desirable principles, qualities, or aims that guide one's conduct. Members first circle the goals and values that are very important to them, then select five that are their current highest priorities. One at a time, members describe to the group why these five goals or values matter most to them. Members consider how the problem behaviors written at the top of their worksheets impact their values or goals, and what impact their actions would have on their current priorities if they were to change their behaviors.

Broadening Perspectives

Additional activities are designed to broaden perspectives by helping members develop their perceived ability to change, and to evoke members' optimism that their lives can improve.

Graphic Feedback

Based on self-reported assessment information, prepare feedback reports tailored for use with dually diagnosed patients, with information about drinking and drug use (quantity/frequency information, norm comparisons), symptom constellations for psychiatric conditions, risks posed by psychiatric conditions, and medical concerns. Much of the information is presented in graphs or charts to simplify the material. Each member receives a sealed envelope containing his or her report. Ask the members to open their envelopes, then describe the meaning of each item to the group, and inquire about members' reactions to the feedback. Ask them how the information affects their view of their substance use, psychiatric condition, and the interaction of these two problem areas, and reflect any change talk that emerges. Discourage group members from comparing results in order to prevent distraction and to enhance consideration of their personalized information.

Personal Strengths

Prepare in advance a worksheet that lists a variety of personal strengths (e.g., committed, caring, flexible, spiritual, honest, creative), and ask members to write at the top of the worksheet a current behavioral problem they want to change (e.g., poor treatment attendance/participation, medication nonadherence, consuming alcohol). Ask group members to read over the list and circle five personal strengths (personal strengths that currently apply to group members). You may find it useful to read the strengths aloud one at a time while members are selecting them. Next, ask members to think about their five selected personal strengths and describe how they have demonstrated these strengths in their lives. Finally, instruct members to examine the current behavioral dilemma they wrote at the top of the page and describe how they might apply their personal strengths to the problems they have had difficulty changing.

Thinking Out of the Box

Ask members to write down a current problem that thwarts their dual-diagnosis recovery, and that they want/need to change but feel unable to address because they either do not know how to manage it, or they lack the skills or supports necessary for problem resolution (e.g., not having transportation to get to appointments, having children at home and no child care available, not trusting professionals in the mental health field). Members place their dilemmas in a box supplied by the leader. Mix the dilemmas, draw one out, and have the member who wrote the dilemma describe it in more detail to the group. Then lead a brainstorming activity in which all members call out possible ways to address the problem to help the member "think out of the box," recording all ideas on a board. The member then goes to the board, crosses out any suggestions he or she will not consider, and circles items that are likely possibilities. The member then discusses the steps he or she might take to enact these suggestions.

Past and Future Success

Ask members to write down two areas of success: (1) something they have already achieved and are quite proud of (e.g., college degree, raising children), and (2) something they would like to achieve in the future (e.g., employment goals, a stable and loving intimate relationship). Members are asked to write down both successes as if they have already happened. Next, members read the two areas of success to the group, and group members guess which success is past and which one is desired in the future. After some discussion, the members reveal the proper categories, then discuss what skills they have applied to achieve past successes and how they might use these skills for future accomplishments. Members find the game-like activity engaging and often are heartened when other group members are surprised by their past achievements or assume they have already demonstrated certain successes.

Looking Forward

Ask members to think about the ways their substance use and psychiatric conditions have affected their lives. Next, ask them to consider how they envision their future 1 year from now under two different conditions: (1) not attempting to change their dual-diagnosis problems; and (2) making efforts to change them. Members then discuss these two different pathways as the leader writes the respective set of comments on the board. Conclude the activity by asking members about their preferred pathway and the steps they can take to work toward a future marked by greater psychiatric stability, nonhazardous substance use or abstinence, and improved functioning.

Fostering Improved Mental Health

Begin the session by asking members to volunteer instances when their alcohol or drug use worsened or complicated their psychiatric problems. Next, explore any past instances when they experienced stable or improved mental health by asking an open-ended question, such as "Tell us about a time when you felt mentally healthy and emotionally stable"; "What did you notice when your mental health was better?"; "What types of activities were you doing when your mental health had improved?"; or "What was life like at the time that things were going better for you?" Group members typically recite instances in which they participated in healthy activities in a period of better functioning, such as exercising, going to church, taking medication as prescribed, regularly visiting a 12-step program sponsor, holding a job, maintaining a stable marriage, keeping appointments with treatment providers, or not using alcohol or drugs. Members then consider how they could renew healthy activities to improve day-to-day functioning, the capacity to not drink or use drugs, and overall mental health.

Importance and Confidence Rulers

Using a board, draw two rulers scaled 0 (*not at all*) to 10 (*extremely*) that represent the levels of importance and confidence members attribute to their own behavior change efforts. Ask members to think about a current problem that affects their dual-diagnosis recovery (e.g., a member who has a history of complex anxiety disorders and prescription benzodiazepine dependence infrequently attends the program, because she fears the psychiatrist might alter her medication regimen), then to go to the board one at a time and write their initials by the number that best represents how important trying to change this problem is and how confident they feel in changing it. Members explain their positions (e.g., "I gave it a 9 in importance, because if I don't go to this program, I can't get help, but I put a 2 in confidence, because I'm afraid the doctor will take me off Klonopin and I won't be able to handle my anxiety"). Then addressing each dimension separately, ask the group members two questions: (1) why they didn't place themselves at 0, evoking the relative importance of change and confidence in one's ability to change (e.g., "This program helped me learn ways to cope with my anxiety in the past"); and (2) what would need to occur for them to move one scale point higher, generating a discussion about additional skills, supports, or resources that might increase their confidence to change (e.g., "I would want to know what other medication options I have before I agree to taper down on Klonopin"). When members indicate a 0 on either scale, explore this position briefly, then focus on the second question.

Moving into Action

The moving into action phase is unlikely to apply to all group members in acute care dual-diagnosis specialty programs, particularly when many of them have been referred to the group precisely because they have not been taking action on the problems related to their dual disorders. However, in the latter part of most "broadening perspectives" activities, ask members specifically to identify steps they feel ready to take toward behavioral change. Use your discretion, however, to determine whether moving toward action might be premature and cause members to backtrack motivationally. Also, many dual-diagnosis programs already have other groups that address planning and implementing change. Because of this, MI groups may focus more on bringing people to the point that they are ready to make and implement plans regarding treatment goal setting, relapse prevention, and symptom management.

Group Facilitation Issues

Several group facilitation issues arise during the group activities. First, given the diversity of potential behavior change targets (substance abuse, psychiatric conditions, medication or treatment adherence, relationship problems, medical issues), you can ask members to select the behavioral areas they want to address in group. Emphasize the elicitation of member change talk as it applies across behavioral domains.

Second, you should actively involve all group members in the activities and prompt them to consider how the issues might apply to their circumstances. You can accomplish this by (1) asking open questions, such as "How does what [member's name] said apply to other people's situations?"; (2) reflecting member's change talk to the larger group as a way to encourage other members to elaborate about similar change-promoting beliefs; and (3) inviting group members to speak within the activities to encourage members who otherwise tend to be silent, anxious, and detached.

For example, a patient named Joe in his mid-20s was referred by probation to a dual-diagnosis program. He elected to attend MI groups. Joe had a history of gang-related trauma, likely posttraumatic stress disorder, and polysubstance dependence. In his introduction, Joe noted that he did not need to be in treatment and remained silent throughout most of the group. After the leader presented the "mixed bag" activity, Mike, another young man, volunteered to participate in it. Mike had self-described "odd experiences" of auditory hallucinations, difficulty thinking clearly, racing thoughts, limited sleep, and a prior manic episode, complicated by frequent use of marijuana sometimes laced with angel dust (PCP). Mike was ambivalent about attending the dual-diagnosis treatment program. His reasons not to participate follow: (1) He was not sure he had a psychiatric condition; and (2) he thought he could stop smoking marijuana on his own and that his odd experiences would abate with marijuana and PCP abstinence. Mike's reasons to participate were as follows: (1) His odd experiences persisted weeks after drug abstinence; (2) some of his drug-using associates told him he was "whacked" and "crazy"; (3) he had been smoking more marijuana in the last few weeks to relax, but he was sleeping less and becoming more anxious; (4) he had dropped out of college due to his unusually poor academic performance and thought it might be a sign that something was wrong with him; and (5) his own efforts to help himself had not been successful. The leader offered a summary reflection of Mike's change talk to the group:

LEADER: (to group) So Mike's discomfort is becoming worse. It's not going away, even when drugs are out of the picture. Other people notice changes, and important areas of Mike's life are falling apart. Mike is beginning to wonder if treatment might help. [The leader notices that Joe has been listening attentively to what Mike has said and seems even more engaged following the summary reflection, though Joe did not spontaneously respond to it.] (to Joe) Joe, something seems to have struck you about Mike's situation. If you would be willing, tell us what you are thinking?

JOE: I can kind of relate to what Mike is going through. I mean I don't have the same type of issues as Mike, but I also struggle with things that I try to blow away with drugs, and that's when I blow off treatment. Hey, Mike. Why don't you try the program for a week and see how it goes?

MIKE: Yeah, I guess.

LEADER: (to Joe) So it seems Mike isn't so sure. How about you, Joe? When you think about your situation, where are you in terms of coming to this program?

JOE: I'll keep coming. I just don't like the fact that my probation officer has a gun to my head about it. I have my own reasons for coming.

These facilitation efforts maximize the opportunities to elicit change talk among as many members as possible within a time-limited and shared group setting.

Third, when members interact in MI-inconsistent ways (e.g., direct confrontation, unsolicited advice), you can safeguard the MI spirit of inter-action by reminding members about the group ground rules and reframing MI-inconsistent statements as possible expressions of genuine concern and intention to help others. For example, Carmen gets upset with Mary, who is ambivalent about entering a 5-week women's residential dual-diagnosis program. Mary is being monitored by a state protective family services worker because of allegations of child neglect. Mary has bipolar disorder and alcohol–cocaine dependence. She is reluctant to enroll in residential treatment, because it would mean being without her two young children and having to ask her mother to take care of them. Carmen, who lost her parental rights several years ago secondary to drug dependence and a poorly managed psychotic disorder, offers unsolicited advice:

CARMEN: You have to go to that program. You have to put your recovery first. If you don't, you could lose your kids. Take it from me. I know. I've been there and I did lose my kids, and I hate myself for it. You still have a chance.

LEADER: (to Carmen) Carmen, it seems like you want to help Mary prevent what happened to you from happening to her. That's really supportive. However, telling Mary what she needs to do, when she hasn't asked for advice, may make it less likely that Mary will hear what you have to say. Would you be willing to ask her if she's up for hearing sugges-tions at this time? And if she is, would you then make your suggestions without telling Mary what decision she should make?

CARMEN: (to Mary) Sure. It's just that it's hard for me to get over my own loss, and it seems like the only thing I can do is to try to help someone else not go through the hell I experienced. Mary, can I tell you what I think about your situation?

MARY: Sure. Go ahead.

Carmen explains that she had opportunities for intensive treatment and did not take them. She then recommends that Mary balance her immediate desire to be with her kids with her longer-term goal of becoming psychiat-rically stable, alcohol and cocaine free, and fully capable of parenting her children. Mary is receptive to this input.

Finally, implementing an MI group may differ in an inpatient setting from implementing it within an intensive outpatient program. In inpatient settings, patients typically attend only one or two MI group sessions near the last days of their stay, when they are less impaired by acute psychiatric or substance abuse symptoms. Discharge planning and referral to continuing treatment and recovery support become central concerns of patients. Thus, motivation for aftercare often is a common behavioral target for inpatient MI groups. It may be useful to hand out a sheet that summarizes the various treatment options available in the community and discuss in the group when patients seem ready to take action. In addition, because severe psychiatric symptoms may continue to impair patients' functioning, more provocative group activities (e.g., warm seat) or those that require substantial mental flexibility (e.g., on the fence) or abstraction (e.g., past and future success) may or may not be appropriate with these patients.

> *Motivation for aftercare is a common behavioral target for inpatient MI groups.*

Research

Evidence related to MI groups with patients who have severe dual psychiatric and substance use disorders is limited, and most research has involved individual applications of MI for this patient population. Randomized controlled trials of individual MI have demonstrated some benefits for improving referral engagement (Steinberg, Zeidonis, Krejci, & Brandon, 2004; Swanson, Pantalon, & Cohen, 1999), treatment attendance patterns (Bellack, Bennett, Gearon, Brown, & Young, 2006; Martino, Carroll, O'Malley, & Rounsaville, 2000), and reduction in drinking days and daily alcohol consumption (Graeber, Moyers, Griffith, Guajardo, & Tonigan, 2003); others have failed to show effects (Baker et al., 2002; Martino, Carroll, Nich, & Rounsaville, 2006). The strongest MI treatment effects have occurred when MI was combined with other treatment approaches over a 6- to 12-month period (Bellack et al., 2006; Barrowclough et al., 2001) or accompanied by multiple booster sessions (Kemp, Kirov, Everitt, Hayward, & David, 1998). MI may work best with psychotic patients when clinicians use it periodically to promote engagement and retention in other dual-diagnosis treatment, as the patients' motivations for behavior change and treatment adherence wax and wane (Bellack et al., 2006).

Only one controlled clinical trial specifically tested the effectiveness of MI groups for dually diagnosed patients. Santa Ana, Wulfert, and Nietert (2007) compared MI group sessions to standard group sessions focused on psychoeducation and discharge planning. Overall, while the MI group did not result in a greater proportion of patients attending aftercare treatment or being completely abstinent, those who had been in the MI group who attended at least one aftercare session attended a greater number of sessions. Similarly, among patients who drank or used drugs at least once, those who participated in the MI group had significantly fewer drinks per episode and fewer binge-drinking episodes and drug-using days at the follow-up.

Two studies examined the effectiveness of outpatient group treatments for dually diagnosed patients that combined MI with cognitive-behavioral therapy. In an uncontrolled evaluation, Bradley, Baker, and Lewin (2007) found that patients who participated in open-ended weekly group treatment in a rural area showed significant improvements in substance use, psychiatric symptoms, treatment adherence, and overall psychosocial functioning over time (average number of groups attended was 28–29 over 3 years). In a controlled experiment, James and colleagues (2004) tested the effectiveness of six weekly outpatient group sessions for patients with psychosis. Relative to the control group, patients in the combined group had significantly greater reductions in drug use, severity of dependence, global psychopathology, antipsychotic medication dose, and rate of hospitalization at a 3-month follow-up. As with individual MI for dually diagnosed patients, MI in a group format may work best when it is integrated with other treatments and used in more than one to two sessions.

Conclusion

MI groups have become a practical reality in a dual-diagnosis service system dominated by group treatment interventions. MI groups offer an opportunity to create a synergy between group therapeutic factors and core elements of MI spirit that might maximize motivation for dually diagnosed patients. The use of structured activities designed to elicit change talk among group members is necessary when MI groups are implemented in acute care settings. Beyond the practical and conceptual appeal, preliminary data suggest that MI groups may help patients adhere to dual-diagnosis treatments, reduce problematic substance use, and improve their psychiatric functioning. Thus, MI groups appear promising for motivating dually diagnosed patients to address their complex problems, and implementing MI in group is a useful practice within the patients' overall treatment program.

References

Baker, A., Lewin, T., Reichler, H., Clancy, R., Carr, V., Garret, R., et al. (2002). Brief intervention for substance use within psychiatric inpatient services: Findings from a randomized controlled trial. *Addiction, 97,* 1329–1337.

Barrowclough, C., Haddock, G., Tarrier, N., Lewis, S., Moring, J., O'Brien, R., et al. (2001). Randomised controlled trial of MI, CBT, and family intervention for patients with comorbid schizophrenia and substance use disorders. *American Journal of Psychiatry, 158,* 1706–1713.

Bellack, A. S., Bennett, M. E., Gearon, J. S., Brown, C. H., & Yang, Y. (2006). A randomized clinical trial of a new behavioral treatment of drug abuse in people with severe and persistent mental illness. *Archives of General Psychiatry, 63,* 426–432.

Bradley, A. C., Baker, A., & Lewin, T. J. (2007). Group intervention for coexisting psychosis and substance use disorders in rural Australia: Outcomes over 3 years. *Australian and New Zealand Journal of Psychiatry, 41,* 501–508.

Drake, R. E., Essock, S. M., Shaner, A., Carey, K. B., Minkoff, K., Kola, L., et al. (2001). Implementing dual diagnosis services for clients with severe mental illness. *Psychiatric Services, 52,* 469–476.

Drake, R. E., & Mueser, K. T. (2000). Psychosocial approaches to dual diagnosis. *Schizophrenia Bulletin, 26,* 105–118.

Foote, J., DeLuca, A., Magura, S., Warner, A., Grand, A., Rosenblum, A., & Stahl, S. (1999). A group motivational treatment for chemical dependency. *Journal of Substance Abuse Treatment, 17,* 181–192.

Goldsmith, R. J., & Garlapati, V. (2004). Behavioral interventions for dual-diagnosis patients. *Psychiatric Clinics of North America, 27,* 709–725.

Graeber, D. A., Moyers, T. B., Griffith, G., Guajardo, E., & Tonigan, S. (2003). A pilot study comparing MI and an educational intervention in patients with schizophrenia and alcohol use disorders. *Community Mental Health Journal, 39,* 189–202.

James, W., Preston, N. J., Koh, G., Spencer, C., Kisely, S. R., & Castle, D. J. (2004). A group intervention which assists patients with dual diagnosis reduce their substance use: A randomized controlled trial. *Psychological Medicine, 34,* 983–990.

Kemp, R., Kirov, G., Everitt, B., Hayward, P., & David, A. (1998). Randomised controlled trial of compliance therapy: 18-month follow-up. *British Journal of Psychiatry, 172,* 413–419.

Kivlighan, D. M., & Holmes, S. E. (2004). The importance of therapeutic factors: A typology of therapeutic factors studies. In J. L. DeLucia-Waack, D. A. Gerrity, C. R. Kalodner, & M. T. Riva (Eds.), *Handbook of group counseling and psychotherapy* (pp. 23–36). Thousands Oaks, CA: Sage.

Martino, S., Carroll, K. M., Nich, C., & Rounsaville, B. J. (2006). A randomized controlled pilot study of motivational interviewing for patients with psychotic and drug use disorders. *Addiction, 101,* 1479–1492.

Martino, S., Carroll, K. M., O'Malley, S. S., & Rounsaville, B. J. (2000). Motivational interviewing with psychiatrically ill substance abusing patients. *American Journal on Addictions, 9,* 88–91.

Miller, W. R., & Rollnick, S. (2012). *Motivational interviewing: Preparing people for change* (3rd ed.). New York: Guilford Press.

Minkoff, K. (2001). Developing standards of care for individuals with co-occurring psychiatric and substance use disorders. *Psychiatric Services, 52,* 597–599.

Moyers, T., & Martino, S. (2006). *Personal values card sort for dually diagnosed patients.* Available online at *www.casaa.unm.edu.*

Santa Ana, E. J., Wulfert, E., & Nietert, P. J. (2007). Efficacy of group motivational interviewing (MI groups) for psychiatric inpatients with chemical dependence. *Journal of Consulting and Clinical Psychology, 75,* 816–822.

Steinberg, M. L., Zeidonis, D. M., Krejci, J.A., & Brandon, T. H. (2004). Motivational interviewing with personalized feedback: A brief intervention for motivating smokers with schizophrenia to seek treatment for tobacco dependence. *Journal of Consulting and Clinical Psychology, 72,* 723–728.

Swanson, A. J., Pantalon, M. V., & Cohen, K. R. (1999). MI and treatment adherence among psychiatrically and dually diagnosed patients. *Journal of Nervous and Mental Disease, 187,* 630–635.

Walters, S. T., Ogle, R., & Martin, J. E. (2002). Perils and possibilities of group-based motivational interviewing. In W. R. Miller & S. Rollnick, *Motivational interviewing: Preparing people for change* (2nd ed., pp. 377–390). New York: Guilford Press.

Yalom, I., & Leszcz, M. (2005). *The theory and practice of group psychotherapy* (5th ed.). New York: Basic Books.

Zeidonis, D. M., Smelson, D., Rosenthal, R. N., Batki, S. L., Green, A. I., Henry, R. J., et al. (2005). Improving the care of individuals with schizophrenia and substance use disorders: Consensus recommendations. *Journal of Psychiatric Practice, 11,* 315–339.

CHAPTER 17

Motivational Interviewing Groups for People with Chronic Health Conditions

Claire Lane, Susan Butterworth,
and Linda Speck

Chronic health conditions often develop in the context of long-term health behavior habits and choices. In the United States, for example, even moderate lifestyle improvements would prevent 40 million chronic disease cases, saving over $200 billion in treatment costs annually (DeVol & Bedroussian, 2007); estimates are similar in other countries. Prevention is better than cure.

Once conditions such as heart disease and emphysema develop, they often can be managed but not cured. Optimizing lifestyle behaviors can prevent progression, reduce severity, and decrease functional limitations. Health recovery and maintenance cannot be provided by the medical system but are instead behavior changes that can only be successfully implemented and maintained by patients themselves, either on their own or with the support of the health community.

Motivation and Ambivalence in Health Issues

Many people do not make changes to their lifestyle or health habits when they develop chronic health conditions. Health behavior change is just one of many challenges they face, along with the shock of diagnosis, role changes, and competing commitments. Returning to work is often a concern. Some avoid exercise due to the fear they will harm themselves. Often, several risky behaviors must be changed simultaneously, challenging people's belief in their ability to change. Many argue that they are "feeling well," and don't see how making changes would result in additional benefits. Some believe that chronic disease is not a concern following surgery or treatment, even after receiving information about how lifestyle changes can prevent future acute events, or they do not believe that steps they take will make a difference (Hibbard, Mahoney, Stock, & Tusler, 2007).

Psychological factors that can be addressed in treatment include perceptions of illness, health beliefs, depression, anxiety, and denial (Bennett, 2000). Family and social factors also play an important role in managing acute and chronic health conditions. Poor social support during recovery may lead to poorer psychological prognosis (Pedersen, Middel, & Larsen, 2002). Socioeconomic factors also play a role; those with socioeconomic deprivation often experience difficulties accessing health care, affording healthy foods, and using leisure and exercise facilities (Dowler, Turner, & Dobson, 2001).

Why MI and Why Groups?

Many people with a chronic illness manage their own care and make most of the decisions that affect their long-term health. Self-management groups for those with chronic disease improve clinical indices and reduce health care costs (Bodenheimer, Holman, & Grumbach, 2002). Meta-analyses of interventions to reduce risk factors for chronic disease suggest that effective interventions are those that change health behavior, rather than increase knowledge (Jepson, 2000). Advantages of group interventions with patients with chronic conditions include cost-effectiveness and social support between members experiencing the same condition, which can provide psychological benefits and improved self-efficacy for managing chronic conditions (Classen et al., 2001).

Patients themselves make most of the decisions that affect their long-term health.

MI is congruent with improving self-efficacy and patient activation, which are key factors for managing chronic illness. MI shows promise for helping people reduce their health risk factors, both individually and in groups (Butterworth, Linden, & McClay, 2007; Knight et al., 2003; Linden, Butterworth, & Prochaska, 2010; Rubak, Sandboek, Lauritzen, & Christensen, 2005). In this chapter, we describe MI groups for chronic disease populations. We use several case examples that are generic to any chronic condition to illustrate the strategies used in the four phases of MI groups. Our examples include MI groups that focus on early disease detection and management, as well as restoring function and reducing disease-related complications of an established condition.

Facilitating MI Groups for People with Chronic Health Conditions

Engaging the Group

MI health groups focus on not only behavior change but also on physical symptoms, side effects, knowledge about the condition, medications or equipment, what to do in emergency situations, exercise, reviewing clinical laboratory tests, and understanding disease. Despite these information provision goals, you can incorporate participatory elements into every meeting, fostering mutual support among members and avoiding the idea that motivation is a topic to be addressed once before focusing on information. For example, you might include a planned "feedback" time within every session, during which members share their experiences since the last session, including progress toward goals and both positive experiences and challenges, and raise health topics they wish to discuss with their clinicians. Topics may include lifestyle changes, emotional aspects, symptoms, concerns about progress, and positive–negative experiences during the past week. Keep a record of these on the wall, as a reminder of topics requested and addressed. Encourage members to keep a diary about issues they might want to raise, but respect their personal choice if they prefer not to do so.

Exploring Perspectives

While continuing to build engagement among group members, you might begin to explore how people feel about changing health behaviors.

Exploring Lifestyles and Looking Back

The MI strategies of exploring lifestyles and looking back explore members' perspectives. Often members who have enjoyed their unhealthy habits until now are less interested in changing. This is commonplace with chronic diseases and important to address in order to normalize these kinds of feelings. It also demonstrates respect for the autonomy of group members and helps to establish a good rapport with the group. In the following example, the group facilitator respects this member's ambivalence, emphasizing that the choice to make any changes is his. As you read this, think what the consequences might have been if this facilitator insisted that the member give up his unhealthy behaviors.

FACILITATOR: We've discussed the identified risk factors for your condition. It's clear that many of you are aware of lifestyle changes within your control that could decrease the chances of having further problems. Who would like to share the risk factors that you feel might be important to address? [engaging members; eliciting an assessment of importance; focusing on the topic of change]

ALAN: I suppose I've done everything I shouldn't have in the past. You name it, I've done it . . . and loved every minute of it! *(laughter)*

FACILITATOR: Okay, Alan, perhaps you'd like to tell us a little bit about it, but let's stick to the risk factors, shall we? [using humor but focusing on change at the same time]

ALAN: Well, I've always enjoyed life, but now I'm told that everything I enjoy is bad for me. I used to smoke and drink, and the only exercise I got was watching a game of football, and I enjoyed my food. There's nothing I liked better than steak and chips [fries] and then 10 pints of beer on a Saturday night in the local club with my mates. But now you're going to tell me that I have to give it all up—what a boring life this is going to be!

FACILITATOR: You expect I'm going to tell you that you have to give everything up, even if that would mean losing all enjoyment in your life. But in fact, it's up to you, and perhaps making lots of changes at the moment would be extremely difficult to do. What do you think you *could* do? [expressing acceptance and compassion; eliciting a response that reinforces confidence and activation]

ALAN: Yes you're right . . . I suppose I could think about drinking less. That may not be too difficult, as I haven't been able to get out to the club for ages anyway.

Exploring Ambivalence

One of the fundamental goals of MI is to explore and resolve members' ambivalence:

FACILITATOR 1: So, we're all here because we have problems with our hearts [or kidneys, blood glucose, etc.], and I'm guessing that some of us have been told about changes we should be making. But in this group, we are not here to try to force you to change. Any changes you decide to make are up to you. Our role is to help you explore possible changes that you identify. [supporting autonomy]

FACILITATOR 2: It's quite normal to feel two ways about changing. In fact, you might have mixed feelings about being here today. (*Group members chuckle.*) On the one hand, you might think making some changes would be a good idea, but on the other, it might seem hard and you want things to stay the same. I'm wondering how you are feeling about taking a look at things you could change to improve your health? [normalizing ambivalence and focusing]

JIM: Yeah, I suppose I have mixed feelings about the whole thing.

FACILITATOR 2: Mixed feelings? [eliciting]

JIM: Well, I'm here because my family wants me to be. I know they're worried and don't want me to have another heart attack, and neither do I, obviously. But I know a lot of stuff already, and to be honest, I like what I eat, what I do, what I drink. I don't want another heart attack, but I don't want a life I don't like living either. So, yeah, I feel two ways, but I'm willing to give it a go.

FACILITATOR 1: So although you weren't sure you wanted to come here, your health is important enough to give it a try. [using double-sided reflection to respond to the change talk and affirm the effort that has been made]

JIM: Don't get me wrong, I'm happy to be here, but I'm not sure about it still.

FACILITATOR 1: Thanks for sharing that, Jim. How do other people feel? [affirmation and continuing to focus with the group]

OLIVIA: Well, I'm very happy to be here. I want to try to change things as soon as I can. I've already made some changes.

FACILITATOR 1: And why do you want to make those changes? [evoking]

OLIVIA: . . . [change talk]

FACILITATOR 2: So some people feel more ready for changes than others, and in fact you have already made some changes. [affirmation]

OLIVIA: Yes.

FACILITATOR 1: That's fantastic. Who else is feeling two ways? [affirmation; evoking]

ELSIE: This is going to sound a bit strange, but even though I know some of the things I should be doing, and I want to do, when it comes down to actually doing it, it's another story.

SUZIE: That's me, too. I tell myself to have an apple, but I have cake instead.

ELSIE: I know that feeling, and I wish I could be better. It's hard isn't it?

JIM: You see, I've got the other problem. I think I probably could change things, but I don't know if I really want to, because I like them. I think

I'm determined enough that if I truly wanted to change them I would, but I don't know how much I want to.

FACILITATOR 2: And it's completely normal to feel these ways. Over the next few weeks, we're going to be talking about making changes to different areas of our lives. If some of you decide that a change is not right for you, then that's all right, too. It's up to you to decide what to do. [maintaining engagement by normalizing ambivalence; supporting autonomy and expressing acceptance]

In this example, the facilitators present ambivalence as normal, and they affirm member successes, no matter how small. They respect autonomy and demonstrate respect for the diversity of perspectives within the group. They encourage members to discuss the different ways they experience ambivalence. The facilitators express understanding and help members explore ambivalence through open questions and reflective listening statements.

Exploring Values

Quite often, other things are more important to people than making health behavior changes. In the example below, the facilitator uses an exploring values exercise to explore how doing more exercise fits with a member's other concerns. This is a useful way to investigate ambivalence about change, giving you opportunities to elicit and reflect change talk.

FACILITATOR: We've discussed exercise in some detail today. What changes to your exercise levels would be good for you? [eliciting change talk with an open question]

CHRIS: I've always liked exercise and I used to play a lot of football when I was young, but I may need to do a bit more, and more regularly, than I've done lately.

FACILITATOR: So, exercise has always been an important part of your life. [reflecting change talk]

CHRIS: It certainly has, but over the years other things have got in the way. I haven't had the time to do it regularly. Perhaps I need to find another sort of exercise that I can do on my own.

JENNY: For me the problem is that I don't have the time. I know that lack of exercise must have affected me and contributed to my heart attack . . . but how do you fit it in when you've got two young children who need their mother's attention? At the moment they're my priority!

FACILITATOR: It might be useful to consider what it is that your children need from you right now . . . [validating and evoking, supporting autonomy and working in partnership]

JENNY: Well, they need their mother, for lots of different reasons. They're young; the oldest is only 10 and Tom is only 6. They need me to give them good meals, to make sure they have clean clothes, just everything! How do I fit in exercise and manage a job when I'm well again?

GEORGE: What if you weren't there Jenny? How would they cope then? They need you.

JENNY: I really don't know; I have to recover, for them even more than myself (*a few tears*).

FACILITATOR: What *could* you do to make a good recovery? [eliciting change talk]

JENNY: I know that I have to keep taking the medication and that's easy. But I really need to live a healthy lifestyle to be there for my children. I've got to find time for it somehow.

FACILITATOR: So you think it's important to exercise, but fitting it in while looking after the children is standing in your way. [double-sided reflection to express acceptance]

JENNY: Let me think about it more this week and see what I can figure out.

Here, the facilitator guides Jenny to consider how doing more exercise might fit in with the most important thing in her life—her family—and reinforces that she is in control of her choices, without pressing for change.

Broadening Perspectives

Exploring Importance and Confidence

MI groups allow patients to explore how they feel about different health behaviors, and share this with others in the group. *Exploring importance and confidence* when information about health behavior change is imparted works well in MI groups. It helps members explore how ready they feel to make changes and provides another opportunity to evoke change talk. In the next example, the facilitators highlight different members' positions with regard to the importance of and their confidence about making particular changes.

FACILITATOR: Where might you place yourselves on a scale of 0–10—how important is it to you to exercise [or monitor blood sugars, etc.]? [evoking importance]

JOHN: Well, I think I'd place myself right up there on 10.

FACILITATOR: For you it's really high priority. Someone else? [maintaining group engagement]

ANNE: Only 5 for me, as I know I need to exercise but finding the time is difficult.

FACILITATOR: Perhaps we need to separate out how difficult it might be from how important it is. How important is it for you, without considering its difficulty? [clarifying; evoking]

ANNE: Well, I'd rate it at 9 for importance, if I ignore the obstacles I'd actually have if I tried to exercise regularly.

Discussing importance and confidence can be challenging, especially when some members are unable to grasp the separate nature of these aspects of motivation. In this example, the facilitator addresses this, and encourages the member to understand the difference between them.

Exploring Strengths

"Feedback" provides opportunities to *explore strengths* within a group setting, with the opportunity for other members to assist in the process. This can elicit change talk from group members and support their self-efficacy. The example below illustrates one kind of topic that may be raised in feedback:

ROBERT: When it comes to food, I like everything that's bad for me. I don't have willpower.

FACILITATOR: So eating healthy is difficult for you. [validating challenge; maintaining engagement]

ROBERT: Definitely, especially as I've given up smoking since my heart attack.

FACILITATOR: How do you feel about having given up smoking? [evoking]

ROBERT: That was quite difficult as I'd smoked for over 30 years!

FACILITATOR: It certainly is something that many people find difficult. I'm sure others here would be interested to hear how you managed it. [validating; evoking change talk]

MICHAEL: Giving up smoking is *really* hard, so you have willpower, even if you don't see it.

ROBERT: Well . . . having a heart attack was quite a shock, and the doctors and nurses in hospital said that smoking contributed to it and . . . you're right, it did take a lot of willpower.

The facilitator focuses on the member's successes with other behavior changes rather than dwelling on what has not yet been achieved. The input from another member in the group affirms this achievement and encourages the client to relate this to his present challenge.

Change Success Stories

It is useful to affirm even small changes. This is especially helpful for members who have feelings of frustration and reduced motivation about not reaching their goals. Encouraging group members to share *change success stories* can build hope for change.

FACILITATOR 1: Last time we talked about some things about our lifestyles that we are unhappy about. Some people said that they were going to try and eat more fruits and vegetables. I'm just wondering how that went? [evoking]

JIM: Not that well. I did give in a bit on Sunday—I had a dessert after dinner.

FACILITATOR 2: Sounds like you enjoy dessert. [expressing acceptance]

JIM: Yeah, it's my biggest weakness—a big piece of chocolate cake with whipped cream.

OLIVIA: Oooooh, my favorite! Was it good?

JIM: (*Laughs.*) Yeah, a bit too good. I just couldn't resist it—you know what it's like.

OLIVIA: I'm with you on that! I make the best chocolate fudge cake! I won a prize for it once.

FACILITATOR 1: Wow—a prize-winning cake maker in the group—how about that? I'd like your recipe Olivia, if you'll share it. [affirmation; engaging]

FACILITATOR 2: A little of what you fancy does you good every now and then, right Jim? [validating; maintaining focus]

JIM: It wasn't exactly a little. . . . (*Group laughs.*)

FACILITATOR 2: Even though you enjoyed it, you don't feel very good about it. [reflecting ambivalence]

JIM: No—I feel like I let myself down a bit.

FACILITATOR 1: But Jim, you never said you were going to give up chocolate cake. (*Group laughs.*) How have you done with your plan to have a bit more fruit and vegetables this week? [evoking]

JIM: I don't think I managed my five a day, but I did have fruit with my breakfast, fruit or vegetables with lunch, and vegetables with my evening meal.

FACILITATOR 2: So, you managed more fruits and vegetables than last week. [providing affirmation; reflecting change talk]

JIM: Yeah—I suppose I did. I definitely managed to fit more in.

FACILITATOR 2: Congratulations! [affirmation]

JOHN: How did you find it, Jim? Was it hard?

JIM: Actually eating it, no, not really. But remembering to do it was. I mean, since my heart attack, other than a big piece of cake and a few dollops of whipped cream here and there (*laughs*), I've stopped eating fried stuff and fatty stuff as much. But I never used to eat fruit and vegetables. I want to now, because I know it's good for your heart, but sometimes it can be easy to forget to have some. I get my wife to remind me.

JOHN: Yeah, there really aren't that many vegetables I like, and I hate most fruit, too.

FACILITATOR 1: So increasing the amount of fruit and vegetables you eat probably wasn't what you wanted to do differently, John. [expressing empathy and acceptance]

JOHN: No.

FACILITATOR 1: What is it that you thought about last week, and how did it go? [evoking; shifting focus]

In this example, Jim does not recognize the significance of the changes he has already made. The facilitators draw attention to this and highlight the discrepancy between a behavior that he simultaneously liked and disliked. They keep the interaction on track in a lighthearted manner, as members begin to digress from the main discussion (as can be the case at times within group sessions).

Information Exchange

Sometimes it is essential to provide members with chronic disease information. Rather than simply providing this to the group, rendering the group members passive, you can *exchange information* with the group, using the elicit–provide–elicit framework. This enables you to get important information across, and check group members' understanding, so that they process the information in a meaningful way.

FACILITATOR: I'm wondering what you all know already about alcohol and your heart? [eliciting; demonstrating partnership; engaging and maintaining a focus]

OLIVIA: It's bad for you, isn't it?

FACILITATOR: In what way, Olivia? [eliciting]

OLIVIA: Well, it's no secret that people who spend their life in the pub have more heart problems than those who don't.

JIM: Yes, but I remember I saw on the news that alcohol can be good for your heart.

FACILITATOR: Tell us a little bit more about that, Jim. [eliciting]

JIM: People who drank red wine had fewer heart attacks than those who didn't, I think.

OLIVIA: But that really doesn't make sense.

JIM: Maybe not, but I did see it on the news a few years ago.

FACILITATOR: What else do you know? [eliciting]

JOHN: Alcohol isn't good for your blood pressure. It makes it high. My doctor used to go on at me about that.

FACILITATOR: Anything else? [eliciting]

SUZIE: It's confusing. All the time we're told, don't drink, but from what Jim said, perhaps it is good for you.

JIM: I think they said moderate drinking was good for you. I think if you drink a lot it's bad—and it was definitely red wine that was good. Perhaps other things aren't so good.

FACILITATOR: So there's some conflicting information out there. What else? [expressing acceptance; eliciting]

JOHN: I think alcohol does something to your cholesterol, too—but I'm not sure what.

JIM: Oh, that's odd, because I don't think there is fat in alcohol, is there?

JOHN: Don't know. But that's what I was told.

JOAN: It makes you fat—look at the beer bellies people get—it must have a lot of calories.

ELSIE: My husband has diabetes. It's bad for that. It can make his blood sugar go low, so we don't drink a lot at home.

JOAN: Oh, that's strange. It definitely makes you fat, so you'd think it would have sugar in it, rather than make his sugars go low.

FACILITATOR: So, in this room we have a lot of expertise in this area. You know a lot about alcohol. Still, some of these messages are a little bit confusing. Would it be all right if I told you a little bit more about alcohol? [affirming; asking for permission to share] (Group signals agreement.) Okay, well, to start with Jim's point, you're absolutely right. There has been some evidence that moderate consumption of alcohol—and it doesn't have to be red wine—can be good for your heart. [providing] Now, what is moderate consumption? [eliciting]

SUZIE: Is it about a glass of wine a day?

JIM: I would have thought a couple of pints a couple of times a week is alright.

FACILITATOR: You're both sort of right. Evidence has shown that one to two units of alcohol per day, though preferably not every day, can be beneficial for the heart. However, men who drink more than three units, and women who drink more than two units per day are putting more strain on their heart, and this can raise your blood pressure significantly. And drinking a lot of alcohol at once can damage the heart. So, what does that tell us? [validating; providing; eliciting]

JOAN: That if you want to drink a bit, that's all right, but drinking a lot really isn't that good for your heart. So really, you should try not to do it too much.

FACILITATOR: Yes. Drinking a little is unlikely to do you a lot of harm, but the more you drink, the more you increase your risk of further heart problems. Remember though, it's everyone's own choice to decide what to do with their own drinking. All I'm doing today is making sure you understand the risks and benefits. What you choose is up to you. [validating; providing; supporting autonomy]

JIM: So, when you say units, what's a unit? Is that like a pint?

The interaction continues, and then at the end of the session, the facilitator asks:

FACILITATOR: So, we've talked a lot about alcohol this afternoon. What messages will you take home today? [eliciting; focusing]

OLIVIA: A lot of the benefits you see from alcohol, you can get from exercise. It would be easy for me to accidentally drink too much, but I don't think I'll accidentally exercise too much. (*Group laughs.*)

FACILITATOR: You think exercise will work better for you. [reflecting change talk]

JIM: I need to check how much alcohol is in the beer I drink. I was surprised to find out some of our beers can be far more than one unit per half pint, and I may have been drinking more than I should. I think I need to be a little more careful.

FACILITATOR: So, healthy drinking for you. [reflecting change talk]

JIM: Absolutely.

ELSIE: I think I understand how alcohol lowers blood sugar, and that some drinks contain more sugar than others. I know why my husband has to eat some starchy foods and carry dextrose to have a drink now.

FACILITATOR: So, along with how alcohol affects our hearts, you have learned a bit more about your husband's diabetes. What else? [expressing empathy; eliciting]

The facilitator begins by *eliciting* the existing knowledge in the group. The members have some knowledge, and the facilitator reflects the apparent contradictions in their understanding when *providing* information. Later, the facilitator *elicits* by asking what messages they are taking home, providing an opportunity for them to personalize the information.

Moving into Action

Getting Started with Action

At this point in the group, it is time to shift from eliciting preparatory change talk (*importance and confidence*) to mobilizing change talk (*moving into action*). The following example, *getting started with action*, demonstrates how you can encourage members to focus on things they would like to change and begin to plan how to go about changing them.

FACILITATOR 1: We've talked about a few things you would like to be different. So, what small changes would you like to make? [focusing on personal changes; evoking change talk]

BRIAN: I'd like to get a bit more exercise.

FACILITATOR 1: Be a little more active. [reflecting change talk]

NANCY: Me, too.

FACILITATOR 1: I'm guessing there are a few other people who might be interested in getting some more exercise. Do you want to give us a wave? That's great. [eliciting]

FACILITATOR 2: What other kinds of things? [evoking change talk]

JOHN: I've cut down on my smoking, but I would like to give it up completely. It's going to be hard.

FACILITATOR 2: So you'd like to make even more changes to your smoking, if you could find the strength to do it. [reflecting change talk]

JOHN: Yeah, I'm not sure I can stop yet, but perhaps I could try cutting down a little bit more.

FACILITATOR 1: How many other people would like to tackle smoking? So, you aren't on your own there, John. What other kinds of things are people thinking about? [validating; evoking change talk]

SUZIE: This sounds a bit stupid—but I actually want to change in terms of getting back to normal. I want to be able to do my housework, like I used to before my heart attack, but I haven't been able to because of my husband.

ELLA: I know exactly what you mean. Life at home is chaos at the moment. They just don't understand, do they?

SUZIE: Exactly. It's driving me mad, and I'm finding it hard to think of anything else at the moment. I'm sorry to be difficult, but that's how it feels.

FACILITATOR 2: That sounds like a lot. Which bit is most important to you at the moment? [expressing compassion; evoking change talk; focusing in on a target behavior]

SUZIE: I think showing my husband that he doesn't need to wrap me in cotton wool would make things feel more normal at home, and easier to make other changes later.

FACILITATOR 2: So, improving that relationship would help things get better at home. [reflecting change talk]

SUZIE: Yes, I think that's highest on the list at the moment.

FACILITATOR 1: So we have quite a few different things people would like to change. Take a few moments to think about what your top thing is. Now, what do you think would be the best three reasons to make that change? [focusing; evoking change talk]

JOHN: Well, I think one reason is that it's no secret that smoking kills you, is it?

FACILITATOR 2: You want to live for as long as possible. [reflecting change talk]

JOHN: And I don't like having to smoke before doing things. Even if I didn't manage to stop completely, if I didn't have to do it as often, that would be good.

FACILITATOR 2: Even cutting down would make life better for you. [reflecting change talk]

JOHN: Yes, definitely.

FACILITATOR 1: Who else wants to share their reasons? [evoking change talk]

EMILY: The thing I want to change is to get more active. I like spending time with my grandchildren, too, but it wears me out. I'd like to be able to keep up with them better.

FACILITATOR 1: So one reason is that you want to feel less tired with your grandchildren. What else? [reflecting; evoking change talk]

EMILY: Well, I suppose that's the main one. But the talk we had from the physiotherapist about how some exercise can be really good for your heart—I really want to try not to have another heart attack if I can help it. And show myself I can do it, get fitter.

FACILITATOR 2: So, you want to help your heart get healthier, and you would like to prove to yourself that you can achieve some difficult goals. [reflecting change talk]

EMILY: Yes. I'll see how I go.

FACILITATOR 1: So, Emily, how might you start on these changes? [evoking change planning]

EMILY: Well, I was thinking when the physio said last week—small changes for big differences. I'm not sure I could find a 30-minute block to go for a walk. But perhaps I could have a little walk 10 minutes before breakfast in the morning, 10 minutes before lunch, and 10 minutes before I put the dinner on in the evening. I could start like that, and then see how I get on.

FACILITATOR 2: You've really thought about how to fit it in with your life. [affirming]

EMILY: Yes, I've been thinking about it for a week or so, how it might work best for me.

FACILITATOR 2: You're ready to give this your best shot. [reflecting change talk]

EMILY: Yes. It's not much though, is it? Not sure how much good it will do me.

FACILITATOR 1: Any change, no matter how small, may make a big difference to your health, especially if it starts some momentum and fits in with life well enough that you can do it. [giving information; respecting autonomy]

EMILY: Yes, that's what I was thinking. At least, I know I could do this.

FACILITATOR 1: That's great. What other ideas do people have about how to make changes? [evoking change talk; planning for change]

In this example, the facilitators elicit change talk from group members by asking key questions, such as "What kinds of changes are people thinking of making?"; "What are the best reasons to make the change?"; and "How do you think you might go about it?" Group members think about their own specific goals after such questions and share their ideas with the group. The facilitators also ask members with similar ideas to identify themselves, which is useful for those who wish to support each other. The facilitators respond to change talk through reflections and guiding questions, rather than telling group members what to do.

Dealing with Challenges and Setbacks

There are times when members experience barriers in relation to their desired behavior changes. The following example shows how you might go about *dealing with challenges and setbacks* in a group situation.

FACILITATOR 1: So, did anyone find things tough at all this week? [evoking]

JOAN: Yes. I don't think I did so well.

FACILITATOR 1: Tell us about that Joan—remind us of your goal this week. [evoking]

JOAN: I was going to try to be a bit more active this week. I was doing quite well. I was going out for my walk in the afternoon, and then on Friday it was raining, and I didn't feel like going out, you know? I hate the rain. Even taking an umbrella—it's just horrible.

FACILITATOR 2: Not much fun. [expressing acceptance]

JOAN: It's miserable. So I told myself that I would do it when it stopped raining, but then it was dark. Then the next day, there was an emergency and I had to rush round and look after my grandchildren, so it didn't happen then. Then the next day it rained again. Then the next day I just thought, what's the point. And now I'm back at square one.

FACILITATOR 1: So, how are you feeling about things, Joan? [evoking]

JOAN: A bit miserable really. I wanted to do better. I've got no willpower.

FACILITATOR 2: Yet you still managed to get out and go for your walk for 3 days this week. You've got some willpower. [affirming; reflecting change talk]

JOAN: Yes, I did.

SUZIE: Some people don't even manage that, right? We can't be angels all the time. (*Smiles.*)

BERT: I hate the rain, too, so you're not alone! I don't think you should be so hard on yourself, Joan. You did get some walking done. When it's raining, I just do something different.

JOAN: What kinds of things?

BERT: Sometimes I go to the museum and walk around there instead. Or I go swimming.

JOAN: Mmmm. I'm not too sure that swimming is for me really.

FACILITATOR 2: You find that these things really work for you, Bert. [expressing empathy; reflecting change talk]

BERT: Yes, I just approached the problem differently.

MARY: One thing I do when it's raining is give my house a good once over. You know, I'll clean out some of the cupboards or I'll vacuum or something. It kills two birds with one stone, because I get to huffing and puffing, and I sort my house out, too.

JOAN: Now, that's something I might try.

FACILITATOR 1: It sounds like you did really well at the start of the week. [affirming; reflecting change talk]

JOAN: Yes, I did.

FACILITATOR 1: What kinds of things might you do differently this week, so that you can do even better? [evoking; planning for change]

JOAN: I might be more energetic with the housework, like Mary said. But thinking about different ways I can be active when things happen might be useful. I need to think about it more.

FACILITATOR 2: You've already given it some thought, and it seems that making some time to think it over will help you be successful in the long run. [affirming; addressing self-efficacy]

JOAN: I think so.

FACILITATOR 1: So, what is your goal for this week, Joan? [evoking; planning for change]

JOAN: Just to do what I can as far as the exercise goes, and make some plans to try out the week after.

The facilitators address the setbacks by focusing on Joan's achievements and encouraging her to draw on her experiences of putting change into practice. The group encourages members to share ideas and to talk about successes with changes they have made. Again, the facilitators reinforce the change talk through reflective listening.

Conclusion

When providing group interventions, it is important to address the complex process of behavior change rather than simply to provide information about what changes to make and how to make them. MI groups can help people become more empowered to manage their disease, relieve some of the burden associated with caseload, and reduce the costs of poor management of chronic conditions. When the groups also provide valuable social support to people who often feel isolated, they make health care services not only more efficient, but also more human.

> *MI groups can help empower people to manage their disease, relieve the burden associated with caseload, and reduce the costs of poor management of chronic conditions.*

References

Bennett, P. (2000) *Introduction to clinical health psychology.* Buckingham, UK: Open University Press.

Bodenheimer, T., Lorig, K., Holman, H., & Grumbach, K. (2002). Patient self-management of chronic disease in primary care. *Journal of the American Medical Association, 288*(19), 2469–2475.

Butterworth, S., Linden, A., & McClay, W. (2007). Health coaching as an intervention in health management programs. *Disease Management and Health Outcomes, 15*(5), 299–307.

Classen, C., Butler, L. D., Koopman, C., Miller, E., Dimiceli, S., Giese-Davis, J., et al. (2001). Supportive–expressive group therapy and distress in patients with metastatic breast cancer: A randomized clinical intervention trial. *Archives of General Psychiatry, 58,* 494–501.

DeVol, R., Bedroussian, A., Charuworn, A., Chatterjee, A., et al. (2007). An unhealthy America: The economic burden of chronic disease—Charting a new course to save lives and increase productivity and economic growth. The Milken Institute. Retrieved September 27, 2008, from *www.milkeninstitute. org/publications.*

Dowler, E., Turner, S., & Dobson, B. (2001). *Poverty bites: Food, health, and poor families.* London: Child Poverty Action Group.

Hibbard, J. H., Mahoney, E., Stock, R., & Tusler, M. (2007). Do increases in patient activation result in improved self-management behaviors? *Health Services Research, 42*(4), 1443–1463.

Jepson, R. (2000). *The effectiveness of interventions to change health related behaviours: A review of reviews.* Glasgow: Medical Research Council Public Health Sciences Unit.

Knight, K. M., Bundy, C., Morris, R., Higgs, J. F., Jameson, R. A., Unsworth, P., et al. (2003). The effects of group motivational interviewing and externalizing conversations for adolescents with Type-1 diabetes. *Psychology, Health and Medicine, 8,* 149–157.

Lindon, A., Butterworth, S. W., & Prochaska, J. O. (2010). Motivational interviewing-based health coaching as a chronic care intervention. *Journal of Evaluation in Clinical Practice, 16,* 166–174.

Pedersen, S. S., Middel, B., & Larsen, M. L. (2002). The role of personality variables and social support in distress and perceived health in patients following myocardial infarction. *Journal of Psychosomatic Research, 53,* 1171–1175.

CHAPTER 18

Motivational Interviewing Groups for Weight Management

Erin C. Dunn, Jacki Hecht, *and* Jonathan Krejci

Who Struggles with Weight Issues?

Brianna's struggle with weight began when she injured her knee playing soccer during her first year in college. Surgery left her immobile for many weeks. Prior to her injury, Brianna never gave much thought to her weight. After surgery, however, she began to feel anxious about weight gain and loss of fitness. At first she cut back on junk food, but ultimately she began to restrict calories, weigh herself multiple times per day, and exercise excessively, losing 40 pounds in a few months. Her athletic trainer urged her to seek help. She ultimately agreed to treatment, worried that she might jeopardize her good standing with the coach.

Larry is a 46-year-old businessman who quit smoking 6 years ago and has gained about 70 pounds since. He used to play tennis several times a week, but his schedule now gets in the way. He recently learned that his blood pressure and cholesterol are elevated, and he will have to go on medication if he doesn't lose weight. He can't see how he can change his eating or join a weight loss program given that he conducts many business meetings in restaurants and travels frequently.

The Weight Management Spectrum

The biological purpose of eating is to provide sustenance for daily living, but eating also serves psychological, behavioral, cultural, and environmental needs that influence consumption. Problematic eating occurs on a spectrum: from underweight individuals, who restrict food intake and expend calories by exercising; through average-weight people, who binge-eat then purge to compensate; to obese people, who binge-eat chronically, without compensatory behaviors to regulate weight. Disordered eating contributes to serious physical and psychological consequences, mood disorders, low self-esteem, and limited social activities. Obesity increases risk for the most common chronic illnesses: type 2 diabetes, hypertension, cardiovascular disease, and cancers. Anorexia and bulimia often result in serious physical complications, as well as increased depression and suicide risk, anxiety, and substance abuse (Kaye, Bulik, Thornton, Barbarich, & Masters, 2004; Keel et al., 2003).

Treatment Goals for Weight Management

A standard treatment goal for overweight individuals is to lose 5–10% of body weight, which is associated with significant health benefits (National Institutes of Health, 1998). Successful outcomes are often the result of learned behaviors rather than willpower. Many weight loss programs outline specific calorie and exercise goals, and behavioral strategies to reach them. These include routine weighing, consuming calories and fat grams within a target range, increasing physical activity, and self-monitoring behaviors in a daily journal. Although the basic formula for maintaining weight loss is to establish balanced and routine eating and exercise patterns, this simple formula can be difficult to follow, and many drop out of treatment and regain the weight they initially lost (Fabricatore & Wadden, 2006).

Typical treatment goals for anorexia and bulimia include reducing problematic behaviors (e.g., dietary restriction, compensatory strategies, and preoccupation with weight), while also normalizing eating, enhancing adaptive coping strategies, and improving body image using combinations of cognitive-behavioral therapy (CBT) and family therapy. Similar to treatment for obesity, relapse following treatment for anorexia and bulimia is common, suggesting that new approaches are needed to enhance treatment outcomes for these conditions (Treasure & Schmidt, 2008).

Use of MI in Weight Management Treatment

Those struggling with weight management often experience significant ambivalence. Studies of MI for weight management have been promising (Treasure & Schmidt, 2008). Preliminary studies indicate that MI groups for weight management also show promise (Feld, Woodside, Kaplan, Olmstead, & Carter, 2001; Minniti et al., 2007; Stahre, Tarnell, Hakanson, & Hallstrom, 2007; West et al., 2010).

MI Groups for Weight Management

This chapter outlines our method of working with weight management issues in groups founded on MI principles. We outline a sequential approach to group treatment, based on an unfolding process in ongoing groups with stable membership. In the first phases of MI groups, *engaging the group* and *exploring perspectives,* MI strategies and techniques build group rapport by creating an empathic and autonomy-supportive environment and focus on exploring members' experiences, goals, and motivation for change. The third phase, *broadening perspectives,* helps group members develop options for change and enhances their confidence by reflecting upon past successes and personal strengths. The final phase, *moving into action,* helps members to specify, plan, and implement changes that are personally relevant to their goals.

Engaging the Group

Engaging members and helping them maintain their commitment to treatment can be difficult. Members may choose to be vocal or quiet for different reasons. In obesity treatment, some members who lose weight are eager to share their achievements, while others are concerned that this will be perceived as bragging. In treatment groups for anorexia or bulimia, members may excitedly share their victories when they decrease bingeing or purging, while those working on weight gain may be embarrassed to discuss their increased caloric intake. Social comparison presents another challenge in group treatment: Members who continue to struggle with making changes sometimes feel they aren't as good as more successful peers. As a result, they have difficulty discussing their ongoing struggles. Sometimes members in this position eventually stop attending altogether. With such complex group dynamics, it is helpful to rely on guiding principles to elicit engagement and cohesion.

Setting the Frame: Establishing a Safe and Productive Group Environment

After member introductions it is useful to review group guidelines and expectations (e.g., the importance of attending group and notifying the leader in advance of missed sessions, policies around making up missed groups, and completing homework assignments). Next, we recommend orienting group members to the MI approach and interactional style:

> "This group may be a little different than other groups you have been part of. We don't spend a lot of time teaching new skills or information. What this group tries to do is help you better determine what you might like to change, what strengths will help you change those things, and what stands in the way of change. In order to do that, we need to establish a few guidelines that everyone will follow, including me. First, not everyone is in the same place, and that's OK. Some people are certain they want to change, while others have mixed feelings. Some people are sure that change is possible; others are not so sure. Each of us can learn from others who are in a different place than we are. The best way we can do that is by really listening to each other and helping each other stay focused on our own goals. For that reason, we try never to give advice unless it is asked for. No one here, including me, should try to make you change; rather, we can best support one another by respecting individuals' decisions. How does that sound to everyone?"

Engagement Strategies

When clinicians rely primarily on accurate, empathic listening and OARS (open questions, affirmations, reflections, and summaries) counseling skills to elicit statements about importance, confidence, and readiness to change, the personal relevance of change becomes more vivid and meaningful for clients. One challenge to implementing MI in a group format is to maintain an individualized, client-centered focus, while remaining attuned to group dynamics and engaging all members. To facilitate this, turn to members who have been successful in areas where others are struggling:

> "Some people are finding it hard to complete food records on a regular basis, yet others are saying that it's the most important tool they are

using. For those who are keeping track, how do you manage to do this?"

This has three benefits. First, by not adopting the role of expert you avoid evoking resistance, while highlighting the successful experiences of other group members. Second, members who hear peers' determination, commitment, and previous successes may shift their own perspectives and actions in the direction of the changes toward which they are striving. Third, eliciting change talk from members who have experienced initial success helps them to consolidate their own commitment to change.

Consider asking the group's permission to establish a guideline whereby you invite each member to comment on a specific topic, while respecting his or her right to refuse. Also, instead of focusing primarily on outcomes (e.g., changes in weight) during the past week, use OARS strategies to elicit members' successes and obstacles with behavioral strategies. This avoids making some members feel inadequate and invites silent members to become actively engaged. When encouraging members to share their victories and challenges, remain aware of how such details may impact other group members. You could suggest that they focus on the frequency or severity of behavior (e.g., "I reduced my bingeing to once per day"; "I added a protein at dinner three times this week"; "I added two walks to my exercise routine this week") rather than share potentially upsetting information such as calories consumed or clothes sizes. Other engagement strategies include dividing into pairs, with instructions to report back to the group, and explicitly addressing the imbalance of sharing within the group by asking quiet members to comment about their decisions to sit quietly.

Encourage members to share their victories and challenges while remaining aware of how such details may impact other group members.

Exploring Perspectives

In MI groups, exploring each member's ambivalence and values helps you to understand their perspective and build a foundation for a later focus on change. Members find it helpful to hear their peers' thoughts on these topics, as it validates their experiences and highlights issues they might have overlooked.

Exploring Ambivalence

One fundamental premise of MI is that resolving ambivalence is a hallmark of behavior change. Clients often are enthusiastic about losing weight in the beginning but still harbor underlying mixed emotions. They may be *desperate* to lose weight and *tentatively hopeful* that things will be different, but simultaneously be *ashamed* about their perceived lack of self-control and *doubtful* that they have the ability to achieve their long-term goals. In addition, different clients have different levels of motivation for specific behaviors. Some find it easy to exercise more but have difficulty reducing caloric intake; others focus on diet but struggle with exercise. Individuals with anorexia or bulimia may desperately want to stop binge eating and purging but be unwilling to limit exercising. They may also feel unable to alter beliefs about their body shape or weight. In groups, clients find it a relief to have their ambivalence acknowledged as a normal and expected part of the process, and to hear that they are not the only ones who feel stuck.

Exploring Functions

Individuals across the weight spectrum often share a lack of insight about the function that overindulgence or restraint serves in their lives. Thus, a focused exploration of factors that influence members' eating decisions can increase both awareness and motivation for change. A conversation about perpetuating factors helps members understand that many of these factors are experienced as positive and thus become barriers to change. For example, members may use food as a way to distract attention from negative emotions, so reducing overeating or bingeing leads to increased emotional pain. Exploring this dynamic and developing alternative strategies for managing negative emotions often help to increase members' readiness to change eating habits.

Another strategy is to discuss the pros and cons of continuing with an unhealthy behavior that many members share in common (e.g., dietary restriction, late night overeating). This is especially helpful for members who have not considered the reasons they continue to engage in harmful behaviors, or who judge themselves harshly for their habits or struggles. Using this strategy in groups helps members recognize that making mistakes, suffering, and personal inadequacy are part of the shared human experience—something that *everyone* goes through—rather than something that happens to them alone.

Exploring Values

To address ambivalence, consider including an explicit discussion of values. Motivation to change any entrenched behavior often arises from a discrepancy between that behavior and deeply held personal values. In our experience, these values often fall into three categories: (1) *roles* (the ability to fulfill important responsibilities); (2) *relationships* (personal connections with others); and (3) *self-concept* (a desire to experience oneself as autonomous, moral, consistent, etc.). Explicitly building the bridge between these values and changes to eating/weight can help to solidify a commitment to change. Ask members to identify their most important values and discuss how problem behaviors fit with those values. Alternatively, do not focus on the problem behaviors themselves, but help members envision a more values-consistent life: "If you woke up tomorrow living your life according to your values, what would your day look like? How would you spend your time?" Similarly, you might have members review how they spend their time, and evaluate the extent to which these activities are consistent with their priorities.

Exploring Importance and Confidence

Another strategy for resolving ambivalence is to examine each of the three elements of motivation using scaling rulers for importance, confidence, and readiness to change eating habits. Even if initial importance, confidence, and/or readiness ratings are relatively high, members are still likely to experience some ambivalence. Stay attuned to this ambivalence by monitoring members' reactions to recommended changes and inviting them to explore discrepancies between their stated values/goals and subsequent actions. This can be done during the initial group check-in, through the topic of the day, and when summarizing and reviewing goals for the coming week.

Broadening Perspectives

Once members have begun to engage in group participation and to explore their current situation and perspectives in a focused way, MI groups elicit members' increased investment in making changes and greater confidence in their ability to try new behaviors. This is typically accomplished through hypothetical considerations of future change possibilities and review of personal strengths and past successes. Evoking members' thoughts on these issues helps to broaden their perspectives and build a stronger foundation for change.

Increasing Importance

Internal motivation can be enhanced when you help members to clearly envision the possibility of change and articulate its personal benefits. One MI strategy, *looking forward,* helps members envision the impact of their change on their long-term goals. For example, many overweight people have specific health conditions they want to improve, such as lowering blood pressure and reducing medications for chronic illnesses. Others focus on social reasons, such as being more active with family or increasing longevity and quality of life. Individuals with anorexia may aim to improve cognitive and physical functioning, whereas those with bulimia may hope to decrease the isolation, shame, or guilt that accompanies their secretive behaviors. The following questions can help members envision the possibility of change:

- "What would you like your life to look like in 5 years? Think about the things that you value and the difficulties you identified; how would these be different?"
- "Let's imagine you decide not to change your eating habits. What do you think your life would be like in 5 years?"

Alternatively, have group members choose their own adventures by writing brief hypothetical scenarios of their lives a year from now. The first paragraph describes what life would be like if they did not change (or if they returned to old habits); the next paragraph describes how things would be if they could totally create their own destiny; and the last paragraph describes what they realistically hope their lives will be like given what they've learned and experienced through group. By comparing the different scenarios, members can examine the consequences of not changing, while also considering how to make their dreams a reality.

> *Have group members choose their own adventures by writing brief hypothetical scenarios of their lives a year from now.*

Building Confidence

There are two primary strategies for enhancing confidence in one's ability to change. The first involves eliciting examples of previous success with changing. The second involves eliciting or highlighting personal strengths that the client can harness in the change process, as in the following example:

LEADER: How many of you have lost weight before? (*Many hands raise.*) Clearly, many of you have experience with this. How did you feel when you lost weight?

RAJ: I felt great. I had much more energy and my clothes fit better. Now they're tight again, and the added weight is really slowing me down.

GINELLE: My blood pressure came down and I was able to manage stress a lot better. I felt good about myself! (*Others comment similarly.*)

LEADER: You felt more energetic, healthier, and proud of the way you looked. (*Many members indicate agreement.*) How have you been able to lose weight in past?

SONYA: I've taken part in other weight loss groups and it really helped. Mostly, I counted calories and kept track of what I was eating. But, that's hard to keep doing and my weight crept back up over the past year.

MARCO: I went to the gym everyday. That's the only way I can lose weight. When I stop, the weight comes back on.

LEADER: For each of you, it sounds like when you really make a commitment to change you do your best to stick with it. Sonya, for you it was helpful to have the group's support and for you, Marco, going to the gym helped you stay committed to your plan.

MARCO: Well, I never really thought about it before, but after I went to the gym I didn't want to blow it by eating junk. So, maybe I was eating less and making healthier choices.

GINELLE: That's definitely true for me. When I go to the gym after work, I wind up eating dinner later and then I don't snack at night.

LEADER: So while it can be hard to get started, committing to an exercise routine really helps you stay on track.

CALVIN: I find that cutting back on sweets really helps me. That's my downfall.

LEADER: So, while different approaches have worked for different people, all of you were able to lose weight by staying focused on your goals. Reducing calories, keeping track of what you're eating, cutting back on high-calorie foods, and maintaining an exercise routine helped you to do this. What would it be like if you strengthened your commitment by combining all of these approaches together?

Helping members connect with a time when they felt good about themselves can reinforce their desire and reasons for change. In this example, the leader affirms Marco's determination and persistence, and relies primarily on reflective listening and open-ended questions to evoke change talk and to help make past successes more vivid. By eliciting personal examples rather than providing information, the leader encourages the group to take ownership of the change process and ensures that the examples will be personally meaningful. The leader also explores members' reactions to engaging in *all* of the described behaviors as a way to consolidate their commitment.

Another way to increase members' confidence is to elicit personal strengths. This can be particularly helpful with members who state that the only thing they are truly good at *is* their eating disorder (e.g., restricting, overexercising). To address this, you might have members list positive attributes about other members, and then share these anonymously, in written form, or verbally, if all group members feel safe, trusting, and agree to this process. Doing this activity anonymously might be introduced in the following way:

> "We've discussed how important it is to focus on things about you that make you amazing, as well as things that you do well, in order to increase your confidence in your ability to make changes and your perception that you are worth making changes for. People often get stuck when asked to list nice things about themselves, but they find it easy to list the positive attributes of others. It's very powerful to hear how others view us, so I'd like to try an exercise where each of you writes down something nice about every other person in the room. It could be something you've noticed in group or something you know about them from outside of group. Please write each member's name and one strength that they possess on a separate scrap of paper. Do not put your name on the paper. When you are finished, please put your papers in the container in the middle of the room. I will read them aloud, so that the comments remain anonymous. I'll give you an example of the type of strengths you might write about someone—I think that [the co-leader] genuinely cares about people."

Once everyone has finished and the papers have been collected, have one co-leader read the papers while the other records each of the strengths on a chart, not attached to anyone's name. Encourage members to write down the attributes their peers see in them:

> "Write down the positive qualities that your peers mention. Use this list to affirm yourself. Carry it with you or post it somewhere you can read it often. Take every opportunity to remind yourself of these positive attributes you have. Be sure to keep adding to this list as you think about other strengths you possess."

When this process is complete, elicit members' summaries of how they see the group at this time, including your own appreciation of their strengths and abilities.

Moving into Action

After engaging group members and focusing on their long-term goals and values, evoking interest in and importance about making changes, and boosting their initial confidence around methods of change they might try, it's time to move into the final group phase: guiding members to specify, plan, and implement changes that are personally relevant to their weight management goals.

Change Planning

Change planning in groups can be tricky because members have different levels of readiness to change. Even when members have high levels of importance and confidence about making changes, some may not be ready to take action yet. In keeping with the spirit of MI, avoid pushing members into action if it is beyond their level of readiness. Nevertheless, you can discuss what they might do if they decide to experiment with making changes.

One change planning exercise involves eliciting ideas about how members could improve their health or quality of life in an elicit–provide–elicit format:

> "We've discussed your goals and values, the pros and cons of making changes, your personal strengths, and past successes with change attempts. Now let's talk about what you could change as you move forward. What ideas do you have about things you could do to increase your health or well-being? "

Group members will likely generate a list of possible changes (e.g., keep food records, control portions, increase social support), but be prepared to offer a few suggestions (with permission) if the group struggles:

> "It can be difficult to figure out where to start when making changes. It can be overwhelming to pick one thing to work on. Or maybe you know exactly what you want to do but aren't sure what the first steps should be. We have some ideas we can share with you, if you are interested."

If members seem uninterested or lukewarm about hearing your ideas, acknowledge their autonomy and invite them to approach you if they are interested in further discussion. If they express interest, offer some ideas about changes individuals might make. After providing information, elicit feedback from the group about this process: "What do you think about these suggestions? How might these work for you? What else do you want to add?" Write all ideas on a chart and review them verbally at the end of the exercise.

Well-meaning members often offer unsolicited advice or try to coerce another member to change. This can be addressed by using the *reframe, remind, return* framework:

JULIE: I know I should, but I just can't seem to bring myself to tell my boyfriend to stop bringing cookies into the house. I've tried before, but I'm afraid he'll get mad.

MIKE: You just need to make up your mind and do it. Don't worry about what he thinks. If he doesn't support you, he doesn't really love you.

LEADER: Mike, I really appreciate your concern for Julie. [reframe] As a reminder to everyone, we decided to avoid giving advice unless someone asks for it. [remind] Julie, it seems like you are a bit stuck right now. What kind of input would you like from the group? [return]

To avoid putting Mike in the spotlight, the leader directs the reminder to the entire group, then focuses on Julie. Alternatively, the leader could return to Julie by asking her to expand further on her concerns about her boyfriend, her own ambivalence about keeping cookies in the house, or the pros and cons of not being assertive with him.

Strengthening Commitment to Change

It can be useful to introduce members to the concept of *commitment language*: discussing how personal speech influences actions, reviewing the range of commitment verbs (Amrhein, Miller, Yahne, Palmer, & Fulcher, 2003), and encouraging members to pay more attention to the commitment strength of their speech. For example, a member who severely restricts her caloric intake describes her desire to challenge her fear of eating out:

ALEJANDRA: I was thinking about having a sandwich when I went out with friends the other night, but when I looked at the menu I panicked and ordered something that felt "safe," a salad with low-fat dressing on the side. Afterwards, I was mad at myself.

LEADER: You wanted to try something new, but you were scared, and afterwards you felt disappointed.

ALEJANDRA: Yeah, I really wanted to see what would happen if I ate something more challenging, but I guess I was too afraid.

LEADER: What could you do next time to make it easier to follow through on your plan, so that you can find out what will happen?

ALEJANDRA: I could decide what I will order ahead of time and not even look at the menu. If I order first, before everyone else, I won't be able to change my mind as easily.

LEADER: I wonder how this fits for others. When do you feel pulled back and forth, when is your commitment is tested? What can you do to maintain your commitment?

In this segment, the leader uses a double-sided reflection ("You wanted to try something new, but . . . ") to highlight Alejandra's ambivalence, then reflects back underlying emotion (" . . . you felt disappointed") to accentuate the discrepancy between behavior and goals. She uses an open-ended question to elicit Alejandra's ideas about how to maintain commitment despite ambivalence, then she expands the conversation from Alejandra back to the group to reengage everyone and link members together in their quest to change.

Getting Started

Once the group has generated a list of possible areas to focus on, and commitment to making changes has been solidified, it's time to help members specify their goals and implement changes. However, it is still possible that some members will not be ready to take action. It can be helpful to remind members that treatment is an experiment, and that they do not have to be *completely* ready to change in order to start the process or see how small changes feel. You can start with a general discussion about goal setting and what makes a good goal:

> "Today we are going to discuss effective goal-setting techniques and strategies. We'll start by reviewing the most important aspects of a goal. Can anyone tell me what makes a goal 'good'?"

Remind members that treatment is an experiment and that they do not have to be completely ready to change in order to start the process.

Providing information about the importance of making goals specific, meaningful, and realistic helps members. It is also useful to discuss the possibility of making their goals public and reviewing them frequently:

> "For some people, making their goals known to others can increase their commitment and increase the support they receive. Regular review can point out goals that might be revised in order to increase the likelihood of success. What do you think about sharing your goals and revising them along the way?"

Eliciting examples of times in members' own lives when they set successful goals versus ones that did not work well for them can be illustrative and also increase confidence of those who have effectively set (and attained) goals in the past. Finally, move into a discussion about specific goal setting: "Now that we have a sense of what makes a good goal, what goals are you interested in setting for the upcoming week?"

Most members should be able to set one realistic goal for the upcoming week. If some members remain silent or state that they are not yet ready to make changes, normalize their ambivalence, then open a general discussion about it:

> "Not everyone is ready to make changes at this time, which is fine. Sometimes our current behaviors serve a powerful function; other times we're not yet feeling confident about making changes. Can those of you who are not yet ready to make changes help us understand more about how you feel?"

After a brief discussion about the barriers to making changes, inquire about whether there is *any* goal that these members could set for the upcoming week:

> "Even if you're not ready to set an action goal, you may consider setting a goal that would increase your importance, confidence, or readiness rating by a point or two. What types of things might it be helpful to focus on?"

Examples may include completing a pros–cons list or revisiting the higher values exercise. Individuals who lack confidence might set a goal to reread their positive attributes card or journal about times when they were able to make changes or attain goals. Another possibility is to set a goal that focuses on improved quality of life (e.g., decrease isolation) or changing another, related health behavior (e.g., sleep, smoking, drinking).

Enhancing Ownership of Change

Avoid the expert trap of believing that your role is to provide expert guidance and advice. While this role can be a comfortable one for you and for members alike, it carries the risk of establishing passive members who are witnesses rather than agents of their own change. To enhance ownership of change among members, consider discussing the role of personal choice in making changes, and exploring times in their lives when they made changes for themselves versus others. Group members generally agree that they are more committed to making changes, and maintain change longer, when they change for themselves (e.g., because they want to feel better) rather than someone else (e.g., because a loved one gives them an ultimatum).

Another way to enhance ownership for change is to foster problem solving when members have difficulty meeting their goals. Review their records of weight, food intake, and physical activity frequently, offer comments, and return the records to members. Offer written, open-ended questions or reflective statements that encourage members to come up with their *own* ideas and solutions:

> "As you look over your food record, what patterns do you notice during the week compared with the weekend?" or "Your nighttime eating has increased, what might be contributing to this?"

You can also bring these issues back to the group, to enhance feelings of shared experience, as well as generate additional ideas:

> "Some people are having difficulty eating small meals or snacks every 3–4 hours. What kinds of things might help with this?"

Encouraging members to offer their own reflective comments and next steps in their weekly records and group discussion can enhance confidence and ownership. One member noted:

> "At first I was disappointed that you asked us to write our own comments in our books, but after reflecting upon my week, I discovered that I really *can* problem-solve on my own and that I have made a lot of progress."

Sustaining Change

Group members often expect their new healthier habits to replace former ones completely and feel discouraged when old habits creep back in. Help members establish realistic expectations by affirming their efforts and reminding them of the progress they *have* made. Members can also reinforce hope by reminding each other of how far they have come, the changes they have already made, and the reasons why these changes are important to them.

Over time, some may focus on perceived deficits or past failures, or on the return of familiar patterns that leave them feeling hopeless and worried that they will never fully recover. Avoid the trap of implicitly colluding with members' sense of themselves as flawed and inadequate by avoiding a premature focus on concrete problem-solving, education, and remedying perceived deficits. Instead, use open questions and affirmations to create a culture of openness and sharing, to engage members and build rapport, to explore strengths and challenges, and to affirm members' efforts. By persistently affirming and highlighting members' strengths, you can enhance their confidence and commitment to change.

JULIANA: The thought of having to keep food records forever is getting me down. I was doing well at first, but I don't know what happened . . .

LEADER: All this monitoring is starting to make you feel a little discouraged.

JULIANA: Yeah, I always seem to forget. Or when I do remember I can't find my book, and then it's too hard to catch up later.

LEADER: I really appreciate that you brought this up. In some ways it would have been easier to stay quiet, but I'll bet other people in the group are having the same struggles.

ALEX: I feel the same way. I started off great, but then I began taking shortcuts and stopped writing things down. Now I'm back in old habits rather than eating healthy meals.

LEADER: *(noting others nodding)* Several of you are struggling right now. You really want to stay on track, but it's hard to keep the momentum going. What might help?

LEENA: I agree. It clearly helps me, because I'll think more about my food choices and portion sizes if I know I'm writing it down. Without it, I'm back to old habits.

LEADER: That makes a lot of sense to me. I hear a lot of strength and determination in what everyone is saying. Even though it sometimes feels draining to stick with self-monitoring, you believe that it's important to help you normalize your eating and manage your weight.

Here, the leader engages the group around a frustration initially expressed by one member. By linking this to similar experiences from other members, the leader normalizes Juliana's experience, affirms her honesty and determination, and redirects her to focus on a solution. Rather than confront the behavior or problem-solve for the group, the leader uses an open question ("What do you think might help?") and affirmations ("That makes a lot of sense to me. I hear a lot of strength and determination . . .") to tap into the collective wisdom of the group and to consolidate their commitment.

Dealing with Challenges and Setbacks

Motivation to change is not synonymous with motivation for specific treatment strategies. Importance, confidence, and readiness may vary considerably across different behaviors, and may wax and wane over time. In the following example, an overweight group member considers dropping out because she does not want to self-monitor. The leader affirms her for expressing her discomfort, reminds the group of the multiple avenues for success, and offers her options:

CARLA: I just can't write everything down. Maybe I shouldn't be in this program.

LEADER: Keeping track isn't working for you.

CARLA: I do want to lose weight, but writing everything down seems pointless.

LEADER: I'm really glad you brought that up. There really is no single correct way. Let's start with something that makes sense to you. One possibility is to start with an exercise plan. Another would be to create an eating plan that doesn't involve monitoring everything that you eat. Which of those sounds possible for you?

CARLA: I could work on an exercise plan. I don't have to keep track of my eating in this program?

LEADER: Keeping track can help people become more aware of what they're doing. But if it's keeping you from reaching your goals, it's not serving its purpose. People change in different ways. The most important thing is finding what works for you.

Many individuals with disordered eating habits dislike keeping food records and will drop out of treatment if it is mandatory. Discussing the pros and cons of self-monitoring is one way to address this common complaint. Individuals who are encouraged to make their own informed decision about keeping food records often stay in treatment and eventually find self-monitoring to be very helpful.

It is also possible to harness the collective wisdom of the group when exploring a menu of options. Group members are often quick to offer solutions, especially to others who are feeling stuck. To avoid evoking resistance, inquire about the member's ideas first and ask the member's permission before enlisting the group in providing options: "What other strategies could help you stay on track? Would it be helpful to do some brainstorming with the group?" If the member agrees, avoiding generating too many ideas all at once. Write each idea on a chart before asking which idea(s) the member prefers. Give the member the chance to ask others about their experiences with the strategies:

> "We've generated a great list of potential alternatives to keeping food records. Carla, how might these options fit for you? Do you want to hear more about others' experiences with these alternatives? Which ones might you explore?"

Finally, there are many reasons why people stop coming to treatment. A common reason is the embarrassment and shame associated with slipping back into old behaviors. Calling members to express your concern can reengage them. Once reached, these members often confess the frustration and/or humiliation they feel about reverting back to old behaviors, and their fear of facing their fellow group members again. Normalizing these feelings can make it safe for them to return to group:

"It sounds like you're disappointed with how things have been lately; this isn't the direction you want to keep going in. It's common for people to avoid sessions when they feel like they're not doing well, yet that's often the time they can most benefit from the group's support. We also miss your contributions to the group. What would you think about returning?"

Conclusion

Millions of people struggle with weight issues; many will seek group treatment. New approaches must meet the needs of the individual, as well as the group, to enhance and consolidate commitment to change. MI groups can support clients through their weight management efforts. Identify perceived benefits of behavior change, while you highlight strengths and past successes, to renew enthusiasm and reduce the shame that often accompanies repeated disappointments and relapses to old behaviors. Help clients to understand the connections and discrepancies between their deeply held values and eating and exercise habits to solidify their commitment and motivation for change. Finally, use open-ended questions, affirmations and reflections, to help *clients* make the argument for change, and thereby enhance perceived importance, confidence, and readiness for change.

At the heart of the group is your client-centered attitude and interactional style. Clients often report that the unconditional regard, positive reinforcement, and nonjudgmental support offered by leaders of MI groups help them to persevere in the face of demoralization and fading motivation. As one member told her MI group leader:

"You never criticized me for skipping group or coming up with reasons why I didn't change my eating. I was waiting for someone to judge me, so that I could drop out and blame it on the program. Instead, you called and said 'We missed you in group today!' and that made me realize that it was up to *me* whether I was going to continue to make excuses or finally change."

References

Amrhein, P. C., Miller, W. R., Yahne, C. E., Palmer, M., & Fulcher, L. (2003). Client commitment language during motivational interviewing predicts drug use outcomes. *Journal of Consulting and Clinical Psychology, 71*(5), 862–878.

Fabricatore, A. N., & Wadden, T. A. (2006). Obesity. *Annual Review of Clinical Psychology, 2,* 357–377.

Feld, R., Woodside, D. B., Kaplan, A. S., Olmstead, M. P., & Carter, J. C. (2001).

Pretreatment motivational enhancement therapy for eating disorders: A pilot study. *International Journal of Eating Disorders, 29,* 393–400.

Kaye, W. H., Bulik, C., Thornton, L., Barbarich, N., & Masters, K. (2004). Comorbidity of anxiety disorders with AN and BN. *Archives of General Psychiatry, 161,* 2215–2221.

Keel, P. K., Droer, D. J., Eddy, K. T., Franko, D., Charatan, D. L., & Herzog, D. B. (2003). Predictors of mortality in eating disorders. *Archives of General Psychiatry, 60,* 179–183.

Minniti, A., Bissoli, L., Di Francesco, V., Fantin, F., Mandragona, R., Olivieri, M., et al. (2007). Individual versus group therapy for obesity: Comparison of drop-out rate and treatment outcome. *Eating and Weight Disorders, 12,* 161–167.

National Institutes of Health. (1998). Clinical guidelines on the identification, evaluation and treatment of overweight and obesity in adults—the evidence report. *Obesity Research, 6,* 51–209.

Stahre, L., Tarnell, B., Hakanson, C., & Hallstrom, T. (2007). A randomized controlled trial of two weight-reducing short-term group treatment programs for obesity with an 18-month follow-up. *International Journal of Behavioral Medicine, 14*(1), 48–55.

Treasure, J., & Schmidt, U. (2008). MI in the management of eating disorders. In H. Arkowitz, H. A. Westra, W. R. Miller, and S. Rollnick (Eds.), *Motivational interviewing in the treatment of psychological problems* (pp. 194–224). New York: Guilford Press.

West, D. S., Gorin, A. A., Subak, L. L., Foster, G., Bragg, C., Hecht, J., et al. (2010). A motivation-focused weight loss maintenance program is an effective alternative to a skill-based approach. *International Journal of Obesity, 35*(2), 259–269.

CHAPTER 19

Motivational Interviewing Groups for Men with a History of Intimate Partner Violence

Ann Carden *and* Mark Farrall

"It wasn't my fault. My wife just won't listen to reason. It's always got to be her way. Nothing is ever good enough for her."

"I work hard and put up with a lot of crap on my job. Then I come home and the place is a mess. She knows how crazy that makes me. She just doesn't care."

"It happened just like that (*snapping his fingers*)! One second I was just trying to get her to listen to me, and the next thing I knew, she was on the floor. I feel really bad about it, but it's not like I meant to hurt her. I don't know what comes over me."

When you hear statements like these from men mandated to domestic violence intervention programs, you might assume their violent actions were driven by a sense of male entitlement, a view of women as lesser beings in need of correction, or an addiction to power and control in relationships. You might conclude that the best way to stop a man from abusing is to get him to change his attitudes toward women, and manage his anger and aggression. You might assume that swift and severe negative consequences will prevent him from engaging in future violence. These views reflect only one aspect of male-to-female intimate partner violence and abuse (IPV), a highly complex behavioral pattern with multiple determinants and dimensions. While it is true that, in some cases, violence against an intimate partner represents a conscious and premeditated attempt to control the partner, it can also be an emotionally reactive response to a situation that the man experiences as confusing, painful, or threatening.

Whatever underlying dynamics may be involved in committing violent acts, the behavior pattern can take on the nature of an addiction. Men who become violent with their partners generally *know better*, but something in their internal organization prevents them from *acting better*. For these men, therapeutic intervention is more likely to lead to meaningful and enduring change than confrontational approaches aimed at convincing them of the need to overcome their "violent nature," "aggressive tendencies," and "self-serving beliefs." An emphasis on competencies rather than deficits; an empathic, nonjudgmental, collaborative stance; and respect for autonomy (essential elements of the MI approach), may be more effective at reducing relationship violence than education or punishment (Carden, 1994; Dutton, 2006; Gondolf, 1997).

Resistance, Ambivalence, and Motivational Issues

Most of the men in domestic violence programs are mandated to attend treatment. Given their frequent negative perceptions of the social service agencies, judges, or family members who referred them, they often expect to be treated with disrespect in our programs. Many resent being forced to attend and make no attempt to hide that resentment. Their defenses are high, their underlying fears are strong, and their motivation to engage in treatment or to change their behavior is based more on external consequences (jail time, social services' control of their families, threats of divorce, or loss of loved ones' respect and trust) than on internal motivation. At their initial interview, they tend to maintain a defensive posture rather than risk the shame and rejection they fear will result if they engage in honest self-examination. In responding therapeutically to them, we view their defensive posture as a sign of psychological "stuckness" rather than pathology or personal deficiency. We intentionally avoid using labels such as "batterer" and "perpetrator." Our goal is to help them build on their positive attributes and opportunities, not to pressure them into change.

To minimize resistance in our first meeting with a new participant, we make every effort to engage him as quickly as possible in co-creating a positive working relationship. We make it clear that we respect his right to choose whether to be involved in our program. We collaborate with him in framing what happened to get him here, and engage him in exploring personal values and life goals. No matter how violently a participant may have behaved, we approach him with the attitudes that define MI spirit—respect for his autonomy, genuine interest in his perspectives, and a desire to help him figure out how to achieve a positive transformation.

When we establish a strong therapeutic alliance, we find that participants are more likely to become actively involved in treatment, and to adopt attitudes and behaviors that improve the quality of their lives (see Dutton, 2003; Gondolf, 1999).

Structuring and Facilitating MI Group Services

Start with a Pregroup Assessment and Orientation Meeting

Before referring a participant for group work, we administer a comprehensive biopsychosocial assessment (Carden & Boehnlein, 1997). In addition to information about physical and psychological health, the assessment addresses the violent episode that precipitated the referral, the history of other violence, the current status of the couple's relationship, alcohol and other drug use, and lethality potential. We provide assessment feedback in an *elicit–provide–elicit* style. We begin by *eliciting* the participant's reactions to the assessment process so far—his thoughts and feelings about the questions we have asked, and his expectations about how the results might be useful to him. We listen and empathically reflect what we learn, encouraging him to elaborate and clarify as needed. Next, we *provide* a nonjudgmental review of the assessment results, inviting him to comment as we present each item. We end by again *eliciting* his thoughts and feelings about the process, and the significance of his results to him personally.

Using the core MI communication skills—<u>O</u>pen questions, <u>A</u>ffirmation, <u>R</u>eflection, and <u>S</u>ummaries (OARS)—we focus each client on the discrepancy between how he would like his life to be and how things currently are. Within the ambivalence he expresses about the importance of considering changes in his attitudes and behaviors, and his confidence about making those changes if he so chooses, we elicit elaboration and clarification of any signs of motivational potential. We then collaborate on developing a violence cessation plan and nonviolence contract as a prerequisite to group work. Next, we provide an orientation to the group process—again, in an *elicit–provide–elicit* style.

- *Elicit:* We ask each participant to describe his expectations and concerns about group (e.g., "What kinds of things do you already know about how group therapy works?"; "What are your thoughts about being part of a group that looks at the issues we've been discussing?"). We reflect his reactions, encouraging him to "unpack" the deeper meanings of his expectations and concerns (e.g., "You're having a hard time seeing how this might be useful to you"; "You're not comfortable with the idea of talking to a group about this part of your life").

- *Provide:* We follow this exploration with a detailed description of our group program.
- *Elicit:* We invite his reaction (e.g., "What else do you want to know about the program?"; "How do you feel about giving this a try?"; "How do you see this working for you?").

Assuming that he is willing to participate and able to benefit from group work, the referral to group is made. Most men are ready to move on to group intervention after these individual sessions. But for those who aren't, we provide one-on-one counseling as a precursor to group work.

Use Co-Leaders

We believe that MI groups for men with a history of IPV are more effective when facilitated by two skilled practitioners. Co-leaders can model the core elements of MI spirit (*partnership, acceptance, compassion,* and *evocation*) with each other, as well as with group members. Each leader tends to elicit different responses from group members. A co-leader team has greater flexibility and creativity in those moments when an MI strategic response such as *reframing* or *shifting focus* is needed to deal with unexpected group dynamics. Given the emotionally charged nature of many group discussions, having two leaders allows for individual support of a troubled member, and provides an added measure of safety should a group member become agitated. After each session, co-leaders can compare impressions of members' strengths and needs, and of group dynamics as a whole, then revise their approach. They can record change talk they hear in group and devise a plan to monitor and strengthen such talk in future sessions. They can note signs of resistance between themselves and a particular group member, and discuss reflective and strategic responses to minimize it. A male–female team provides opportunities to model healthy male–female interactions and explore different perspectives on relationships. Both leaders should be proficient MI practitioners with expertise in domestic violence and abuse, mental health, substance abuse, and group process.

Provide Brief Monthly Individual Sessions

Brief monthly individual MI sessions (more frequently, if needed) provide a valuable supplement to weekly group sessions. These monthly sessions provide opportunities for each member to assess his own progress; receive feedback from group leaders; and explore concerns, values, or goals that he may not feel comfortable addressing in group.

Use the Four Processes of MI

Miller and Rollnick (2013) frame MI as including processes of engaging, focusing, evoking, and planning. In our groups, we focus more on connecting and guiding than on informing and explaining (engaging). We collaborate with group members to create a safe atmosphere within which each member can explore core values and life goals, and disclose details of past aggressive behaviors—including the thoughts and feelings that preceded and followed violent acts (focusing). In this nonjudgmental environment, members can acknowledge their past actions and begin to consider the importance of change at their own pace and in their own way. With a focus on their strengths, and affirmation for their accomplishments, no matter how small, they can come to believe in their ability to choose another way of being in relationships (evoking). Based on this new awareness, each member can develop a specific individualized change plan (planning).

Use an Elicit–Provide–Elicit Group Protocol

The *elicit–provide–elicit* communication format shapes our MI group process. At the beginning and end of each session, we invite member feedback on the group's work.

- Opening questions include "How are you feeling about being here today?"; "What did you learn last week that you'd like to comment on tonight?"; "What are some things you did this week that helped you get closer to what you want in your life?"
- Closing questions include "In what ways was the discussion useful to you?"; "What stood out for you in this session?"; "What are some of the things you plan to do this week to get closer to what you want in your life?"; "What would you like us to do differently in group sessions?"

MI Groups for IPV

We turn now from *how* we do it, to *what* we do. We provide a sense of what our groups are like in action. The four subsections that follow address what we do to engage group members, explore their personal perspectives, broaden those perspectives, and move into action.

Engaging the Group

The old adage "You only get one chance to make a first impression" is supported by empirical evidence of the significance of the first encounter to the quality of the therapeutic relationship and the eventual achievement of clients' goals. We keep this in mind as we facilitate our opening sessions. After the introductions and a review of basic issues, a typical opening in a first session might sound something like this (Jon and Maria are the group leaders).

MARIA: Thanks to all of you for coming tonight. You've all had a chance to meet Jon and me individually at your intake sessions, and learn a bit about what we do here. We're wondering what your thoughts are about coming tonight. . . . What do you already know and what else would you like to know about the program? [respectful welcome; open question]

JAKE: What I know is that this whole thing has gotten blown out of proportion. I'm not a violent person and I really resent that judge telling me I have to come here for the next 6 months. No offense, but I should be spending this time with my wife and kids, and spending the money this is costing me on things for my family.

COREY: At least you have a family. I got thrown out of my own house, and now I can only see my kids with some nosey social worker watching my every move. I can't take them anyplace or do any fun things with them.

JON: You guys are upset about this whole thing—the judge telling you that you have to come here. You don't think this is something you should have to do, Jake. Corey, you're upset about not having time for fun with your kids. And, on top of that, this is costing you your hard-earned money. Pretty frustrating! [empathic reflection; acceptance]

The leader acknowledges members' negative reactions to this perceived threat to their autonomy, interference with their family life, and drain on their finances. In this first empathic reflection, he establishes a nonjudgmental tone, conveying interest in understanding the men in the group and his respect for their perspectives on their situations. After a few exchanges in which both leaders further reflect these negative attitudes and emotions, the conversation continues:

COREY: You know it really wasn't that big of a deal! This is all so stupid! My wife is a real troublemaker! I barely even touched her.

ANDRE: Well, I guess I can see some reason for them thinking I needed to come here, and I for one plan to completely change the way I deal with my girlfriend. I can't lose her!

MARIA: You feel like this whole thing has just gotten blown out of proportion, Corey. And some of the rest of you seem pretty frustrated about having to come here. And then Andre—you have a different take on this. You can see some benefit to being here—including that you won't lose your girlfriend. That relationship is really important to you. What ideas can anyone give Andre about how coming here and talking about ways to react when he feels upset or backed into a corner might help him not lose his girlfriend? [collecting summary; open question; partnership]

Here, the leader offers a brief *collecting summary*. She contrasts Corey's and Andre's perspectives without judging either, and briefly reflects the concerns of other men who have commented. When she invites members to explore possible benefits to Andre of coming to these sessions, she demonstrates trust in the group process and respect for members' opinions. A little later in the interview, the leaders gather up some threads of the group's conversation:

JON: Some of you feel insulted about being told by strangers what you can't do in the privacy of your home. And on top of that, you have to pay for this program. And some of you want to learn about getting your needs met without getting in further trouble. In spite of the stress and frustration you've been experiencing, you each made a decision to come here tonight. You might have been expecting us to put you down or try to force you to talk about things you're not ready to talk about at this point. And you might have been wondering what the other men in the group would be like. A part of you might not have wanted to show up tonight . . . to just take your chances with the court or with your wife or girlfriend. [collecting summary; affirmation]

COREY: Yeah, but I learned that I can't trust the people at the court, so I figured I'd take my chances with you guys.

ANDRE: I don't think that would have gone over real big with Christina.

MARIA: So, while a part of you might have preferred not to come, another part was thinking about a worse situation that might happen if you decided not to show up. How are you feeling about the decision you made? [double-sided reflection; open question; shifting focus]

One leader has summarized group members' communications (verbal and nonverbal) so far. He affirms them for coming to this first session, and starts to shape a double-sided reflection of the dilemma in which some of the men appear to feel caught. They let him know that they're feeling heard. The other leader completes the reflection and shifts to exploring members' impressions of the group so far.

Respectfully emphasizing each member's personal choice and control over how he wants to live, and whether he wants to participate in the program acknowledges the truth: No one else can make choices for him, or change for him. This strengthens the therapeutic alliance and minimizes the "wrestling" effect with which we are all too familiar in mandated services.

Coming alongside and *emphasizing personal choice and control* (as the leaders did in this initial session) is a productive way of relating to group members. It encourages them to take control of their lives at a time when they're feeling relatively powerless. It demonstrates nonjudgmental respect for their perspectives at a time when they're feeling discounted and misjudged. And it establishes a nonthreatening environment in which change is more likely to occur over time.

Exploring Perspectives

Exploring members' perspectives on the incidents that led to referral to the group offers an opportunity to separate the observation "I did a bad thing" from the conclusion "I am a bad person," and separate the belief "It just happened" from the realization "I chose to do it." Openly processing these insights in a supportive environment enhances motivation to make choices that are more consistent with their core values and life goals.

In exploring personal perspectives, the group is a valuable tool. The camaraderie, peer identification, and role modeling in group provide a powerful resocialization experience. The group becomes a safe space where they can explore feelings, have their accomplishments acknowledged and their successes celebrated, and try out new ways of being in relationships. The sense of community in groups breaks the isolation in which many of these men have been living.

The sense of community in groups breaks the isolation that many of these men have experienced.

Evocative questions such as "If you could pick two or three things that matter most to you in the way you want to live your life, what would those things be?" provide an opportunity for members to focus on their core values. Following an in-depth group discussion of their responses to this question with a request for each member to review quietly in his own mind the incident(s) that led to his referral allows time for group members to begin to develop insight into the discrepancy between their most deeply held values and the behaviors that have been shaping their lives.

Framing models commonly used in domestic violence treatment

programs can serve as insight boosters. The "Power and Control Wheel" model (Pence & Paymar, 1986) describes negative patterns commonly observed in dysfunctional intimate relationships. We present this model as one possible way members can consider what has happened in their lives. We begin with a group discussion of the commonalities and differences between members' personal experiences and the behaviors described in the model. Rather than conduct successive one-on-one interactions, we engage the group as a whole in dialogue around an open question designed to elicit change talk (e.g., "What are some problems this has caused between you and your wife/partner?"; "What could you imagine happening if you decided not to do this?"). The center of energy is within the group, not with the leaders, or with a few highly involved members. We listen for change talk, invite elaboration and clarification when we hear it, and affirm members' courage in addressing the difficult issues that arise.

The Power and Control Wheel focuses on patterns in dysfunctional relationships that members can change. Its counterpart, the "Equality Wheel" (Pence & Paymar 1986), focuses on positives and healthy relationships, and helps define what members might move toward, such as nonthreatening behavior, negotiation and fairness, trust and support, honesty and accountability, and so forth. It enables members to envision what their changed future behavior might look like, and allows further development of the discrepancy between members' current status and their values and goals. It can serve as a follow-up to the power and control wheel, or be used alone, when you wish to focus more on building a positive future than on processing past negative events. With either model, we use the MI strategic responses *shifting focus, reframing,* and *agreeing with a twist* as needed to defuse defensiveness.

The "Cycle of Violence" model (Walker, 1984) describes a cyclic pattern of behavior that progresses from tension buildup, to aggression, to apologies and promises, and back to tension buildup. While the pattern may not fit all members' experiences, the model provides a launching point to review the sequence of internal and external events that preceded and followed members' past aggressive behaviors. As we walk with group members through painful memories, we look for opportunities to support their self-efficacy by highlighting and affirming times when they chose actions that were consistent with their current nonviolence goals. We also encourage them to identify opportunities to choose nonviolent solutions to conflict in the future, perhaps drawing from ideas in the equality wheel.

When models like these are presented in a traditional educational format, they can arouse defensiveness, discourage exploration, strengthen investment in the status quo, and block movement toward motivation to change. As models, they carry assumptions that may not be accurate, and presenting them as "truth" invites defensiveness. Presented provisionally, they can encourage exploration and help members move away from investment in the status quo toward motivation to change. Addressing such challenging material within a respectful, calm, nonpunitive interpersonal environment generates self-reflection in some, plants seeds in others, and allows each member to feel valued and less defensive.

Broadening Perspectives

Looking at past attitudes and behavior helps members come to terms with *what has been*. Looking at future choices helps them envision *what can be*. The former enhances members' sense of the importance of change. The latter impacts their belief and hope that another way is possible. Having supported members in taking an honest inventory of the reasons for their referral, we turn our focus to envisioning a future without change ("Where do you see yourself a year from now if you decide to keep doing things the way you've been doing them?"), and a future with change ("How might things be different if you make some changes in the way you deal with feelings of frustration and disappointment?").

In the following vignette, group members explore the pros of change (i.e., choosing nonviolent approaches to resolving conflict and releasing tension in their intimate relationships). The leaders use OARS and three MI strategic responses—*shifting focus, reframing,* and *emphasizing personal choice and control*.

JON: What do you gain when you relate to her respectfully? [open question]

ANDRE: Well, Christina is happier with me and our relationship is a lot better when I do.

MARIA: And that's something you're willing to work to make happen. [affirmation] In what ways would your relationship be better? [open question]

ANDRE: It won't be so stressful all the time. We'll probably do more things together and be more romantic.

JON: You have a good vision of what things could be like for you two. [reflection] What do others think? What might happen in your relationships if you were to make nonviolence a real priority? [open question eliciting change talk]

COREY: I might be able to convince the judge that it's safe for me to have unsupervised visitation with my kids.

MARIA: They're really important to you. [reflection]

COREY: Yeah, and they're just little. They need me in their lives.

JON: It's really important for you to be a good father to them. [affirmation]

COREY: And I could be, if that judge didn't have it in for me. I need him to give me back my parental rights! He had no right to take them away. They're *my* kids!

JON: And being able to spend time with them alone again would mean a lot to you. [reframing] What's the first thing you want to do with your kids when you do get to see them on your own again? [open question; shifting focus from blaming to envisioning the future]

Reflecting Corey's change talk leads initially to more change talk from Corey. But, responding to the leader's affirmation about his desire to be a good father to his children, Corey shifts his focus, angrily blaming the judge for his situation. The leader reframes Corey's complaint by reflecting Corey's earlier statements about unsupervised visitation with his children. The leader follows up with an open question to shift Corey's attention from blaming to thinking about and verbalizing what he wants to have happen.

COREY: I think I'd like to make them pancakes. They really like my pancakes.

WILL: My son's out of the house, on his own, into drugs . . . never calls or comes to see me. I wish I had another chance like you to do it differently.

COREY: Yeah, it's good to get another chance, but the judge just won't give it to me.

IVAN: You gotta earn it, man!

MARIA: So, Corey, you really want your visitation rights back. You know you can be a good father and it's not good for your kids that you're not in their lives. It's hard to understand why the judge won't give you back unsupervised visitation right now. Will, you think Corey's lucky to have the chance you wish you still had with your son. And Ivan, you figure there just might be a way for Corey to get the chance he wants. But, I get the impression, Corey, that you're thinking it's hopeless. That judge is never going to see things your way no matter what you do. [collecting summary closing with an amplified reflection]

COREY: Well I know he'll be looking at whether I keep coming to group, and he'll be getting reports from my PO [parole officer] that I'm staying clean.

MARIA: So you see a few practical things within your control that you can do to help get what you want. That puts the ball in your court! [reflection; emphasizing personal control] What good things might happen for the rest of you if you find new ways to solve problems and resolve tension in your relationships? [open question]

In her summary, the leader is selective in choosing what to reflect and what to intensify. She intentionally overstates Corey's concerns about the judge in the amplified reflection "hopeless") to give him an opportunity to think about what he might do to get what he wants from the court. He responds with change talk. She acknowledges his insight and returns to the group to elicit others' ideas about change. Before the session ends, the leaders engage the whole group in revisiting highlights of the discussion.

> "Before we wrap up, how about taking a minute to think quietly about what you might gain by changing the way you deal with frustrations and tensions in your relationship. Think about some of the benefits we just talked about and maybe some others that weren't mentioned. Write down some of your ideas if you like."

After allowing time for quiet reflection, the leaders invite further discussion, allowing the group process to predominate. This wrap-up time gives each member another opportunity to think about and articulate what he values and wants in his life. Some of the precommitment change talk we hear when we do this exercise includes the following:

- *Desire:* "I want my kids to look up to me and trust me"; "I want to prove to my wife that I can be trusted"; "I want her to love me"; "No way do I want to go back to jail"; "I want to get my kids back"; "I want to be in control of my emotions"; "I want to get rid of this court monitoring."
- *Ability:* "Now I know a few ways to keep it together when I'm feeling really stressed out"; "I know I can do what it takes to stay out of trouble"; "I'm a loving person and I know I can become a better father and husband if I really try."
- *Reasons:* "I'll keep getting into trouble with the law if I don't stop doing this"; "My wife said she would leave me if I can't get my act together"; "When my kids grow up I want them to be good people, so I need to set a good example for them."
- *Need:* "I need my family"; "If my wife took the kids, I don't know what I would do"; "I need to keep my job and this arrest doesn't help"; "I can't let this happen again or I could lose it all."

Our objective is to broaden each member's perspective in ways that allow him to

- See more clearly discrepancies between aggressive actions and his goals and values.
- Envision his future with new behavioral choices and new consequences.
- Increase awareness of his ability to make choices that lead to what he wants in life.

As the men get a clearer sense of the gap between their goals and values, and some of their past attitudes and behaviors, the *importance* of change increases. As they learn and practice new behaviors, their *confidence* increases in their ability to make changes that will bring them closer to what they value and desire.

Moving into Action

Our programs require a nonviolence contract for admission into the group. The challenge for group leaders is to facilitate the evolution of that contract from an externally reinforced statement to an internally driven, personally meaningful commitment to change. Because each member's pace and path to commitment are unique to him, leaders must rely on their clinical judgment in deciding when to transition from *building motivation to change* through broadening personal perspectives, to *strengthening commitment to change,* by moving into action.

> *Facilitate the evolution of a nonviolence contract from being an externally reinforced statement to becoming an internally driven, personally meaningful commitment to change.*

As soon as we notice signs of readiness to develop individual plans for moving into action, we go with this energy. We begin a transitional summary with a comprehensive recapitulation in "you" language ("Some of you . . . ," "Many of you . . . ," "All of you . . . ") of the change talk statements we've heard over group sessions. We take turns reflecting the most powerful examples, strategically omitting others to give group members a chance to restate them. We address blocks to change, and review sustain talk we've heard in earlier discussions. Intermittently throughout the summary, and again at the end, we ask for verification of its accuracy and completeness, and encourage group discussion. If no one has picked up on the omitted change talk, one of us will add it before we move on. After the men have had time to process, correct, and expand on our summary, we ask a key question—again in "you" language (e.g., "What exactly do you want to change in your life right now?"; "What's one change you could start to work on right away as a step toward your goal?").

We use MI reflective and strategic responses to help each member identify and articulate a specific change goal he is ready to make at that moment, however large or small. Then, we distribute a change plan worksheet with the following seven prompts.

1. "One thing I want to change in myself starting right now. . . . "
2. "On a scale of 0 (*not at all important*) to 10 (*extremely important*), this change is a ____ for me because. . . . "
3. On a scale of 0 (*not at all confident*) to 10 (*highly confident that I can make this change*), I would rate myself a ____ because. . . . "
4. "What I'll actually do, and when I'll actually do it to make this change happen. . . . ".
5. "_____ can help me as I make this change by. . . . "
6. "Some challenges that might keep me from succeeding with this, and some ways I can deal with these problems. . . . "
7. "I'll know I'm making progress when I see these things happening in my life. . . . "

Addressing one item at a time, we ask members to work alone on their thoughts about just that item. We spend a few minutes on this solitary exercise, then have members pair up and share their thoughts on that particular item with their partner. To avoid any negative interpersonal dynamics, we preassign pairs. Before they begin, we remind them of Thomas Gordon's (1970) twelve "roadblocks" to listening (which we review often in our group sessions). We ask them to listen with the intention to understand and learn—not to fix, criticize, agree or disagree, correct, persuade, and so forth. We tell them that they will describe their partners' thoughts on that item when the group reconvenes. When we bring the group back together, we ask each member to describe his partner's response to the items, and each partner to verify, correct, or expand on that description. We encourage them to make whatever changes they want to on their worksheets. We use dyads frequently to provide opportunities for each member to explore the positives of change and to practice listening with the goal of understanding another person's perspective—a crucial skill for their future relationship interactions. We circulate to ensure that conversations are on-task and positive, and to provide coaching and redirection as needed.

Toward the end of the session, we ask members to review their plans, make any changes needed, and sign them. We invite discussion and refinement of these change plans in our monthly individual sessions. In the group sessions that follow this one, members celebrate their successes and talk about their struggles in putting their change plans into action. We explore a range of possible strategies for dealing with setbacks and role-play situations that are especially challenging for them at home or in their work or social settings. Here are two examples of the goals, challenges, and successes we have witnessed.

> Dave, a 47-year-old factory floor manager, attended group sessions under court order for 1 year and then attended voluntarily. In his 14th month, one of his working goals was "to listen to others with the intention of understanding their perspective." He expressed a strong commitment to adopting this at work and in social settings, as well as at home, where he had already experienced some success implementing it. Dave also attended a 12-step recovery group. He saw this goal as parallel to the 12th step of Alcoholics Anonymous, which suggests practice of the principles learned in the first 11 steps "in all our affairs." One evening Dave described an encounter he had the day before with a line worker, who questioned a decision Dave had made about a production protocol. Remembering his goal, he overrode his initial impulse to insult the worker and reject her feedback. He heard her out and, in the process, discovered an important detail he hadn't considered. Leaders and group members affirmed his success. The group then explored the sequence of events that led from the worker's message to Dave's initial thoughts and feelings about that message and its messenger, to his awareness of his change goal, to his decision to act on that goal, and to his thoughts and feelings right after the incident. Dave came to a clearer understanding of his impulse to defend himself aggressively from perceived insults to his competency (tendencies with which many men in our programs can identify). He acknowledged that the questioner being female increased his urge to discount her feedback. Dave pinpointed two turning points when (1) the importance of accomplishing his goal overrode his emotional reaction, and (2) he made a conscious decision to act on his goal.

> Eric, a 24-year-old roofer, was referred by the court after assaulting Brenda, the mother of his three young children, at her parents' home, where she had moved with the children a few days before. Although this was not Eric's first arrest for domestic violence, it was his first referral to treatment. Eric grew up in a chaotic family in which he was physically abused by his father and two older brothers. In his second month in treatment, Eric's goal was to "get Brenda to come home," which we guided him to revise into "demonstrate to myself and to Brenda that it's safe for her to live with me again." One evening, Eric reported in an agitated tone that he had left Brenda several phone messages and she had not returned his calls. The leaders responded empathically, reflecting

the frustration and disappointment in Eric's voice, and expressing curiosity about his goal in making the calls. They guided the
group discussion away from advice and judgment toward Eric's
feelings of frustration, and his perspectives on the situation.

Eric is typical of many in our programs who, before discrepancy has
been adequately developed, desperately want the problem situation in
which they find themselves to disappear, and things in their lives to go back
to the way they were. They feel despondent about their loss, certain that
they have "learned their lesson," and they want their partners to "forgive
and forget" (as many have done repeatedly in the past). They sometimes
have an unrealistic view of the negative consequences of their actions and
of the time it will take for trust to be rebuilt and relationships repaired,
and they have difficulty shifting their focus from others' behaviors to their
own. One advantage of groups is that members who have moved past the
struggle to control others become living examples of the brighter future
that significant change can bring.

Conclusion

Although research on MI groups with men who have been violent to their
partners is only beginning to develop, there is some evidence for individual
MI with this population (Morrel, Elliott, Murphy, & Taft, 2003). Similarly,
the MI conditions of empathy, sincerity, warmth, and respectfulness are
significantly and consistently associated with positive outcomes for groups
in the criminal justice system (Marshall & Serran, 2004). When members
feel listened to, understood, and respected, they drop their defensiveness
and engage in self-examination. Many men who at first deny aggression
eventually view the behaviors that led to their referral as abusive and even
disclose other violent acts (Carden, 1993). Many group members voice
relief that the way we treat them is not what they expected and feared.
They express gratitude that we support them in examining their lives and
finding their own answers. They especially appreciate that although their
aggressive behaviors may not be accepted, they, as individuals, are.

Empathy, sincerity, warmth, and respectfulness are consistently associated with positive outcomes for groups in the criminal justice system.

Most men who have been violent toward their partners experience
high levels of ambivalence. They are
deeply troubled by their behavior
and are at the same time, reluctant
to give up the reinforcement it provides. They often have few meaningful social supports. This combination

of ambivalence and social isolation makes MI groups an excellent fit with their therapeutic needs. Empirical data and clinical observations (Carden, 1994; Dutton, 2006; Hamel & Nicolls, 2007; Morrel et al., 2003) support our view that an MI group approach represents a promising treatment for this population.

To maximize the effectiveness of our group intervention, we rely on MI *spirit, principles,* and *strategies* to create an interpersonally dynamic therapeutic environment within which each group member can (1) identify his core values and life goals; (2) examine his past attitudes and actions, including strengths and past successes; (3) consider the discrepancies between what he wants in his life and what his current attitudes and behaviors have created; (4) develop a strengths-based change plan; (5) work through blocks to success; and (6) celebrate strengths and achievements.

Given the potential for danger inherent in domestic violence, our group leaders must hold in vigilant balance a sincere respect for each member's autonomy and a sober awareness that some members' cognitive distortions may threaten the safety and well-being of others. We thoughtfully and cautiously counter all statements supportive of the status quo with reflective and strategic responses. And we remind ourselves, especially when the work becomes difficult (which it often does), that the essential element in facilitating change lies in the accepting and empathic relationship between group members and group leaders.

References

Carden, A. (1993). *Characteristics of men in a diversion treatment program for spousal abuse/violence: A gestalt/ecological perspective.* Dissertation, Kent State University, Kent, OH.

Carden, A. (1994). Wife abuse and the wife abuser: Review and recommendations. *Counseling Psychologist, 22*(4), 539–582.

Carden, A., & Boehnlein, T. (1997, September). Intervention with male batterers: Continuous risk assessment. *Ohio Psychologist,* pp. 9–16.

Dutton, D. (2003). Theoretical approaches to the treatment of intimate violence perpetrators. *Journal of Aggression, Maltreatment and Trauma, 7*(1), 7–23.

Dutton, D. (2006). *Rethinking domestic violence.* Vancouver, BC: University of British Columbia Press.

Gondolf, E. W. (1997). Patterns of re-assault in batterer programs. *Violence and Victims, 12*(4), 373–387.

Gondolf, E. W. (1999). A comparison of four batterer intervention systems: Do court referral, program length and service matter? *Journal of Interpersonal Violence, 14,* 41–61.

Gordon, T. (1970). *Parent effectiveness training.* New York: Wyden.

Hamel, J., & Nicolls, T. (Eds.). (2007). *Family interventions in domestic violence: A handbook of gender-inclusive theory and treatment.* New York: Springer.

Marshall, W. L., & Serran, G. A. (2004). The role of the therapist in offender treatment. *Psychology, Crime and Law, 10,* 309–320.

Miller, W. R., & Rollnick, S. (2013). *Motivational interviewing: Facilitating change* (3rd ed.). New York: Guilford Press.

Morrel, T. M., Elliott, J. D., Murphy, C. M., & Taft, C. (2003). A comparison of cognitive- behavioral and supportive group therapies for male perpetrators of domestic abuse. *Behavior Therapy, 24,* 77–95.

Pence, E., & Paymar, M. (1986). *Power and control: Tactics of men who batter: An educational curriculum.* Duluth: Minnesota Program Development.

Walker, L. (1984). *The battered woman syndrome.* New York: Springer.

CHAPTER 20

Motivational Interviewing Groups for Men with a History of Aggressive Sexual Behaviors

David S. Prescott *and* Marilyn Ross

People often enter treatment for sexual aggression under constraints, and experience treatment as punitive. While some desire to change, many settle for treatment as an alternative to prolonged incarceration. For those on probation or parole, the possibility of a return to prison remains a lingering threat. Practitioners are often obligated to report when a client is having difficulty with treatment. It is hardly surprising when clients then perceive clinicians as an extension of police power. Nevertheless, while clients may initially notice only the legal mandates, MI groups provide the opportunity for members to resolve ambivalence and lay foundations for making significant changes in sexual attitudes and behavior.

Research suggests that warm, empathic, supportive, and directive approaches help individuals change aggressive sexual behaviors (Marshall, 2005). While earlier models emphasized the importance of therapists controlling treatment, a less controlling approach helps clients develop balanced and self-determined lifestyles.

Ambivalence about Change

People who have sexually abused are often vilified. Though few may fit the profile of dangerous predators, it is commonly perceived that all are beyond redemption. When individuals enter services, they may feel over-whelmed by the stigma of their new status and have difficulty reconciling their sense of self with the common view of a sexual offenders. Many experience profound losses that can include their life savings, career, immediate family, and sense of identity, and, if not incarcerated, find that maintaining employment and housing are ongoing challenges. Many face a lifetime of public registration as sex offenders and ongoing restrictions in daily life.

In treatment, ambivalence occurs all along the pathway to change. Initially, clients weigh a desire to be open against concerns about the consequences of doing so given the stigma involved and the freedoms lost (freedom of privacy, autonomy). Once engaged in treatment, clients often experience ambivalence about coming to understand their lives differently, examining the harm they have caused, and developing new attitudes and beliefs. While working toward changing, clients frequently experience ambivalence about whether they truly desire to learn and rehearse new skills, give up comfortable behavioral patterns, and—in many cases—abandon their sexual fantasy repertoire and sometimes sexual expression itself.

Group Treatment for Sexual Aggression

For practical reasons, group treatment is the modality of choice with this population (Jennings & Sawyer, 2003; McGrath, Cumming, & Burchard, 2003). A group can provide support, acceptance, mentorship and, for some, the only time that they feel heard. Treatment for sexual aggression is often up to 2 years or more. The consistency of such a program can help clients establish meaningful relationships within the group, providing a sense of safety about addressing sensitive issues.

Treatment focuses on decreasing the likelihood of future harmful behavior. This requires group members to describe sexual arousal and behaviors normally viewed as too personal to discuss. The warm, supportive, and directive environment of the MI approach provides the safety to allow members to explore these issues. Specifically, by honoring rather than challenging clients' accounts of themselves, conveying a nonjudgmental attitude in exploring discrepancies, and accepting clients who initially avoid taking full responsibility for their actions, you create an atmosphere of mutual respect within the group that promotes self-disclosure.

A focus on change and a safer future is fostered by developing improved relationships and the capacity for feeling competent within them, exploring and clarifying beliefs about sexual behavior, and increasing clients' skills for decision making and managing daily life. They may also include redirecting sexual interests and patterns or eliminating them altogether. The established effectiveness of cognitive-behavioral therapy (CBT); Hanson et al., 2002; Reitzel & Carbonell, 2006), provides a good rationale to combine MI and CBT elements in groups.

Comparatively little attention has been given to clients' goals. Clients often hope for many of the same things that others want: a sense of competence, inner peace, purpose, and belonging within their community. With an MI group approach, members explore their personal goals and integrate them into plans for change, often increasing their commitment to other aspects of treatment. An *approach orientation* helps group members focus on what they are moving toward, not just what they are forbidden to do (Mann, Webster, Schofield, & Marshall, 2004), supporting their autonomy and self-determination.

MI in the Treatment of Sexual Aggression

People who have sexually abused others have a reputation of resisting treatment. In addition to any defensiveness that they may feel about their actions, they likely encounter a poor fit between traditional treatment techniques and their life circumstances (Ward & Maruna, 2007). People who experience the profound life changes that accompany incarceration, probation, or parole benefit from an opportunity to tell their story as they see it. While confrontational approaches settle for compliance within the treatment setting, the MI perspective shifts the focus to internal changes that endure beyond therapy. An MI group can provide an affirming, warm setting in which they can begin to examine uncomfortable behavior.

MI focuses on resolving ambivalence about change, and people in treatment for sexual aggression often have mixed feelings about much of their experience (Levenson & Prescott, 2009). People who have engaged in sexual aggression typically respond better when therapists avoid stigmatizing language such as denial, admission, offense, or "sex offender" (e.g., Coffey, 2010). Encouraging group members to identify themselves as "*people* who have committed sex offenses" can foster hope for a different future, leaving room for members to develop a sense of a "new me," free from offending.

Pretreatment Groups

Early treatment helps clients identify factors that led to their aggressive behavior and explore the extent of their misconduct. Some are initially unprepared to take these steps, and deny the offense with which they have been charged or have difficulty claiming responsibility for their abusive behavior. It is important to engage all clients positively, including those who maintain they have not committed harmful behavior. While denial is not a risk factor for recidivism per se, treatment expulsion *does* correlate with higher risk of future harm (Hanson & Bussiere, 1998).

Integrating such individuals one at a time into a treatment group can create an atmosphere that encourages thinking about change. If that is not possible, if those groups constitute a poor fit, or if the groups may be threatened by these clients' presence, consider providing a pretreatment or "exploration" group specifically for those who deny responsibility for the actions that led them to be accused or convicted by the court. The goals of this group are to engage participants in a context that does not require admission of wrongdoing or a "fast forward" into committing to or taking action, and to prepare them to participate later in offense-specific treatment. Individuals entering this group need a sampling of treatment components in a format that is warm, accepting, and free of demands to acknowledge offending behavior. For example, you might allow them to complete any mandatory historical review assignments in a hypothetical manner, "as if" the charges made against them were true. In this way, group members privately notice the discrepancy between their stated position and the likely reality of their situation, without being forced to take a stand or shift their position publicly. We recommend that you limit the time and scope of these groups with a clear finish date. The treatment goal for this group is to help group members examine their thinking in specific ways, not to change their position.

MI Groups

Engaging the Group

Members are probably highly ambivalent about attending. The more apparent the spirit of collaboration and support for autonomy, the better their chances of success. Accepting members as individuals regardless of the positions they take, can minimize resistance from new clients (Marshall & Marshall, 2007; Serran & O'Brien, 2009).

Minimize resistance by accepting new members as individuals regardless of the positions they take.

Eliciting group rules from members is one way to promote engagement, particularly if you have a closed group. If needed, you can suggest other MI-consistent rules. You may also wish to describe the OARS (open questions, affirmations, reflections, summaries), focusing members on the first three and providing summaries yourself that productively frame group themes. Seek permission before giving feedback, and encourage the group to provide affirmation before giving one another feedback. This becomes reinforcing for members over time, and some come to eagerly anticipate the understanding and acceptance the group provides, and how the positive environment fosters self-exploration and consideration of change.

By eliciting members' support and encouragement of one another, you help the group become more cohesive and ultimately more helpful. Your behavior sets the tone for the group. Group members see the way you handle conflicts as a model for behavior and learn to be more accepting of one another, as in this exchange:

HAL: This group is fine for the rest of you, but I don't belong here. I haven't done half the things you guys did.

LEADER: It doesn't feel like this is the right place for you.

FRANK: I really appreciate you telling us how you feel. I felt that way when I started as well.

Handling Challenges

Successfully managing resistance is important in mandated groups, where clients are often defensive about requirements imposed on them. Some research suggests that resistance is inversely related to treatment progress (Levenson & Macgowan, 2004). While engaging the group, it may be best to accept any resistance, and find points of agreement to keep the group moving toward exploring perspectives:

ROBERT: I was forced to be here. Otherwise, you can bet you would never have seen me.

LEADER: You're pretty unhappy that you have to be here now, to say the least.

ROBERT: That's right. You're not going to change me with this group.

LEADER: Sure. People change when they decide to change.

Exploring Perspectives

As group members become more comfortable and trusting around one another, you can more sharply focus on the issues that brought them to group. Early group work gives clients the opportunity to explore their ambivalence about their actions and accept responsibility for them. Having the time and freedom to explore their ambivalence rather than feeling immediate pressure to reject their past thoughts and actions helps lay a foundation for developing autonomous motivation to change that can be longer-lasting than externally pressured change.

As you work with members who deny committing an offense or see little reason to change, other than to avoid further punishment, you will hear much *sustain talk* (defenses of their past behavior, arguments against the need for change, etc.). While it may not be necessary intentionally to elicit discussion of the negative side of ambivalence, directly challenging sustain talk early on can prevent an honest and open consideration of change, and prevent the development of a cohesive group atmosphere. When members explore the "negative side" of their ambivalence early on, they are simply sharing with you what they already think, and preventing them from doing so may lock them into a defensive position that makes it harder for them to consider new ways of thinking. Sustain talk can also reveal important obstacles to change for later consideration while developing change plans, and preventing expression of it simply keeps you in the dark about these factors, reducing your ability to help members work past them later.

Once the negative side has been vented a bit, and members feel understood and begin to develop a sense of shared identity rather than feeling like a group of strangers, it may be time to pivot toward positive change as the opportunity arises. You can focus on assessing the DARN factors (Desires, Abilities, Reasons, Needs) to foster those opportunities.

LEADER: I understand your position regarding the charges that got you here. At the same time, I'm wondering what positive things might come from being in this group?

ROBERT: It might show people that I'm doing what I'm asked and staying out of trouble. And I might learn a few things and show others that I'm not the monster they think I am.

You may also consider *coming alongside* such as "Some parts of this could be hard for you to accept if you did acknowledge engaging in this behavior." It might also take the form "Some of the consequences of acknowledging this may not seem like they're worth it right now." Your goal is to demonstrate sensitivity to the client's situation. While you may feel urgency to challenge negative perspectives, it is important to avoid eliciting resistance. Change talk can seem elusive when you feel pressure to produce results, especially when clients experience that pressure. You can selectively use reflections to influence the direction of the session and allow members to make their own case for change. In the following example, the leader first reflects a member's emotions using a metaphor, then takes a "half-step" ahead, uses a *continuing the paragraph reflection,* and finally affirms him:

JIM: Look . . . I know I put myself here . . . in this place.

LEADER: This has been a hard road for you.

JIM: I don't want to lose my family . . . again.

LEADER: You're thinking it's time to make things right for yourself and others.

JIM: Yeah. I hurt a lot of people.

BILL: We've all been there. What helped me was just biting the bullet and facing up to it.

JIM: I know I have it in me. I just don't want to end up in even more trouble.

LEADER: It's impressive how seriously you're taking this.

This member spontaneously mentions an important value he holds (e.g., being part of his family again). Members' values can serve as guideposts to help them discover a direction forward, and exploring them can help increase members' motivation to change:

LEADER: You want to find your place in your family again.

JIM: Yes. There's nothing more important to me.

LEADER: What can you do that might help make that happen?

JIM: I don't know. I need to earn their trust back.

LEADER: You want to be trustworthy.

JIM: I don't know if they'll ever trust me again. I can't believe it's come to this. I don't even know if I trust myself. I just wish I could do something to get them back.

LEADER: It's overwhelming, but you want to try. You want to be able to trust yourself again, and be someone your family can trust. You want to be a part of your family, not standing on the outside looking in.

JIM: More than anything. I just don't know how.

You can explicitly invite a discussion of members' values, helping them focus on prioritizing what's most important to them. With their values clarified, you can either explore the fit between their values and their actions, or use those values to help them define how they want to be and act going forward.

For most mandated clients, treatment dropout is a minor issue, but revocation of conditional release looms large. Meaningful early treatment engagement can help decrease compliance-related problems that lead to revocation. It can be helpful to give new clients opportunities to say what they think about the treatment program. Often they state that it is different from their expectations, and they are finding other group members to be more like themselves than they expected. This allows them to voice change talk about accepting the group as a resource that may have something to offer. Sometimes group members privately express the feeling that they are quite different from the remainder of the group. This perspective may come from beliefs that they hold about themselves ("What I did was not so bad") and others ("A lot of these guys have done far worse things than I have"), and often dissipate over time.

Handling Challenges

Occasionally the group dynamic may turn negative, threatening the group's progress. The following example shows how you can help get the group back on track using MI strategies.

BRIAN: If I had just been a little younger or she a little older, this would never have come to trial. (*Becomes tearful.*)

GEORGE: (*jumping in*) That's not right, man. They shouldn't have done that to you. [affirming member's position as the victim]

PHIL: The system's always out to get folks. They don't care about what really happened, just the letter of the law. [affirming presenter's position as the victim]

LEADER: You're having a hard time understanding why she complained.

BRIAN: It seemed like we were getting along fine. I even gave her my cell phone number.

LEADER: You're confused why the police, DA [distrcit attorney], and the judge all honored her complaint.

BRIAN: Exactly.

LEADER: You were on the same page at the beginning; then she called the police on you.

BRIAN: Well, I did tell her I was going to get beer, but I really just wanted to get her into my car. After she thought about that, maybe she felt that I took advantage of her.

TIM: You did a good job with that. That's really honest.

LEADER: (*to Tim*) That really reflects the spirit of this group.

JIM: It's hard to put yourself out there like this in front of the group. I've noticed a change in the way you see things from the time that you first came into group.

By ignoring the MI-inconsistent statements and reflecting some of the members' thoughts, you help the group return the focus to affirming and reflecting to guide toward change.

Exploring perspectives may include looking at discrepancies between the official version of "what happened" from an offense report and the client's perspective. You may wish to handle this sensitive material in individual sessions. When you discuss it in group, you can engage clients in exploring discrepancies by keeping an open, pleasant, and matter-of-fact demeanor. Fellow group members may be particularly encouraging at this point as they describe the initial difficulties they had in making full disclosures and reiterate their commitment to be nonjudgmental.

> *Help the group regain the momentum toward change by ignoring sustain talk and reflecting positive thoughts and feelings.*

Broadening Perspectives

Over time, group members bond with one another. This helps minimize any differences between them as they recognize that they share common goals. It is not unusual for clients to report that their first meaningful friendships are with other group members. The processes of sharing, and being accepted and gently encouraged to reconsider past actions in light of personal values and goals helps most members to acknowledge past actions, accept some degree of responsibility, and become more ready to look forward.

An important task is imagining a different future. As members practice the skills they learn, it becomes easier for them to believe they can be successful. Explicitly asking them to look forward and envision a future they want to create, even if they cannot see a path to getting there, can help solidify a future focus that pulls them forward. Whether you ask group members to envision the future on their own, in pairs or as a whole group, you are communicating that they are worthy of investing in themselves and their future, and able to create a better path forward than the one on which they have been.

With the necessary focus on past misdeeds, it can be challenging to balance a focus on things they need to change about themselves and keep a positive energy that allows them to make those changes. Two MI strategies that help with this are *exploring strengths* and *eliciting change success stories*.

When group members have lost much of their previous lives, they may have difficulty identifying the relevance of past successes. However, you can help members to do so by asking them to discuss a time when they were successful in the past, then eliciting the specific skills they utilized in order to reach past goals. As they identify their skills, you can encourage them to think of ways that these skills could be useful in the present. Group members may actively engage in feedback at this point to encourage, affirm, and brainstorm new ideas.

If your group has members who enter at different times, those further along in the process serve as models for the newer members and can help them to identify strengths. For example, when Arturo entered the group he was very quiet and seemed extremely nervous. As time passed, he began giving good feedback to other members. The following suggests some ways you as leader may wish to affirm this.

> "I always appreciate the feedback that you have for others. It shows how carefully you listen. How does that skill help you in other areas of your life?"

Alternatively, you may frame feedback to members in terms of looking back and then forward.

> "You've come a long way since you began group. You used to sit without speaking when you first came. How will this change help you in the future?"

You can also use scaling questions to assess confidence and elicit change talk:

ARTURO: I haven't always listened so well to others, particularly my girlfriends. My anger used to get in the way a lot more.

JOHN: You listen really well. I've noticed you really take the time to think. It's helped me.

LEADER: Thank you. Arturo, as you look forward to the rest of your life, on a scale of 0–10, how confident are you that you can keep using your listening skills?

ARTURO: Maybe a 7. I guess I have come a long way. Still, it's not hard to imagine problems trying to keep a job when I'm on the registry and manage a relationship, trying to stay in touch with my kids and be a good father.

LEADER: With all of these challenges, that's pretty high! What makes your confidence a 7 versus a lower score like 0 or 4?

ARTURO: Slowing down and listening is something I've gotten really good at. When I slow down, I can give people good feedback, like you and John said. Being able to listen and give people feedback feels really good. I want to keep getting better at this. I know what you're going to ask me next: The way I get to 9 is to keep practicing. That's what I need.

Handling Challenges

This phase of MI group work can be challenging. At times, group members present themselves as instantaneously changed. They voice commitment to being different before they learn the tools to support that change. Fortunately, MI strategies that are effective with individuals are also useful to address this and build group cohesion. The overall spirit of the group reflects warmth and acceptance. We use a collaborative, nonexpert style of interaction.

JASON: Believe me, after all I've been through, I'm not going to do that ever again.

LEADER: You've learned a lot from your experience.

JASON: That's right. I would be a fool to come near a minor again in that way.

HARRY: I thought it would be easy when I first came to treatment, but I found that I still had a lot to learn about myself, and a lot of struggles to go through.

LEADER: I wonder what tools are most helpful to make sure you remain safe.

Group treatment poses unique challenges and opportunities for dealing with clients. In an MI group, members may experience anger from situations outside of the treatment setting, but overt expression of anger occurs rarely. At times, however, members may become overly directive and even confrontational. This can escalate into an argument if leaders do not carefully manage it, as in the following example:

DOUG: With all the restrictions that I have, there's nothing I can do. I just sit around my house thinking about how my wife left me and feel depressed.

PAUL: You could go for a walk. [expert/providing solutions trap]

DOUG: I don't know all the child safety zones that I need to avoid.

RYAN: You could go for a bike ride.

DOUG: I don't have a bicycle, and I don't have the money to get another one.

CHRIS: How about renting a movie?

DOUG: I don't have a DVD player.

The interaction continued like this, with all members becoming increasingly irritated as group members inadvertently fell into the expert trap. The leader tried to steer the group onto a more productive focus, but failing, then attempted to break the seriousness of the growing negativity with paradoxical light humor:

> "Okay, guys. Your job (*looking at group*) is to continue suggesting things that he can do and, your job (*to Doug*) is to reject each person's idea."

Two group members then offered suggestions and Doug continued to disagree with relish, while everyone laughed. The group understood the need to abandon attempts to set things right and stopped behaving defensively. By highlighting the no-change aspect of Doug's ambivalence (with humor and no aggression), the members allowed him to explore and resolve it. The group's mood improved, and Doug agreed to develop his own list of leisure activities.

Moving into Action

As treatment progresses, group members begin to make plans for avoiding a return to problematic behaviors. This can be a very positive time as they begin to see and experience rewards for the work they have done. These rewards may take the form of increased privileges or a clearer vision of a positive future. When this occurs, clients remain more focused on commitment to change.

One nonthreatening approach is to develop a menu of changes members might consider going forward, or consider changes in a hypothetical manner. For example, you may encourage the group to discuss intimacy, self-management, or other risk factors and imagine how positive changes in those areas would alter their future. It may help to focus on the horizon, to the time after they get off community supervision or out of incarceration, with an eye toward eliciting commitment to change:

LEADER: What might you do when you're no longer involved with the legal system?

JOHN: Probably have a beer. It's been a long time. I can't decide, though. A part of me has been following these rules so long, I'm not sure whether I will do anything different.

RICK: What are some good and not-so-good things that could happen if you do?

JOHN: It would just be nice to be able to drink a few and not have somebody breathing down my back about it. But, really, I don't want to lose what I've worked so hard for.

LEADER: A part of you thinks it would be nice to have a beer and another part of you thinks it would be good to keep doing what has kept you straight so far.

JOHN: Yeah, a beer would be nice, but I'm not sure that it's worth it, if it's a start toward trouble. That slippery slope, you know. (*Laughs.*)

RICK: Buddy, we all know about that slippery slope. (*Group laughs, agrees.*)

LEADER: How does drinking fit in with your goals?

JOHN: It really doesn't. The fact is that I've come too far to go backwards now. I want to feel free to do what I feel like, but I guess it's not really helpful to even start down that path again. I know my judgment goes down when I drink, so why risk it?

LEADER: How do the rest of you think about balancing freedom to do what you want and the risk that some of those things might distract you from the life you're building or start you down that slippery slope?

(*Discussion continues.*)

Change planning with men who have committed sexual offenses is generally quite involved, and beyond the scope of this chapter. As members move toward discharge, they complete assignments identifying personal risk factors for continued aggression and plans for preventing their recurrence. They also develop broader change plans, beyond simply avoiding risks, building on new or expanded visions of themselves. In MI groups, members share their developing plans with one another, gather input from other group members and the leaders, and continue to revise their plans to be increasingly comprehensive, multifaceted, and resilient in the face of temptations, threats, and obstacles. Input can be given using the elicit–provide–elicit format of information exchange, and processing of plans is not approached in a confrontational way, even when members seem to be avoiding topics or minimizing risks. While some hierarchical elements may be inevitable given the dual commitment of leaders both to help members and protect the public, any feedback you give should be evenhanded, address behaviors or situations, and should not be presented in a way that members may perceive as a personal attack. When you hear what may be minimizing or distorting, it can sometimes be useful simply to mention that something in a member's plan seems missing or underdeveloped, identify what it is and whether the member seems defensive in any way, and suggest that the group not get sidetracked but keep moving forward with other members' plans, and that the member keep revising his plan as he hears ideas he likes from others.

Change planning involves identifying goals, steps toward those goals, personal strengths and interpersonal supports for change, potential challenges to the plan, and plans for noticing and addressing those challenges, as well as any other relapse risks. Some anxiety and tension can develop during the process of developing and reviewing change plans, because ambivalence may resurface about some of the losses and challenges involved, and members' confidence becomes vulnerable. How well you manage this phase of treatment can make the difference between members who are well-prepared, open-minded, and realistically confident to face the challenges ahead and those who are underprepared, defensive, and either overly self-confident or overly self-doubting.

Handling Challenges

Although moving into action can foster significant change, watch for continuing ambivalence and signs of resistance. Resistance may occur when members receive feedback about ongoing behaviors and choices, or make changes that feel threatening to other group members who are less ready to change.

In recent years, programs have experienced increasing pressure to assess client truthfulness, risk, and patterns of sexual arousal. Many of these measures are physiological, and clients perceive them as intrusive. Those administered after the individual has started a program may place a client in a risk pool that requires greater surveillance, more concentrated treatment, or other factors the client may not have anticipated and about which he may become defensive. Frame these measures in terms that underscore the value of identifying factors that relate to future success, and allow the client to demonstrate how well he is doing in treatment. When discussing these assessments in group, members can add affirmations for their successful completion or, when this is not the case, gently inquire about the desire, ability, reason, and need to change in order to create a more successful outcome in the future.

Client truthfulness is a serious concern in treatment for sexual aggression. While MI can be extremely useful, do not allow it to become a means of shaping unverifiable client self-report. Given the high stakes involved in treating this population, it is likely you will be in a position to verify client sexual history and compliance with probation conditions with a polygraph examination. While this can appear intrusive, one study found that three-quarters of those participating in polygraph examinations experienced the process as helpful, and that 90% of the participants agreed with the examiner's findings (Kokish, Levenson, & Blasingame, 2004). You can frame these measures positively by suggesting that they are opportunities for clients to show that they are truthful and following their conditions of community supervision.

People may commit technical violations of their conditions of probation or parole, or a nonsexual law violation. Changing laws may result in new consequences being applied to individuals, some of whom were nearing the end of treatment. In each case, clients can be very worried about what may happen next.

JOE: When I went to register, they gave me this brochure outlining changes to the laws. It looks like instead of registering once a year, we will have to register four times a year.

(*Group members pass around the brochure.*)

RON: They can't make that retroactive on us, can they?

JIM: Yes, they can.

PETE: That burns me up. There's always something new they put on us.

LEADER: You're angry and worried about what the changes might mean to your particular situations.

(*The group continues to discuss the changes.*)

LEADER: How do you think you will handle it if these changes do go into effect?

You can continue to shape the group's response from grievance (sustain talk) toward action (change talk) by posing DARN-CAT questions followed by reflections.

Potential Traps in Facilitating MI Groups for Sexual Aggression

There are many potential difficulties that you might experience while providing MI group services:

• *The group supports the no-change position.* Feelings expressed in a group can become amplified. Members may begin to resonate with individuals who are angry about conditions of community supervision, or who blame others for their own behaviors. You can handle this by practicing reflective listening, asking DARN-CAT questions, and affirming pro-change statements.

• *The leader is mandated to use MI-inconsistent material.* You may be required to use a curriculum with components that are at odds with the MI approach. If possible, you might change the language of the curriculum when doing so does not change the content, eliminating labels such as "criminal" or "offender" and forced-change wording (i.e., "you should" or "you need to"). Other elements may be handled by universalizing them. For example, it is customary for treatment manuals to focus on "thinking errors." If you identify these as common to everyone and point out a few of your own, it can help group members to feel more comfortable in discussing their own thought patterns.

• *Not sticking with the style.* Group members can present numerous challenges, whether directly (e.g., through intimidation) or indirectly (e.g., by only appearing to participate meaningfully). You may experience an urgency to "fix" clients or respond harshly to wrongdoing. Sometimes novice MI practitioners quickly find themselves saying, "I tried an MI approach and it didn't work," only to subsequently experience heightened resistance. This may be particularly true when attempting MI in the complexity of a group format. It may be useful to introduce elements of MI in a sequential manner into the group, until you and group members are comfortable and proficient with it.

• *The group engages in the righting reflex.* At times, group members will give unsolicited advice in an attempt to fix another member's problem. This can result in resistance and frustration. Using OARS can help prevent these problems. When such instances occur, the leader may comment on the group's desire to help with the member's problem, and the member's apparent desire to address the problem himself.

• *Loss of the correspondence between individual and community goals.* Treating people who have sexually abused balances honoring the needs of your clients and those of society at large. It is easy to side with the client against society, or the opposite—to treat the client in a harsh, punitive manner. Explore with group members how their interests and community interests are the same—neither they nor the community wants them to do further harm. When clients agree to this from the outset, they can focus on living as part of a community where members do no harm. Because groups often amplify the feelings expressed within them, this focus is particularly crucial.

Evidence for MI-Based Approaches

Historically, many professionals have considered strongly confrontational responses to sexual assault to be appropriate, even necessary, despite evidence to the contrary (Matravers, 2003). Sometimes, this has meant excluding individuals from treatment unless they are clearly amenable (Laws, 2003). Instead, using MI, you can be more effective when you expect resistance. In viewing resistance as a natural part of the change process, you can better understand and address its underlying ambivalence. Although no controlled trials of MI have yet focused on this specific population, MI is consistent with current thought in other areas of working with adjudicated clients (e.g., Walters, Clark, Gingerich, & Meltzer, 2007). Many of the same aspects of successful treatment addressing general criminal behavior also work with those who have engaged in sexual abuse (Hanson, Bourgon, Helmus, & Hodgson, 2009).

Conclusion

Group treatment for sexual aggression requires patience, skill, and knowledge of the issues that brought group members into treatment. Clients may enter treatment hoping to appear compliant with short-term legal requirements, yet enact long-term change in response to the group's culture. By avoiding labels and focusing on the individual, an MI-consistent group signals the importance and worth of each person. People have the opportunity to look at difficult pieces of themselves in an atmosphere of acceptance that gives them a safe, nonshaming basis for reflection. MI group treatment exemplifies the values of a nonabusive lifestyle: collaboration instead of intimidation, guiding instead of mandating, and support for the right of people to make their own choices as they move toward a more socially responsible lifestyle. The result can mean no more victims—benefiting both the client and society.

> *MI groups exemplify the values of a nonabusive lifestyle: collaboration instead of intimidation, guiding instead of mandating, and support for people to make their own choices.*

References

Coffey, P. (2010). Public policy and juvenile sexual offending: What should we call the boy next door? In D. S. Prescott & R. E. Longo (Eds.), *Current applications: Strategies for working with sexually aggressive youth and youth with sexual behavior problems* (pp. 95–116). Holyoke, MA: NEARI Press.

Hanson, R. K., Bourgon, G., Helmus, L., & Hodgson, S. (2009). The principles of effective correctional treatment also apply to sex offenders: A meta-analysis. *Criminal Justice and Behavior, 36,* 865–891.

Hanson, R. K., & Bussiere, M. T. (1998). Predicting relapse: A meta-analysis of sexual offender recidivism studies, *Journal of Consulting and Clinical Psychology, 66,* 348–362.

Hanson, R. K., Gordon, A., Harris, A. J. R., Marques, J. K., Murphy, W., Quinsey, V. L., et al. (2002). First report of the collaborative outcome data project on the effectiveness of treatment for sex offenders. *Sexual Abuse: A Journal of Research and Treatment, 14*(2), 169–194.

Jennings, J. L., & Sawyer, S. (2003). Principles and techniques for maximizing the effectiveness of group therapy with sex offenders. *Sexual Abuse: A Journal of Research and Treatment, 15*(4), 251–268.

Kokish, R., Levenson, J. S., & Blasingame, G. D. (2004). Post-conviction sex offender polygraph examination: Client reported perceptions of utility and accuracy. *Sexual Abuse: A Journal of Research and Treatment, 17,* 211–221.

Laws, D. R. (2003). Harm reduction and sexual offending: Is an intraparadigmatic shift possible? In T. Ward, D. R. Laws, & S. M. Hudson (Eds.), *Sexual deviance: Issues and controversies* (pp. 280–296). Thousand Oaks, CA: Sage.

Levenson, J. S., & Macgowan, M. J. (2004). Engagement, denial, and treatment progress among sex offenders in group therapy. *Sexual Abuse: A Journal of Research and Treatment, 16,* 49–63.

Levenson, J. S., & Prescott, D. S. (2009). Treatment experiences of civilly committed sex offenders: A consumer satisfaction survey. *Sexual Abuse: A Journal of Research and Treatment, 21,* 6–20.

Mann, R. E., Webster, S. D., Schofield, C., & Marshall, W. L. (2004). Approach versus avoidance goals in relapse prevention with sexual offenders. *Sexual Abuse: A Journal of Research and Treatment, 16,* 65–75.

Marshall, W. L. (2005). Therapist style in sexual offender treatment: Influence on indices of change. *Sexual Abuse: A Journal of Research and Treatment, 17*(2), 109–116.

Marshall, W. L., & Marshall, L. E. (2007). Preparatory programs for sexual offender treatment. In D. Prescott (Ed.), *Applying knowledge to practice: Challenges in the treatment and supervision of sexual abusers* (pp. 124–142). Oklahoma City: Wood'N'Barnes.

Matravers, A. (2003). Setting some boundaries: Rethinking responses to sex offenders. In A. Matravers (Ed.), *Managing sex offenders in the community: Managing and reducing the risks* (pp. 1–28). Cullompton, UK: Willan.

McGrath, R. J., Cumming, G. F., & Burchard, B. L. (2003). *Current practices and trends in sexual abuser management: The Safer Society 2002 Nationwide Survey.* Brandon, VT: Safer Society Foundation, Inc.

Reitzel, L. R., & Carbonell, J. L. (2006). The effectiveness of sexual offender treatment for juveniles as measured by recidivism: A meta-analysis. *Sexual Abuse: A Journal of Research and Treatment, 18,* 401–421.

Serran, G. A., & O'Brien, M. D. (2009). A treatment approach for sexual offenders in categorical denial. In D. S. Prescott (Ed.), *Building motivation to change in sexual offenders* (pp. 96–117). Brandon, VT: Safer Society Foundation, Inc.

Walters, S. T., Clark, M. D., Gingerich, R., & Meltzer, M. (2007, June). Motivating offenders to change: A guide for probation and parole. Washington, DC: U.S. Department of Justice National Institute of Corrections (NIC Accession Number 022253). Retrieved February 22, 2008, from *http://nicic.org/downloads/PDF/Library/022253.pdf.*

Ward, T., & Maruna, S. (2007). *Rehabilitation.* New York: Routledge.

CHAPTER 21

Motivational Interviewing Groups for Adolescents and Emerging Adults

Sarah W. Feldstein Ewing,
Scott T. Walters, *and* John S. Baer

Half of the adolescents are sitting expectantly, hands on knees, eyes up and alert. The rest have their arms folded across their chests, heads back, eyes prepared to roll.

"I don't even know why I'm here," Paco says.

"Nobody has let you know why you have to be here today," responds the counselor, in a warm, empathic tone.

"No, I know why I'm here. But it wasn't up to me to come."

"You're being forced to do something that you don't want to do," states the counselor in a genuinely curious manner.

"Yeah, that's always true for us," says Mark. "You wouldn't understand."

Adolescents and emerging adults rarely seek treatment. Often, they are enrolled in programs *despite* their level of interest and may be ambivalent about participating. MI provides a rationale and set of strategies for conducting groups. It allows adolescents and emerging adults to state their opinions openly and comfortably. An MI approach values their thoughts (particularly those of the reluctant ones), and considers them an important foundation for respectful and active therapeutic interactions.

> "You are absolutely right," says the counselor, joining with the adolescents. "I haven't lived your life, and I haven't walked in your shoes. And I appreciate your thoughts on how you feel about being here. Today, we're going to talk about some behaviors that can get in the way of a healthy lifestyle. Rather than telling you what to do, I'm interested in you talking about your experiences, because you are the experts on your own lives. Let's get started."

Adolescence, Emerging Adulthood, and MI

Growing interest in using MI with youth stems from the need for brief, effective interventions with these age groups. Adolescents and emerging adults are different from adults in important ways; programs developed for adults cannot be adopted wholesale for younger generations. Before describing MI groups with youth, we note some important developmental considerations and describe why MI groups are a good fit for adolescents and emerging adults.

Adolescence is a developmental stage characterized by significant changes in biological, psychological, and social systems. Adolescents grow rapidly, develop secondary sex characteristics and higher-order cognitive abilities, and adopt adult social behaviors. They begin to reason hypothetically, to contemplate others' points of view, and to learn how to make complex choices about their future. One task of adolescence is developing an identity separate from parents, and an increased sense of personal autonomy. During this period, peer interactions and influences increase. Most adolescents transition to adulthood without any sustained adjustment problems. Still, healthy individuation involves testing rules and challenging authority.

One mark of the closure of adolescence is when an individual is self-supporting and has assumed adult roles. People's risk behaviors often increase in their 20s. Arnett (2000) suggested an intermediary developmental stage of "emerging adulthood" for those approximately 18 to 25 years old who are demographically, subjectively, and psychologically distinct from younger and older age groups. Identity explorations for emerging adults in the areas of love, work, and worldview go beyond adolescence but stop short of adulthood. Emerging adults stay in educational systems longer, delay marriage and parenthood, and engage in more serial preparatory employment experiences or extended professional training. Health risks increase as emerging adults explore their identities and roles by engaging in risky behaviors (i.e., substance use, risky driving, risky sexual behavior). Most emerging adults naturally reduce their health risk behaviors between their mid-20s and 30s. Effective prevention and intervention programs that enhance this natural process of adopting positive and prosocial behaviors, reduce the harm of health risk behaviors, and fortify strategies for deviating from high-risk group norms are particularly beneficial.

MI is a promising approach that explores ambivalence in youth, connects decision making to their autonomy, supports and promotes their self-efficacy, and catalyzes motivation for change. The flexibility of MI makes it easy for adolescents and emerging adults to engage in the process. Finally, the sensitivity of youth and emerging adults to their peers makes group work a powerful strategy for health risk prevention and intervention work with these populations.

Clinical Considerations in MI Groups with Adolescents and Emerging Adults

Several features differentiate MI groups from other common approaches, such as norms education, health information, or psychoeducational groups. The first difference is the core purpose of the group. In an MI group, the goal is to generate a conversation that *will ultimately lead to behavior change,* in contrast to an education-based group, in which the goal is to impart information or knowledge,. The main way of catalyzing behavior change in MI groups is to elicit and reinforce members' change talk. Your goal is to elicit statements such as "I will reduce my drinking"; "I will use condoms"; "I will not drive after drinking."

The second distinction of MI groups involves the decision rules that guide group leaders. While all good youth-based groups seek to share ideas with participants in a comfortable environment, MI groups seek to provide a safe, judgment-free atmosphere that *will form a foundation for youth to explore their ideas and intentions around behavior change autonomously.* Many youth are used to being told what to do, along with being told what is right and what is wrong. However, they are rarely given the opportunity to explore health risk behaviors in a safe setting, where their opinions are not challenged or corrected. Adolescents and emerging adults thrive on the opportunity to explain their own perspectives—*why* they do things; they want people to understand their story. Thus, in contrast to more traditional group educational approaches, we try to begin and end groups with members' own stories. Specifically, we like to open with adolescents sharing what experiences led them to the group, and end with where they might like to go from here. The purpose of the MI group is not to inform but to explore and change their ideas about risk behavior. Therefore, while we provide some information on normative behaviors, it is done in MI-consistent ways, with the explicit goal of evoking change talk.

Structure and Process in MI Groups with Youth

MI groups are appropriate for many different contexts. Risk behaviors may come to the attention of school staff, medical professionals, or juvenile/criminal justice systems. Within these contexts, youth may attend by mandate, attend in return for a benefit (reduction in a justice or school charge), or attend upon the recommendation of a professional. While this chapter focuses on adolescent health risk behaviors, the target behaviors for MI groups are not limited to health risk behaviors.

Several factors make MI groups inherently different from individual MI, including the interpersonal dynamics, the different experiences and needs of members, and the need for the leader to adjust strategies for multiple members, as discussed earlier in this book. A unique factor is that due to social desirability, youth are likely to behave differently in groups than they would individually, perhaps overreporting or underreporting their true thoughts and behaviors. Additionally, the social pressure (and potential misinterpretation) of statements made in a group context may draw out the need for youth to defend themselves against real or imagined criticism, and to define themselves and their positive (and less positive) accomplishments.

We recommend keeping groups small, with six to eight participants. We prefer to have two leaders. We encourage restricting the age range of participants to 2 years for adolescents (e.g., ages 14–16, 16–18), and 4 years for emerging adults (e.g., ages 18–22), to keep participants' experiences similar. Ideally, we also prefer to keep adolescent groups single-sex, as this can reduce group-unrelated social interactions (e.g., flirting). Emerging adult groups can be more flexible in terms of gender composition. Depending on the setting, adolescent MI groups', duration may be brief, sometimes as little as one session. To encourage positive interactions, you may need to be vocal in fostering and maintaining a positive and judgment-free climate. Finally, and most *important,* most of the content should be generated by the group.

Keep the groups positive and effective. Use strategies for preventing negative processes and outcomes that can occur when grouping high-risk youth together (Dishion, McCord, & Poulin, 1999). How? First, have an established reason for forming the group (and maintain that focus throughout the group). Second, be deliberate about the group's composition. Specifically, it is important that group participants have similar age and experience levels (e.g., it is better to have 16-year-old girls with similar levels of risk behavior than to have relatively immature 14-year-olds through high-risk 18-year-olds together in the same coed group). Third, genuinely view the participants as positive, smart, contributing members of society, who ultimately desire to live in prosocial ways. Taking this perspective is a self-fulfilling prophecy; adults who expect positive, smart, prosocial interactions get adolescents who live up to the task. (Similarly, expecting the negative tends to elicit more negative behavior from a group, leaving you to spend more time controlling the groups than facilitating change.) Fourth, if negative interactions do emerge, you may have to use complementary strategies, in addition to MI strategies, such as reminding adolescents of the established group guidelines, gently guiding them back to the discussion at hand, inviting their assistance in helping to keep the group on-track, and occasionally checking in with struggling participants about the fit of the group for them. While we have not experienced difficulties in conducting MI groups with high-risk adolescents, individual MI sessions may be preferable for those who have difficulty settling into the group process.

The aim of many MI group exercises is to develop discrepancies between current behaviors and current or future goals. These work well, but be aware that questioning youths' beliefs (e.g., that drinking is cool, or that everyone smokes marijuana) may elicit resistance; people who feel challenged may argue against change (either out aloud or silently) to preserve their beliefs. Part of the art of MI is to explore members' beliefs gently, without increasing resistance. We suggest encouraging participation and open exchanges, while rolling with arguments against change. Listen to arguments for and against change, and selectively reinforce the arguments for change.

Conducting MI Groups with Adolescents and Emerging Adults

MI with adolescents and emerging adults can be invigorating. With their new skills in hypothesis generation and evaluation, they are adept at examining situations from different angles. In addition, they are keenly aware of the behaviors of those around them, and how those compare with their own. These two areas of heightened attention make them excellent candidates for various MI strategies. For the sake of providing a practical example, we illustrate one adolescent MI group that focuses on reducing health risk behaviors. MI concepts guide us through several steps—fostering a safe and nonjudgmental environment for discussion by exploring perspectives, seeking to raise doubt about current behaviors, exploring reasons for change, and promoting self-efficacy to support the ability to change, should change be desired.

Engaging the Group

The early part of MI groups with adolescents focuses on establishing a safe environment, setting a lighthearted (even fun) tone, and getting members to begin opening up and interacting with one another.

MI groups emerge for widely varying reasons. Depending on the reason for the group, the opening will be different. It is important to lay out clearly the context and the parameters of the group (i.e., Will the group be confidential? When would confidentiality have to be violated? How long will the group run?). Transparency about these issues facilitates a safe, genuine, and comfortable atmosphere. After laying out the parameters, we like to have members generate group guidelines. This gets them talking, which warms them up for more sensitive topics. It also gives them a sense of ownership and control over the group. To validate their thoughts and contributions, we write, display, and reference the rules that they generate (e.g., on a whiteboard). This strategy also helps us to manage negative behaviors within the group, as members tend to be sensitive to violations of their own guidelines.

> "Thank you for coming today. I know that you have lots of things you could be doing instead. In this group, we'll be discussing health risk behaviors. That means we'll be talking about drinking, drug use, and risky sexual behaviors. This is a private, or *confidential* group, which means that we won't tell your parents, teachers, or anyone else what you say, unless you mention that you are being hurt (by yourself or anybody else) or you are hurting someone else. If that comes up, we have to tell someone to make sure that you and those around you are safe. By *confidential,* we also mean that we don't want you to discuss anything that people say in here with anyone else. It is okay to talk about today's topics with other people once you leave, because these topics are important and we want you to be thinking about them, but it is not okay to say who said what. Meaning you can talk with your friends about how to use condoms, or how to keep yourself safe when drinking, but you can't share Mark's private stories. Can we agree to that? Also, for the group to be a safe, respectful, purposeful place, we need some guidelines about what we'll do and what we won't do in here. What guidelines do you think would be important to have today?"

Rather than telling members our rules, we elicit group guidelines from them. Those might include "no name-calling," "no interrupting," "respecting each person's opinion," and "making sure everybody has a chance to talk." If group members have not considered an important issue when brainstorming guidelines, we raise our concern and invite them to discuss it.

> "You have come up with some great guidelines. I'm impressed. There is one other guideline that we would like to see. We don't criticize anyone else's experiences. What do you think about that as another possible guideline?"

Once guidelines have been established, it is important that group members get to know each other, particularly if they haven't met. We begin by asking members to introduce themselves, say something that they like about themselves, and mention one of their goals for the future. This establishes a positive group dynamic that focuses on self-efficacy, with a foundation for developing healthy prosocial behaviors. It is easiest to model this by having one of us start.

> "Hi, I'm Dr. Sarah. I work with adolescents and adults who have a hard time quitting drinking. One thing that I like about myself is that I always say what I'm thinking. For the future, my goal is to create programs that help people your age stay healthy. Angel, you're next."

When adolescents mention that they don't have anything they like about themselves, you can reflect:

> "You can't come up with something right now. At the same time, you're here and willing to participate in the group which is pretty cool. Let's start with that for now."

If they can't generate a goal, you can reflect:

> "It's hard to know where you're headed. We'll keep talking about what you might like to do in the future. Okay, Paco. You're up. Tell us about you."

As the process unfolds, we write down each youth's response, as they can be relevant for later activities.

Exploring Perspectives

Once group members engage with one another, the next task is to explore their perceptions of the prevalence and social norms of health risk behaviors in their age group. From an MI perspective, our challenge is to encourage young people to consider the information without feeling like they are being told what to do. To compare members' ideas about the prevalence of risk behaviors without raising resistance, we like to explore the behaviors of other adolescents in a nonconfrontational, genuinely curious manner. With health risk behaviors, we start broadly, openly exploring the local rates of alcohol, marijuana, and tobacco use, and sexual risk behaviors. It is critical to provide information about demographically matched comparison groups. With U.S. adolescents, the Youth Risk Behavior Surveillance System (*www.cdc.gov/healthyyouth/yrbs/index.htm*) is an excellent resource for comparison data. In addition, Chan, Neighbors, Gilson, Larilmer, and Marlatt (2007) have information specific to college student drinking behaviors in the United States. For groups in other countries, the World Health Organization offers an excellent database for finding drinking data by age group and region (*www.who.int/globalatlas/dataquery/default.asp*).

> *Encourage young people to consider the information, without telling them what to do.*

Next, we investigate group members' guesses about how many people may be engaged in the target behavior. We begin by saying something like the following:

> "All right. We are curious about how your experience compares with what's happening with other kids like you in this area. So, from what you've seen, how many 16-year-olds like you had at least one drink during the past month?"

Having group members shout out their guesses regarding peers' risk behavior usually generates group dialogue in a nonthreatening and nonconfrontational manner. Youth tend to be quite playful when discussing risk behaviors among their peers (particularly if they are from different social groups), and it sets an excellent foundation for talking about their own behavior.

If no responses are generated, we reflect that. "You don't know how many kids your age are drinking." Adolescents might need time to determine the worth of participating in the group (e.g., "Will my friends still like me if I participate?") It is important to give them time to size up the leaders and their peers, without pushing against their lack of participation. If group members still do not respond after we reflect, we may ask the question another way, or move on to the next behavior.

> "OK. How many people your age do you think smoked marijuana in the past month? How many used tobacco? How many people your age have had sex?"

We encourage their guesses and reflect back their hypotheses.

> "It seems like almost everybody is using marijuana, every day. OK! Who else? Anybody have any guesses that are higher or lower?"

Broadening Perspectives

After establishing the group environment and exploring clients' current perspectives, we focus on broadening those perspectives and eliciting motivation to change. We focus our efforts on three elements: (1) raising doubt; (2) exploring reasons, desires, and need for change; and (3) increasing self-efficacy to change. Within the group environment, this shift is subtle and to prevent eliciting resistance unnecessarily, we do not draw attention to it.

Raising Doubt

Because adolescents arrive at the group with varying levels of ambivalence, we use the raising doubt exercise to check in and gently spark their thoughts and ambivalence. For example, once we have generated a number of guesses about peer behavior patterns, we present a poster showing the rates of behavior from survey responses. We wonder with the group about how the rates on the board compare with their guesses:

> "A few of you mentioned that everybody you know had sex with at least one person before they got to high school. And most of them have had sex with at least five people. Our data show that in this area, most kids—more than nine out of 10—have not had sex before age 14. By the end of high school, less than one out of five has had sex with more than four people. What do you think of this? How does it fit for you?"

Some members question the data or state that the data are wrong. With emerging adults, it may be appropriate to mention some characteristics of the survey (e.g., size, year conducted, referent group). However, we are careful to avoid arguing with the group and instead use the opportunity to reflect the discrepancy:

> "This doesn't fit with your experience. It's really surprising." or "The people you know are different from this. Tell us more about that."

We also use this opportunity to encourage responses from members who may have seen less risk behavior:

"People have lots of different experiences. What do the rest of you think of this?"

We believe that the group is our client; group interactions should not be pulled exclusively toward one person. For example, it can be tempting to spend significant time exploring the behavior or ambivalence of the adolescent with the greatest risk. However, this can polarize the group, inadvertently creating a divide between those who are similar to the high-risk adolescent and those who are not. It can also inadvertently reinforce high-risk behavior by conveying the message that the more risk behavior a member describes, the more attention he or she gets. Instead, it is important briefly and systematically to walk through the experience and ambivalence of each adolescent who wants to share, then summarize the "collective" ambivalence of the group.

"Alisha, you mentioned that you really like drinking, but you've noticed that it's gotten some of your family members into trouble. . . . Christina, you don't know what the big whoop is about drinking. . . . Mary, you talked about the importance of doing the same thing as the people around you. . . . Together, you have had lots of different experiences with alcohol. You've noticed lots of reasons why people your age are drinking: People like the feeling, it helps to fit in, and sometimes it makes you feel better. Also, you mentioned a number of not-so-great things about drinking: People have gotten hurt, it makes it harder to get your diploma, and vomiting is just gross. Great job."

Because the entire group is our "client," we also strive to elicit the thoughts of all members in the group. If only a few members are talking, we encourage others by looking at them when we ask questions, standing by them, or asking them directly to share their opinions. Of course, the goal is not to convince members that their perceptions are wrong or that they should give up all risk behaviors. The goal is to raise doubts and curiosity—about assumptions of what others do, about what is normal, and about choices.

Following the guiding approach of MI, we like to summarize before moving onto the next activity:

"Okay, about half of you know kids who drink every day, and the rest of you know people who only drink once a month. And the local average is somewhere in the middle. In terms of marijuana, about half of you know people your age who smoke marijuana pretty often, and the rest of you don't have friends who smoke regularly. Again, on average, about three out of 10 people your age are regularly smoking weed, so it makes sense that this is more than some of you have seen but less than others of you have seen. It looks like almost all of you have friends who smoke cigarettes. That is a lot more than most people your age in this area. And, almost all of you have friends who are having sex, and with multiple partners. The alcohol and marijuana experiences of your friends are about average, and the cigarette use and sexual experiences of your friends are much higher. Did I get that all right? What else would you add?"

Exploring Reasons and Need for Change ("But All My Friends Drink More Than I Do!")

We also use comparison data to explore ambivalence and discrepancies within the group. After summarizing their peers' experiences, we wonder with members about how the behavior of their peers might compare with their own behavior.

> "So we noticed that the people you know use more tobacco than similar people your age in this area. How does the tobacco use of your friends compare with your own experiences?"

Some members may be reluctant to respond, particularly if the group is being conducted in a criminal justice context. To alleviate concerns, we remind participants that their responses are private and contained within the group. Many participants respond in a polarized way, stating that their friends drink more than they do, or that they are drinking at high levels and have never had any problems.

Once group responses have been elicited, you can explore them.

> "Wow, you have a wide range of experiences. Some of you feel like your friends are drinking a lot more than you, and others feel like you're drinking without problems, and are not quite sure what the big deal is. Which would you like to start with?"

For adolescents whose friends are engaged in greater levels of risk behavior than their own, it is worthwhile to explore peer norms, behaviors, beliefs, and comparisons. Specifically:

> "It sounds like your friends are drinking every weekend. And, that's what people do in your school. What do your friends expect?"

Or:

> "What happens to friends in your group who don't drink? What would happen to you if you didn't drink?"

Genuinely and empathically, we explore all of the angles and are curious about the ramifications of the behavior with the group. Again, in this area we encourage group members to generate ideas among themselves.

> "Paco, what thoughts do you have about Maria's friends' expectations for her to drink?"

If the group is encouraging negative behaviors, then we intervene or move onto the next topic.

> "Okay, so lots of your friends drink. How about the ones that don't drink? What are some of their reasons for not drinking? What are some of the things that happen when people drink?"

Notably, as we describe the steps of group MI, we give examples of question stems we use to start different conversations. However, eliciting these different topics and directing them by reflections is better. Again, the majority of the content of an adolescent MI group should be group-generated comments and reflections by the leaders.

With their relatively brief risk histories, it is not unusual when adolescents have only experienced positive effects of risk behavior. We assume that people use substances and engage in risk behavior for good reasons. These behaviors might help them develop friendships, navigate social settings, or move through the fears that may accompany new relationships. Therefore, we believe that, with adolescents, it is important to explore this side of ambivalence before exploring the negative aspects of risky behaviors.

> "All right, let's switch gears for a moment. Some of you mentioned that you have been drinking without experiencing any problems and don't see what the problem is. What do you think would be the signs that a person is drinking too much?"

If group members are unable to generate ideas, we move on to reflecting potential negative consequences with openness and genuineness.

The messages that adolescents get from adults can help them to see the other side of the ambivalence.

> "So you haven't had anything bad happen when you've had unprotected sex. It's hard to imagine anything scary happening to you or anyone

you know because of sex. Tell us what your parents, teachers, and/or doctors said about having sex. Why are they worried about it?"

Once some negative consequences are generated, we explore how those negative consequences might fit with future goals. Pulling from what the participants said earlier, we might say,

> "Okay, so you haven't had anything bad happen to you or anybody you know after having sex. Your mom mentioned that kids can get sexually transmitted infections and, of course, pregnancy is possible. How might getting pregnant (or your partner getting pregnant) affect your life and plans? How about getting HIV?"

We sometimes also use scaling exercises here:

> "How important is it for you to not get (your partner) pregnant? And what makes you pick a _____ and not a lower number?"

Summaries that collect each contribution from the group are critical to reflect members' reasons for risk behavior. We end with a summary of group member's ideas about the negative consequences of risk behavior, checking in to see if we missed any. We tell the members we're going to come back to this but we'd like to do something else first.

Exploring Ability/Increasing Confidence

Before moving on to the action phase of an MI group, it is important to bolster participants' sense of self-efficacy (LaChance, Feldstein Ewing, Bryan, & Hutchison, 2009). We do this to encourage them to make active decisions (1) not to engage in a behavior, (2) to engage in a lower level of a behavior, or (3) to engage in a different behavior. Each is difficult and likely discrepant from the prevalent behaviors of their peer groups. Before encouraging them to take on these changes, we want to increase members' confidence in their *ability* to enact these changes. We have found that three MI approaches work particularly well in youth MI groups.

The first approach is the Characteristics of Successful Adolescents Sheet (Feldstein & Ginsburg, 2007). This activity can be introduced in the following manner:

> "Dr. Eric and I are going to hand out a sheet of paper. We'd like for each of you to take a moment and circle all of the words on this sheet that describe you."

Once participants have circled the appropriate adjectives, we encourage them to pick five favorite adjectives to share and to describe briefly how each one is true of them. It can be very powerful to write these adjectives on a sheet of paper for the whole group to see. Once all members have shared their descriptions, we can reflect the strength of the room.

> "You're a strong group. You're 'alive,' 'honest,' and 'smart.' You could do almost anything you put your mind to."

While adolescents rarely get to say what they think their strengths are, it is even rarer to hear about their positive attributes from their peers. So we next encourage them to highlight the positive attributes about their fellow group members. Introduce this activity by saying:

> "We each said something we liked about ourselves. Now, we'd like each of you to mention a strength of one of your fellow members. I'll start by saying that at the start of group today, Paco said that he's honest. I think that's pretty cool. I have also noticed that Paco thinks really hard about tough issues. Josh, tell me something you appreciate about Mark."

The third approach, eliciting change success stories, also can be powerful in a group context. In this strategy, members describe a time when they were able to do something they thought they could not do. This is powerful for the speaker and increases self-efficacy throughout the group. We introduce this activity by saying,

> "Now, think about a time when we were able to do something we originally thought we could not do. I'll give us a minute to think about it. We'll have Dr. Eric start, then go around the room sharing our stories."

If a member is not able to generate a success story, we might lower the bar:

> "Mary—no worries. This doesn't have to be a changed-the-world kind of event; it might just be a time that you didn't think that you could get up that morning but you did anyway. Why don't we move on to Christina and come back to you in a minute."

Moving into Action

One of the inspiring aspects about working with adolescents and emerging adults is their great potential for change; they have their whole lives ahead of them! The previous two steps, exploring and broadening perspectives, set the foundation for thinking about change, which is the first important step toward action. With attention to not pushing youth beyond their level of readiness, in this phase we facilitate the next steps for those youth who are ready to move toward implementing change.

Hypothetical Change and Change Planning

As with individual MI, some members of a group may not be ready to make formal change plans, and it is important not to push group members beyond their readiness. However, it is helpful to have the group generate hypothetical ideas of what a person could do if he or she wanted to make any behavior changes. We introduce this approach by revisiting the cons of their current behavior, bolstering members' self-efficacy (by summarizing the strengths of the group members and their expertise in their own lives), and brainstorming potential options.

> "Earlier today, when we talked about drinking, we noticed that half of you have many friends who drink frequently. You also said that while you know that drinking can lead to accidents, like falling off of the roof at a party or getting in a car accident, if you were to stop drinking, you're not sure that your friends would still be your friends. We also know that you are smart and creative. And, you're the experts on how these things go at your school. You're the ones who know these situations best. So, we'd like you to put your heads together and think about ways to manage situations, so that you don't lose your friends and you don't get hurt because of drinking. If you were at a party, and you chose not to drink but all your friends expected you to, what could you do?"

By this time, group members are likely to generate helpful ideas. We like to encourage humorous ideas, or ideas of what they should *not* do, to get the group laughing and talking. It is helpful to have some prepared ideas in the event that the group struggles with generating possibilities. When working with adolescent harm reduction, we are ready to discuss three topics if the group doesn't generate ideas: (1) how to be at a party without binge drinking; *glasses half-full (of soda)*; (2) how to get home from a party safely; *designated drivers and planned (safe) sleepovers*; and (3) how to reduce sexual risk taking; *having friend "chaperones" at parties (particularly for girls)*.

> Encourage humorous ideas or ideas of what they should not do, to get the group laughing and talking.

If members encounter problems

in brainstorming, we go through the three steps of the elicit–provide–elicit approach to facilitate greater discussion.

> "Tell me what you know about how to keep yourself safe, healthy, and in control of your own decisions about having sex . . . so you know when you're at a party and you've been drinking that there are a few ways to keep yourselves safe. You can decide not to go to the party, so that you're not facing that risk. And, you can bring condoms—always a good idea! I have some other ideas about how to stay safe. Can I share them with you?"

If the group does not want to hear our ideas during the *provide* step, we close this activity by reflecting in a genuine manner,

> "You have a pretty good handle on these situations and don't want to hear any other ideas right now about what might work."

If the group consents to hearing our ideas, we go on:

> "Okay, so you want to go to this party, because the boy you like will be there, but you don't want to have sex yet. That can be difficult when you feel like his group of friends is sexually active, and they might encourage you to go further than you want. Here are three other ideas. One, you could have an assigned friend check up on you. Second, you can clearly tell your partner that you don't want to have sex tonight. And, third, you can limit your drinking so that you can really think clearly as the night goes on."

We then elicit their further thoughts:

> "What do you think of these options? It's your choice, so I'm interested in what might work the best for you."

Youth are still developing their problem-solving skills, so working through problem-solving strategies together is worthwhile. The steps include (1) identifying the problem, (2) generating several possible solutions, (3) identifying the top three possibilities, (4) evaluating each option, (5) generating solutions to possible obstacles, (6) updating each possibility with the new information, and (7) firming up the final strategies. Role plays are sometimes helpful in trying out the strategies, to determine the possible obstacles and final strategies. So you might start this activity, saying,

"So the group came up with three ways of getting home from a party when intoxicated. You could call your parents or your older sibling, or walk home. Part of figuring out how these strategies might work is really thinking through what it might be like to do that. Let's do that together. Paco, you mentioned the 'call your older sibling' strategy. Let's have Mark pretend to be you, and you can be your older brother. Let's see how that goes. So, your older brother may be busy with his girlfriend and won't come to get you. And, Josh, you mentioned that you don't have an older sibling to call, so this strategy might be tougher for you. At the same time, calling someone to pick you up is a great idea. What could we do to make this strategy work better?"

At the end of this activity, we write members' ideas on posterboard and verbally review the strategies.

Using MI Groups with Emerging Adults: Additional Considerations

For the sake of providing consistent examples, we have focused on adolescent health risk behaviors, but it is important to consider differences between adolescents and emerging adults. Certainly the demography of drinking is different. Younger groups may contain more "experimenters," while older groups may have participants with more established (though probably still episodic) alcohol and other risk behaviors. As can be expected with age and development, emerging adults may have more experiences and greater comfort in sharing. Motivation for risk behaviors may also be different. Emerging adults may drink and use substances to manage life transitions, such as moving away from home and dealing with new living and social situations. They often have well-formed opinions about why they engage in health risk behaviors. Older group members may need less prodding to engage in serious discussions and often already have mixed views on substance use.

> Emerging adults drink and use substances to manage life transitions such as moving away from home, making new friends, and dealing with new living and social situations.

In terms of group composition and discussion, both age groups, adolescents and emerging adults, include a range of participants, including some who already have chosen not to engage in risk behaviors. Some older group members might speak more knowledgeably because of their experience or leadership status. If one of these natural opinion leaders is supportive of the group aims, it can be helpful to let this person make statements that we as group leaders might otherwise make. Older group members also may generate more complex strategies for remaining safe.

For additional guidance in working specifically with emerging adults, Walters and Baer (2006) provide a useful resource. Specifically, Chapter 7 describes in their book a one- to three-session motivational group for college drinkers that includes setting an agenda, raising ambivalence around drinking, creating individual and group discrepancy, introducing problem-solving scenarios, and managing difficult situations.

Evidence for This Approach

While many practitioners may be using MI groups with youth, research on MI groups with adolescents is relatively new (D'Amico et al., 2011). Qualitative evaluations have indicated that the MI approach resonates with adolescents (Stern, Meredith, Gholson, Gore, & D'Amico, 2007), and that most adolescents will select group, if it is offered, over other types of health risk interventions (i.e., individual and Web-based) (O'Leary et al., 2002). Several pilot studies have explored the use of MI-based groups to improve diabetes management (Knight et al., 2003), and to reduce sexual risk behavior (Schmiege et al., 2009) and alcohol use and related risks (Bailey, Baker, Webster, & Lewin, 2004), with promising improvements in the perceptions and behaviors of MI-group members.

More studies on drinking have been conducted with emerging adults, but with mixed results. Whereas some studies found that a single-session motivational group for college students decreased drinking among heavy drinkers (LaBrie, Lamb, Pedersen, & Quinlan, 2006; LaBrie, Thompson, Hutching, Lac, & Buckley, 2007; LaChance et al., 2009), other studies have not (Walters, 2000; Walters, Bennett, & Miller, 2000; Walters, Ogle, & Martin, 2002). Groups that combine motivational and skills-based strategies found reductions in drinking after heavy-drinking students attended a 6-week, skills-based class and discussion group (Baer et al., 1992). A group that combined motivational and skills elements reduced drinking among both voluntary and mandated students when compared to a student group that did not receive the intervention (Baer et al., 1992). Finally, a series of MI groups for adjudicated college students that focused on social norms education, decisional balance, and expectancy challenge and relapse prevention resulted in overall reductions in drinking (Fromme & Corbin, 2004).

Conclusion

MI in groups is a promising avenue for work with adolescents and emerging adults. However, the work has only begun in this area. Future research on outcomes for MI group participants, particularly relative to group composition, type of content, and delivery, will ultimately help determine what types of MI group approaches are most effective, for which behaviors, and for whom. Future studies should examine group activities, such as raising ambivalence, normative comparisons, and skills building, that almost always are used together in a group format. Research might also compare different group sizes, participant composition, and leadership strategies. In addition, future work on mechanisms of change in MI groups may illuminate why groups work. Furthermore, self-efficacy has been found to be an active ingredient of behavior change in MI group interventions with emerging adults (LaChance et al., 2009). Ultimately, these data will help to elucidate both how and why MI group interventions are effective for adolescents and emerging adults. These data are key to building upon and improving health outcomes through this promising intervention approach.

References

Arnett, J. J. (2000). Emerging adulthood: A theory of development from the late teens through the twenties. *American Psychologist, 55*(5), 469–480.

Baer, J. S., Marlatt, G. A., Kivlahan, D. R., Fromme, K., Larimer, M. E., & Williams, E. (1992). An experimental test of three methods of alcohol risk reduction with young adults. *Journal of Consulting and Clinical Psychology, 60*(6), 974–979.

Bailey, K. A., Baker, A. L., Webster, R. A., & Lewin, T. J. (2004). Pilot randomized control trial of a brief alcohol intervention group for adolescents. *Drug and Alcohol Review, 23,* 157–166.

Chan, K. K., Neighbors, C., Gilson, M., Larilmer, M. E., & Marlatt, G. A. (2007). Epidemiological trends in drinking by age and gender: Providing normative feedback to adults. *Addictive Behaviors, 32*(5), 967–976.

D'Amico, E. J., Feldstein Ewing, S. W., Engle, B., Osilla, K. C., Hunter, S., & Bryan, A. (2011). Group Alcohol and Drug Treatment. In S. Naar-King & M. Suarez (Eds.), *Motivational interviewing with adolescents and young adults* (pp. 151–157). New York: Guilford Press.

Dishion, T. J., McCord, J., & Poulin, F. (1999). When interventions harm: Peer groups and problem behavior. *American Psychologist, 54*(9), 755–764.

Feldstein, S. W., & Ginsburg, J. I. D. (2007). Sex, drugs, and rock 'n' rolling with resistance: Motivational Interviewing in juvenile justice settings. In A. R. Roberts & D. W. Springer (Eds.), *Handbook of forensic mental health with victims and offenders: Assessment, treatment, and research* (pp. 247–271). New York: Thomas.

Fromme, K., & Corbin, W. (2004). Prevention of heavy drinking and associated negative consequences among mandated and voluntary college students. *Journal of Consulting and Clinical Psychology, 72*(6), 1038–1049.

Knight, K. M., Bundy, C., Morris, R., Higgs, J. F., Jameson, R. A., Unsworth, P., et al. (2003). The effects of group motivational interviewing with externalizing conversations for adolescents with Type-I diabetes. *Psychology, Health, and Medicine, 8*(2), 149–157.

LaBrie, J. W., Lamb, T. F., Pedersen, E. R., & Quinlan, T. (2006). A group motivational interviewing intervention reduces drinking and alcohol-related consequences in adjudicated college students. *Journal of College Student Development, 47*(3), 267–280.

LaBrie, J. W., Thompson, A. D., Hutching, K., Lac, A., & Buckley, K. (2007). A group motivational interviewing intervention reduces drinking and alcohol-related negative consequences in adjudicated college women. *Addictive Behaviors, 32*(11), 2549–2562.

LaChance, H., Feldstein Ewing, S. W., Bryan, A., & Hutchison, K. (2009). What makes group MET work? A randomized controlled trial of college student drinkers in mandated alcohol diversion. *Psychology of Addictive Behaviors, 23*(4), 598–612.

O'Leary, T. A., Brown, S. A., Colby, S. M., Cronce, J. M., D'Amico, E. J., Fader, J. S., et al. (2002). Treating adolescents together or individually? Issues in adolescent substance abuse intervention. *Alcoholism: Clinical and Experimental Research, 26*(6), 890–899.

Schmiege, S. J., Broaddus, M. R., Levin, M., & Bryan, A. D. (2009). Randomized trial of group interventions to reduce HIV/STD risk and to change theoretical mediators among detained adolescents. *Journal of Consulting and Clinical Psychology, 77*(1), 38–50.

Stern, S. A., Meredith, L. S., Gholson, J., Gore, P., & D'Amico, E. J. (2007). Project CHAT: A brief motivational substance abuse intervention for teens in primary care. *Journal of Substance Abuse Treatment, 32*(2), 153–165.

Walters, S. T. (2000). In praise of feedback: An effective intervention for college students who are heavy drinkers. *Journal of American College Health, 48*(5), 235–238.

Walters, S. T., & Baer, J. S. (2006). *Talking with college students about alcohol: Motivational strategies for reducing abuse.* New York: Guilford Press.

Walters, S. T., Bennett, M. E., & Miller, J. H. (2000). Reducing alcohol use in college students: A controlled trial of two brief interventions. *Journal of Drug Education, 30*(3), 361–372.

Walters, S. T., Ogle, R., & Martin, J. E. (2002). Perils and possibilities of group-based MI. In W. R. Miller & S. Rollnick, *Motivational interviewing: Preparing people for change* (2nd ed., pp. 377–390). New York: Guilford Press.

Index

Index

therapeutic factors in, 54–55
transtheoretical model of change and (see Transtheoretical model for cocaine abuse)
Motivational Interviewing Treatment Integrity Scale, 114–116, 280
Moving into action phase; see Phase IV: Moving into action

N

Negative reactions, counteracting, 63–64
Nonassertive group member, description, strengths, MI strategy, 157t
Nonviolence contract, 363
Norms, group, 182–185

O

OARS communication style, 38, 41, 42, 54; see also Affirmations; Open questions; Reflections; Summaries
in intimate partner violence groups, 353
in IPV groups, 360–361
mandated group treatment and, 265–266
in MI groups, 54
in TTM groups, 269
using, 68–69
in weight management groups, 336
in women's empowerment groups, 290–291
Obesity, diseases associated with, 333
On the fence exercise, for dually diagnosed patients, 303
OPEN acronym, 169, 273
Open questions, 38–39
for broadening focus, 139–140
in engagement process, 43–44
in intimate partner violence groups, 355
in TTM/MI groups, 273–274
Optimism, centrality of, 64
Orientation, pregroup, 164–166
Outcomes; see Treatment outcomes
Overconfidence, addressing, 136–137
Overly nurturant group member, description, strengths, MI strategy, 157t

P

Pairs, for shaping conversations, 125
Past and future success exercise, for dually diagnosed patients, 305
Perceived task interdependence, 20
Personal strengths; see Strengths
Personal values; see Values
Personality styles, 155
Perspectives
broadening (see Broadening perspectives phase)
exploring (see Exploring perspectives phase)
Phase I: Engaging the group, 43–45, 149–175
in acute care settings, 301–302
in adolescent/emerging adult MI groups, 392–393
in chronic health conditions groups, 316
eliciting member goals and, 172–174
first session closure and, 174
first session facilitation and, 167
first session preparation and, 164–167

group development and, 56, 149–153, 150f, 151f, 152f, 153f
group guidelines and, 170–171
group overview and, 168–170
in groups treating sexual aggression, 372–373
in IPV groups, 352–353, 355–358
in mandated treatment groups, 258–259
meeting space preparation and, 166–167
in MI women's empowerment groups, 288–291
pregroup orientation and, 164–166
session opening and, 167–168
session structure and, 161–164
in weight management groups, 334–336
Phase II: Exploring perspectives, 87, 176–198
in adolescent/emerging adult groups, 393–395
in chronic health conditions groups, 316–320
with dually diagnosed patients, 302–304
group dynamics and, 179–180
guiding principles for, 176–179
in IPV groups, 358–360
leader functions in, 181–187
for fostering client self-awareness, 187
for group norms, 182–185
managing boundaries, 181–182
for managing emotions, 185–187
in mandated group treatment, 259–260
MI strategies in, 187–197
exploring ambivalence, 190–195
exploring lifestyles, 188–190
exploring values, 195–197
positive focus in, 177
progress indicators for, 198
tips and traps in, 197–198
in treatment for sexual aggression, 373–377
in women's empowerment groups, 291–292
Phase III: Broadening perspectives, 199–225
in adolescent/emerging adult groups, 395–400
with aggressive sexual behaviors, 377–380
in chronic health conditions groups, 320–326
for dually diagnosed patients, 304–307
group dynamics and, 203–204
guiding principles for, 200–203
in IPV groups, 360–363
leader functions in, 205–212
in mandated group treatment, 260–262, 377–380
MI strategies in, 212–223
assessment feedback, 217–219
change success stories, 222–223
decisional balance, 220–221
exploring importance and confidence, 221–222
exploring strengths, 223
heuristic models of, 212–217
looking forward/envisioning, 219–220
reexamining expectations, 220
therapeutic factors and, 204–205
tips and traps in, 223–224
in weight loss groups, 338–339
in women's empowerment groups, 292–293
Phase IV: Moving into action, 67–68, 226–248
in adolescent/emerging adult groups, 400–403
in chronic health conditions groups, 326–330
for dually diagnosed patients, 307